DATE DUE

MR 9 04			
DE 13 05			

DEMCO 38-296

TAKING OUR PULSE: THE HEALTH OF AMERICA'S WOMEN

IRIS F. LITT, M.D.

Taking Our Pulse

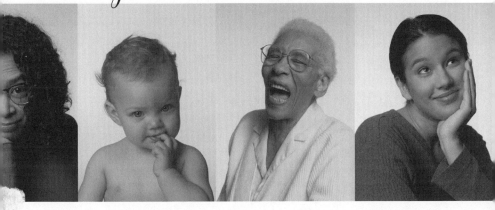

THE HEALTH OF AMERICA'S WOMEN

STANFORD UNIVERSITY PRESS
STANFORD, CALIFORNIA
1997

Stanford University Press
Stanford, California
© 1997 by the Board of Trustees of the
Leland Stanford Junior University

Printed in the United States of America

CIP data are at the end of the book

To M.A., whose long and valiant battle with ovarian cancer (and her doctors) was an inspiration to all who knew her. May she not have died in vain.

To V.C.V., for the love, humor, understanding, and technical support that sustained me through the long period of researching and writing this book.

Preface

Family legend has it that at the age of two, I would tell passersby, "The dolly in the carriage has pneumonia and is being treated with sulfadiazine and aspirin." In later elementary school years, I treasured the Saturday afternoons when, after all the patients left, I emptied the ashtrays in my father's waiting room and set out with him on house calls—he with his worn black bag of instruments and samples of medications, I trying to become invisible in his shadow. Welcomed into kitchens from which emanated strangely seductive aromas and into the bedrooms of the fevered, the elderly, and the expectant, I was introduced to the world of the family doctor, the world I naturally adopted as my own. Often departing with a sample of supper or a loaf of Italian bread, my father and I would descend the stairs deep in conversation about the patient's condition and prognosis. During high school, I became his receptionist during evening office hours, my job being to pacify those who were waiting while I could hear my father joking with the patient in his consultation room.

Why then, after all those years of socialization into the world of medicine, did it come as a surprise to my father when I casually mentioned one day that I planned to go to medical school? Because medicine was "too demanding a life" for a woman, he protested. And later, "Be a teacher, like your mother, and you will have summers free to be with your family." It didn't take too much to bring him around, however. In fact, although I didn't learn about it until years later, he agreed to give my hand in marriage only upon the condition that my husband allow me to pursue my goal of becoming a doctor.

Once resigned to the reality, and perhaps even secretly pleased about it, my father began his own brand of medical education, sharing secrets of the "art" of medicine. From how to lance a boil, to surefire cures for inflammation, to the secret ingredients in his "magical" pink pills, he taught me everything they would never teach in medical school. What I remember most clearly, however, was his view (and undoubtedly that of his medical colleagues) of the health problems of women: they could all be explained as the result of the fact that a woman was before, during, or after her menstrual period. It was that simple!

It's been thirty years since that introduction to the myths and biases about women and their health problems that permeate the practice of medicine. It has been much more recently that I have come to understand their origin and to question and challenge them. This book is about that transition. It is written from my perspective as a woman patient and physician, as an educator of future physicians, as a researcher, and as a student of feminism. Each of these roles has brought special insights, and in their synergy may be a unique synthesis.

Acknowledgments

This book needed four years to complete; it would not have been possible without the support, inspiration, and suggestions of many people. My colleagues in the Division of Adolescent Medicine at Stanford University, Drs. Cynthia Kapphahn and Seth Ammerman, deserve a special thanks for their relief of me during my two minisabbaticals. Sadly, Dr. Norman Schlossberger did not live to see my written thanks, but he surely knew how much he meant to me. My secretary, Ann McGrath, kept the office running efficiently and protected me, interrupting only when necessary, and Sally Schroeder kept IRWG going.

Credit for my formal feminist education and scholarship goes to the Senior Scholars at the Institute for Research on Women and Gender at Stanford (Susan Groag Bell, Edith Gelles, Phyllis Koestenbaum, Karen Offen, Elizabeth Roden, and Marilyn Yalom), as well as my faculty colleagues Myra Strober, Deborah Rhode, Estelle Freedman, Sylvia Yanagisako, and Diane Middlebrook, to name just a few. The work of Deborah Tannen has been invaluable in reorienting my views of the dynamic relationships in the world of medicine. My son Bill, through his legal research, enlightened me about issues of gender discrimination, thus adding to the richness of our interactions. The more experiential part of the educational process has been lovingly shared over the years with my dear friend and colleague, Karen Hein.

My activities aimed at improving the health of women have been encouraged and inspired by fellow warriors, among them Kim Yeager, Marjorie Shaevitz, Karen Johnson, Joan Leiman, Linda Clever, Florence

Hazeltine, Terry Dunn Gross, Vivian Pinn, Bernadine Healy, Helen Rodriquez-Torres, Jane Zones, Kate Karpilow, Karen Davis, and Susan Blumenthal. Many of these have, in the process, become close and valued friends.

Without the encouragement of my friends among the Associates and the National Advisory Panels of the Institute for Research on Women and Gender and of the Office of the Dean of Research at Stanford University (Dean Charles Kruger and Carol Vonder Linden), this book could not have been written. I owe thanks to the students in my class in Stanford's Continuing Studies Program who provided feedback on parts of the early manuscript.

Figure 2.1, showing pelvic floor exercises, is reprinted with permission from the Clinical Symposia, vol. 47/3. Copyright 1995. Novartis. Illustrated by John A. Craig, M.D., and Carlos Machado, M.D. All rights reserved.

A word of special thanks to those women who through their generous philanthropy have supported research on women's health at a time when many believe it's all been done.

My sincere thanks to the staff at the Stanford University Press (Muriel Bell, Laura Bloch, and Lynn Stewart) for their guidance, patience, and editorial assistance over this past year.

No words can express my appreciation to my husband, Victor C. Vaughan III, for his support, encouragement, and love. My mother, Bertha Figarsky, not only believed in me throughout my life, but read an early draft of this manuscript and claims to have learned more from it than from her doctors. To my beloved sons, Bill and Bob, who have grown into respected friends, and my cherished daughter-in-law, Cynthia; to M.S.L. and my stepchildren, Jonathan and Virginia Vaughan, Sarah and Philip Sayre, and Joanna Vaughan, and their children (Joe, Toby, Alex, and Hannah); to my sister- and brother-in-law, Clarice and Warren Vaughan; and to my nephew, Peter Steinerman: thank you all for keeping me focused on the most important thing in life, one's family!

There are many others who have enriched my life and my work during the writing of this book. Space prevents me from naming them all, but they are not forgotten.

Contents

Figures and Tables

TAKING OUR PULSE: THE HEALTH OF AMERICA'S WOMEN

Introduction

Women in the United States live about seven years longer than men. More than half of U.S. expenditures for health are attributed to the care of women. "What, then, is the problem with women's health care?" I am often asked. There are two answers to this question. First, we are seeing sharp rises in some serious health problems among women. For example, over the last two decades, the cancer death rates have risen twice as much for women as for men (6 percent versus 3 percent) (Brody 1995). Second, it is true that women live longer on average, but they spend most of those extra years in a state of disability and dependency as a result of myriad chronic, degenerative illnesses that befall them in older age. Although the absolute life expectancy for women has increased, the "active life expectancy" has actually decreased.

I am not questioning the absolute amount of money spent on women's health in this country, but rather the way in which this money has been spent. Recent evidence suggests that some of the diseases that have decreased women's active life expectancy may be preventable, or detectable early enough to improve their outcomes. Yet relatively little money has gone toward such prevention and detection. The costs attributed to women's health are largely for institutional care and terminal hospital care in the last years of life, for medications, and for time lost from participation in the paid labor force as a result of illness. Very little of this money has gone to research that might ultimately make the current level of these expenditures unnecessary. In fact, in 1988 only 13 percent of the budget of the National Institutes of Health (NIH) went for research on women's health (Kirschstein 1991), although women contribute as many of their tax dollars as men to support this federal research body.

This discrepancy between research on men's and women's health problems has recently been publicized. The heroic efforts of Rep. Pat Schroeder and others have led to the creation of an Office of Women's Health Research at the NIH, a ruling that all NIH research include women when appropriate, and legislation that appropriated additional money to the NIH for research on breast cancer, ovarian cancer, osteoporosis, and heart disease. Together, these efforts are known as the Women's Health Initiative. These are clearly steps in the right direction, but mere drops in the bucket in terms of the magnitude of the problem.

Significantly, except for heart disease, the conditions to be addressed by the Women's Health Initiative are all related to the reproductive status of women. Although these problems are vitally important, the disproportionate emphasis on them is a reflection of the way in which women have traditionally been viewed by the medical profession. Recent evidence reminds us that women are not merely "walking wombs" but are subject to a wide range of medical problems in addition to those associated with their gynecologic systems. The three leading causes of death in all women are the same as those for men: heart disease, cancer, and stroke. For example, last year in the United States, ten thousand more women died of lung cancer than of breast cancer. That is not to suggest that research on breast cancer and programs for its early detection be abandoned. Quite to the contrary, these efforts are critically important and demand more attention and resources. But we also need more investigation of the realities of the full range of women's health problems, more research into their prevention and early detection, a better understanding of the relationship between women's changing roles in our society and their health status, and reeducation of today's doctors to broaden their view and better prepare them to meet the full spectrum of health needs of women.

These challenges require additional expenditures of health dollars for research, medical education and training, and public education directed at the health problems of women. Only after all this is achieved will we really know how many years of women's lives have heretofore been lost or wasted because of their unrecognized or ignored health problems and how many of our country's health dollars have been misspent in the name of improving women's lives.

Attitudes toward women's health need to change among health care providers, the public at large, and women themselves. At present, for example, doctors rarely consider certain "male" diagnoses, such as heart disease, in their women patients, and they often are delayed in recommending life-prolonging treatments as a result. There is also a bias toward considering women to have more emotional diseases than physical ones; this results not only in misdiagnosis, but also in the prescription of more psychotropic medication for women than for men.

Another example of a public bias about women's health that needs to be reexamined also relates to heart disease. Popular belief holds that the recently revealed fact that women have a high rate of heart attacks is a new phenomenon attributable to the stress of their participation in the paid labor force. This interpretation is incorrect; heart disease among women is a long-standing reality that had not previously been recognized.

Finally, women need to critically examine some of the effects of their socialization. They have been wrongly taught to accept some symptoms, such as menstrual cramps, as "inevitable" and emotionally based rather than to recognize their physical origin and to seek medical care for them.

This book is written for women (and their families) who wish to update their knowledge about their bodies and their health, to have the confidence to seek more specific information from their physicians or the literature, and to participate in the process of advancing scientific knowledge as researchers, subjects, or philanthropists. I hope it will be helpful to women in their pursuit of better health care. It is also written for students of nursing, medicine, nutrition, and women's studies, with the hope of enabling them to better understand and serve their women patients. And it is written to focus attention on the gaps in our knowledge, in order to suggest directions for future research and education efforts for both the medical and the consumer communities.

Accordingly, this book not only synthesizes our current knowledge about women's health, but also explores the reasons for the state of women's health today. Its approach is developmental, examining health issues at different stages of the female life cycle.

The first four chapters each examine one of four major life stages: adolescence, young adulthood, the perimenopausal years, and the older years. Key elements of the developmental biology of each stage are discussed, as are health issues of particular importance at that stage. Major health problems that do not fall into any of the succeeding substantive chapters are discussed in the chapter covering the time of life in which they take their greatest toll.

Chapters 5 through 10 go into detail on each of six health issues that are not specific to any one life stage: sexually transmitted diseases, pregnancy and its prevention, mental health, substance abuse, violence against women, and nutrition. Each of these chapters outlines the basic issues important to women of all ages, then discusses the specifics of particular importance at each stage. Thus, for a full discussion of health issues at a particular life stage, the reader will need to check not only the chapter on that life stage, but the substantive chapters' sections on the same stage. The last four chapters take a broader view, addressing the medical care of women in the United States, women as doctors, choosing the right doctor, and research in women's health.

I have sought to make the coverage of this book as broad as possible, but I have not essayed the futile task of even listing, much less discussing, every health issue relevant to women and every disease that can befall them. I have discussed the more significant issues in some depth. However, I have sought not to duplicate readily accessible references on individual topics, but instead to bring together the latest research findings—many of them not so readily accessible—on those topics. On some subjects, which warrant and have received coverage in numerous books of their own, I have noted only a few points, either those of particular importance to women or those that highlight differences between women's and men's health status or health care. The brevity of some of these discussions does not, of course, imply that the topics are insignificant or that little information is available on them.

PART ONE

Life-span Differences in Health Issues for Women

CHAPTER ONE

Adolescence

As we begin our exploration of the special health issues and needs of women throughout the life span, it is appropriate that we first focus on adolescence, when significant health-related gender differences first begin to appear. We will see that gender differences increase with time, and that biologic and psychosocial factors become increasingly intertwined as people age. Accordingly, it is much easier to analyze the independent contributions and directionality of the biologic and the psychosocial early in life than it is later on. Therefore, the biologic and the psychosocial are used as organizing principles in this chapter, but not in the later ones.

After summarizing the biologic and psychosocial changes that occur during adolescence, this chapter addresses some of the most frequent health problems of adolescence, namely, those of the maturing gynecologic system.

Puberty

The most dramatic biological differences between the genders appear in the second decade of life, when we see the transformational power of puberty. At no other time in a woman's life does the entire body grow and change in shape; this development is coincident with marked changes in feelings, with stresses of school performance, and with uncertain societal expectations. The only other time that possibly rivals adolescence in terms of biologic and psychologic upheaval is pregnancy, but the transiency of that stage of life generally renders it less traumatic.

The process of puberty includes all of the changes that occur in response to increased levels of hormones produced in the hypothalamus in the brain. These hormones are produced in pulses and stimulate the pituitary gland to secrete its own hormones, which in turn stimulate other organs in the body, including the ovaries, to produce their hormones (in the case of the ovaries, estrogen and progesterone).

During childhood, the bodies of males and females are rather similar in composition. For both, approximately 7 percent of the body is composed of fat tissue, for example. When puberty is completed, women are generally shorter than men and have more body fat, wider hips, smaller hearts with lower output of blood, less lung capacity, looser ligaments in the arms and legs, and fewer red blood cells. As a result of their lower cardiac output, smaller lung capacity, and lower number of red blood cells, women have less capacity for carrying oxygen in their blood. This appears to be the reason that men have the advantage over women in long-distance running. Lest we fall into the trap of viewing biology as destiny, it should be pointed out that women are rapidly catching up on the playing field and track. Moreover, it is important not to assume (still less embrace) a "deficit model" for the female when sex differences are noted. Clearly, most of the biologic differences that exist at this stage of development are advantageous for the purposes of reproduction. In addition, the greater body fat of women is an advantage in swimming and survival in the cold.

Despite extensive research, it's still not clear why puberty starts when it does. The newborn baby has all the structures necessary for reproduction, and in fact there are "accidents of nature" that cause young children to enter puberty before the usual time. For most girls, puberty begins at about the age of ten, but it may begin a year or two earlier, or up to three years later. One of the most reliable predictors of the timing of puberty is the time that it began in close family members. Although we are not yet sure what triggers puberty under normal conditions, it progresses in a remarkably predictable and orderly pattern.

The process of puberty encompasses four main phenomena: development of secondary sex characteristics, development of reproductive capability, the height spurt, and the weight spurt. Important psychosocial development also takes place.

SECONDARY SEX CHARACTERISTICS

Development of secondary sex characteristics results from the hormones produced by the ovaries and, to a lesser extent, from those produced by the adrenal glands. Secretion of estrogen by the ovaries stimulates growth and development of the breast, whereas adrenal secretion of androgens is responsible for growth of hair on the pubis and axillae, as well as for acne.

Breasts

Breast development begins early in puberty. The increased ovarian production of estrogen stimulates the mammary ducts. Progesterone, produced by the ovaries after ovulation, causes growth of the lobes of breast tissue called alveolae.

The timing of onset can vary considerably across the normal range. Most girls begin to see budding of the breast after their tenth birthday, but it can be normal for this to begin as late as the twelfth year. A number of factors influence this timing—mother's age at the time of her puberty, body weight (higher weight correlates with earlier puberty), exercise (puberty can be delayed in those who exercise vigorously, such as gymnasts), and chronic illness (which can delay puberty), to name just a few.

There are five stages in the development of the breast, sometimes referred to as Tanner stages or sex maturity ratings (SMRs) (see Fig. 1.1). In SMR 1, breast development has not yet begun. In SMR 2, the breast bud appears; in SMR 3, one sees growth of the areola and nipple; in SMR 4, the areola rises above the plane of the underlying breast; and SMR 5 marks the completion of development to the adult breast. These stages are based on the shape, not the size, of the breast. These stages are reached over the course of two to three years in most girls.

The reason it is useful to stage the development of the breast is that these stages (and those of pubic hair, discussed below) are markers for the progress of the entire body's development. Knowing the stage of a girl's breast development can help in predicting when she will have her first menstrual period. For example, 10 percent of girls get their first menstrual period at SMR 2, 20 percent at SMR 3, 60 percent at SMR 4, and 10 percent at SMR 5. Also, many laboratory tests follow stages of breast development more closely than they do chronologic age. For example, the hematocrit, a measure of blood cell number and hence of anemia, falls with each successive stage of puberty in girls.

Few women have two breasts of identical size, but young women are not generally well informed about this. The inequality is particularly likely to be seen before breast development has gone through all its stages. Surgery to correct breast asymmetry (if done at all) should not be undertaken until pubertal development has been completed, both because of the possibility that the asymmetry will self-correct, and because further growth might affect the cosmetic result should surgery be done too soon. For more on cosmetic breast surgery, see Chapter 2.

Another normal variation that often causes concern is retracted or inverted nipples. These often resolve with continuing pubertal development or with pregnancy. For pregnant women wanting to nurse their infants, some recommend daily manual breast pump traction toward the end of the pregnancy if there is not spontaneous resolution before that. For truly inverted nipples, milk cups may be useful, starting as early as the third month of pregnancy.

Skin and Body Hair

The increased production of androgen hormones by the adrenal glands occurs in both boys and girls at puberty, albeit in smaller amounts in the latter. This increased androgen production causes numerous skin changes. The most predictable of these is the development of pubic hair, which, like breast development, progresses through five stages and generates SMRs. SMR 1 denotes the prepubertal or childlike stage. At SMR 2, fine, downy hair appears on the lower part of the mons pubis, the fleshy mound above the "V" formed by the two thighs. At SMR 3, the hair becomes darker, longer, and silky and spreads upward and outward from the lower midline. By SMR 4, the hair has achieved its adult characteristics of coarseness and curliness and covers the entire mons pubis. By SMR 5, it has spread to the inner aspects of the thighs.

The other skin changes in puberty resulting from increased androgen production include the growth of both sebaceous and apocrine glands. The former are the little glands in the skin of the face and back that produce sebum, which is responsible for the oily skin that appears for the first time in adolescence. Sebum is broken down to fatty acids by enzymes produced by bacteria present on all of our skins. In people with a

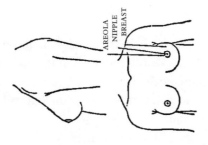

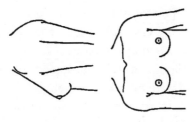

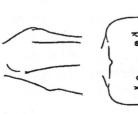

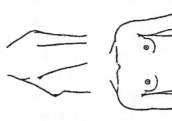

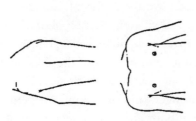

AREOLA
NIPPLE
BREAST

1. The nipple is raised a little in this stage. The rest of the breast is still flat.

2. This is the breast bud stage. In this stage the nipple is raised more than in Stage 1. The breast is a small mound. The areola is larger than in Stage 1.

3. The areola and the breast are both larger than in Stage 2. The areola does not stick out away from the breast.

4. The areola and the nipple make up a mound that sticks above the shape of the breast. (*Note:* This stage may not happen at all for some girls. Some girls develop from Stage 3 to Stage 5, with no Stage 4.)

5. This is the mature adult stage. The breasts are fully developed. Only the nipple sticks out in this stage. The areola has moved back to the general shape of the breast.

FIGURE 1.1. The five stages of breast development

familial tendency to develop acne, however, these fatty acids tend to produce inflammation, causing pimples. Blackheads result when the duct or opening of a sebaceous gland becomes blocked and the sebum accumulates behind the blockage. A blackhead results from oxidation and darkening of sebum upon exposure to the air.

There are many myths about acne. To address three of the commoner ones: Acne is not caused by infection. It is also not caused by dirt. Although we do recommend frequent washing, it is not because of dirt, but rather to rid the skin of the bacteria that make the fatty-acid-producing enzymes. And acne is not caused by chocolate, except in the few teenaged girls who are actually allergic to it. In the absence of such allergy, there is no evidence that chocolate causes or worsens acne.

There are many excellent ways to treat acne that build on the knowledge of its true causes. For example, estrogens decrease the size of the sebaceous follicle and the amount of sebum. Although a physician would never use estrogen for the sole purpose of treating acne (because of its possible side effects and the fact that we have other, less potent treatment methods), its effect on acne is a consideration when choosing a birth control method for a teenager. In other words, all other things being equal (see Chapter 6 for other considerations), a young woman and her physician may together decide that estrogen-containing birth control pills are the best choice for her because of her acne. Once that decision is made, it is important to pick the right kind of pill, one with low progesterone potency, like Demulen. Some combination pills with potent progesterones can worsen acne.

Another good way to control acne is to destroy the bacteria that produce the enzymes that break down sebum into irritating fatty acids. This is done with antibiotics, either taken by mouth (e.g., tetracycline) or placed directly on the skin (e.g., clindamycin or erythromycin). This approach is often misunderstood by parents and teenagers alike because we are all used to thinking of antibiotics as treatments for infections.

Acne is often improved by the use of vitamin A cream (retinoic acid) and/or benzoyl peroxide. Together, these are quite effective, but they often initially cause significant reddening and peeling of the skin, which some feel is worse than the acne. If one can tolerate these effects, the eventual outcome is excellent. A stronger kind of vitamin A (Retin-A) may be recommended for use by mouth for girls with severe, cystic acne.

Although this is very effective, it has many dangerous side effects that may make it unsuitable for some people. For example, it can cause birth defects if the patient is in the early stages of pregnancy, often at a time before she even knows she is pregnant. It can also raise the levels of "bad" cholesterol in the blood (see Chapter 2 under Heart Disease), and it may cause cracking of the skin and mucous membranes of the mouth and vagina, often with significant discomfort.

REPRODUCTIVE CAPABILITY

From the perspective of survival of the species, the raison d'être of puberty is that it results in reproductive capability. For a girl, this means the abilities to ovulate and to nurture a fertilized egg in her uterus. The interaction of hormones produced by the hypothalamus, the pituitary, and the ovaries brings about the necessary functional changes in the ovary and structural changes in the uterus.

As discussed above (see under Breasts), the majority of girls begin menstruating between SMRs 3 and 4 of maturation of secondary sex characteristics. Menarche generally occurs within two years after initiation of breast development and within one year of the peak of the growth spurt. By the time of SMR 5 and the peak of the weight velocity curve, almost all girls will have menstruated, a signal of structural and functional maturity of the uterus. The average age for menarche (first menstruation) currently is about twelve and a half, but the range is quite broad, from about ten and a half to sixteen for healthy girls. There are trend differences among ethnic groups, with menarche occurring earlier in Latinas than in blacks and earlier in blacks than in whites. Even more striking is the consistency of timing of menarche within families. Sisters tend to have menarche at about the same age, which is likely to be within a year of the age at which their mother first menstruated. Because menstruation can occur, and often does, before regular ovulatory cycles are achieved, having reached menarche does not necessarily signal fertility. For most young women, monthly ovulatory cycles are not established until one to two years following menarche. On the other hand, many girls do ovulate regularly following menarche. The occurrence of menstrual cramps is sometimes considered to be a sign of ovulation in that cycle, but this is far from a perfect indicator.

Variability in timing and frequency of menses is discussed below (see under Oligomenorrhea and Amenorrhea).

THE GROWTH SPURTS

The growth spurts in both height and weight occur at an average age of twelve in girls, about two years earlier than in boys, but there is a very wide age range for normal girls. For most girls, the growth spurts are linked to other pubertal events so that the peak of the weight spurt occurs at about the same time as menarche, generally between SMRs 3 and 4 (that is, about two years after breast budding; see above under Breasts). During the year or two of the peak of the height velocity curve, girls grow about 9 cm (3.5 in.) each year, a rate four times that of the prepubertal years. At the peak of the weight velocity curve, the percentage of body fat increases sharply from about 7 percent to 17 percent. By the completion of puberty, this percentage is in the range of 20–25 percent. (In comparison, the percentage of body fat of the male stays constant during puberty or may even decrease slightly, owing to increase in muscle mass.)

The height spurt occurs in orderly progression, starting at the feet and hands, progressing to the long bones of the arms and legs and last to the hips and bones of the trunk. During this period of rapid elongation and widening, bones also increase in strength. As a result, a young woman has the greatest density and strength in her bones at the end of the pubertal growth spurt that she will ever have.

PSYCHOSOCIAL DEVELOPMENT

The pubertal changes in the body obviously do not occur in a vacuum. The context of puberty has serious implications for the way in which it is experienced, especially when it occurs earlier or later than the prevailing peer pattern.

Among the psychosocial tasks that must be mastered during the adolescent period in our culture is emotional separation from the family in preparation for developing independence. Although most earlier studies of this phenomenon focused entirely on the adolescent, it has become clear that puberty plays a bidirectional role in the family's experience of adolescence. For girls, for example, pubertal development often signals fathers to become less physically affectionate. In the absence of open discussion, daughters may experience the resulting paternal withdrawal as rejection. It appears that it is not only parents who are impacted by their teenagers' changing bodies. Clingempeel et al. (1992) found that the more advanced a granddaughter's pubertal development, the less her involvement with her grandfather. In contrast, for pubertal boys, there was increased involvement and greater perceived closeness with both grandparents.

Holmbeck and Hill (1991) examined rule-setting in relationship to pubertal development and found that there were gender differences in rule frequency. Most studies find that earlier-maturing girls are subjected to more rules and curfews, especially in households at lower socioeconomic levels.

Timing of puberty affects school performance as well. For example, Dubas, Graber, and Petersen (1991) found that educational achievement was more strongly associated with the age of onset of puberty than with pubertal status per se. Late-developing boys had the lowest, and late-developing girls the highest, achievement in social studies, literature, and language arts. Timing of puberty may also help determine what type of school environment is best for adolescents. In a longitudinal study, Blythe et al. (1981) found that early-maturing girls who moved to a middle school experienced lower self-image and poorer grades than their early-maturing peers who remained in a K–8 school.

Pubertal timing has also emerged as a critical factor for psychosocial development of adolescents in modern industrialized societies. Within the relatively narrow normal range of onset of puberty (ten to twelve years of age for breast development in females and twelve to fourteen years of age for testicular growth in males), variations in timing appear to have major impact on the way adolescence is experienced in our society. Gender differences are consistently found, with early maturation generally viewed as advantageous in males and midrange maturation more consistent with positive adjustment in females. More specifically, because early maturation in males results in a physique that is taller and more muscular at a time when chronologic peers are still childlike in appearance, the earlier-maturing males tend to be more athletic, more popular, and even more successful academically. Conversely, late-maturing

males have been found to have poorer self-image, poorer school performance, and lower educational aspirations and expectations. Dorn, Crockett, and Petersen (1988) found that boys who were pubertally mature in
the seventh grade had better moods overall and rated themselves better
on impulse control than nonpubertal male peers.

For girls, the effects of differences in pubertal timing are more complex and context-dependent. By the sixth grade, early-maturing girls who
had been well adjusted in the fifth grade had decreasing body image and
reported having been teased (by female peers as well as parents; Brooks-
Gunn, 1984). Brooks-Gunn found that in the fifth and sixth grades, girls
who had early breast development were more likely to have been teased,
with resultant poorer body image. No association between pubertal status
and self-esteem was found, however, in a small, ethnically diverse sample
studied cross-sectionally by Brack, Orr, and Ingersoll (1988).

A landmark report by the American Association of University Women
Education Foundation (1992) described the phenomenon of declining
self-image in girls during adolescence. Although this report did not examine the role of biologic maturation in relationship to this observation,
it is likely, based on the findings cited above, that earlier-maturing girls
were at particular risk.

Because puberty for girls is so closely tied to an increase in adiposity,
girls in contemporary society, which values thinness as the ideal female
form, often react negatively to puberty because of its implications for
their weight. This is particularly so for girls who mature earlier than their
peers. Dorn, Crockett, and Petersen (1988) found that the more physically mature seventh- and eighth-grade girls were less satisfied with their
appearance and weight. These findings were confirmed by Killen et al.
(1994), who found a higher incidence of dissatisfaction with weight
among earlier-maturing females who were followed prospectively from
the sixth grade. Along the same lines, in a reanalysis of data from the National Health Examination Survey, Duncan et al. (1985) reported that the
majority of females became dissatisfied with their weight as they matured. This was particularly true for the early maturers, 69 percent of
whom reported dissatisfaction.

Puberty and its timing can also affect the development of psychological disorders during adolescence. For example, a higher incidence of

psychosomatic symptoms among early-maturing fourteen-to-sixteen-year-old Finnish girls was found by Aro and Taipale (1987). More recent studies suggest that early-maturing girls are also at increased risk of eating disorders, panic disorders, and depression (see Killen et al. 1994).

The development of depression in adolescent girls has been of special interest to researchers. Angold and Rutter (1992) are among those who have studied the relationship between puberty and depressive symptomatology. In their large sample of psychiatric patients, they found increasing rates of depression with age in both boys and girls. Gender differences emerged by sixteen years of age, at which time the girls were twice as likely as the boys to have significant depression. When the researchers controlled for age, however, they found no effect of pubertal status. (See Chapter 7 for further discussion of depression.)

Flannery, Rowe, and Gulley (1993) examined the impact of pubertal status, timing, and age on delinquency and sexual behavior. They found that in girls both delinquency and sexual activity were predicted by the timing and status of puberty, independent of age, with a weaker association in boys. Both boys and girls who matured early had more sexual activity and delinquent behavior than late maturers. In a longitudinal study of the relationship between maturational timing and the development of problem behavior in girls, Silbereisen et al. (1989) found that early maturers studied at fourteen to fifteen years of age had more contacts with deviant peers than later-maturing girls.

The reasons for these differences reflect the complexity of factors that influence adjustment during the adolescent period, when young girls must simultaneously confront their changing bodies, peer pressure, and changing expectations for them in society.

During adolescence, the major health concerns of young women relate to their attractiveness and their normality. They are self-conscious, as are their male peers, and interpret health problems in terms of their potential impact on peer group acceptance. With girls increasingly participating in competitive sports, more recent health concerns include those that may affect their athletic performance. These concerns notwithstanding, the greatest current threat to their health comes from increasing cigarette use, often in order to control weight; more adolescent females than males are now taking up this habit (see Chapter 8).

Gynecologic Problems of Adolescents

Because menstruation begins early in the second decade of life, it is during adolescence that most gynecologic problems begin or are first diagnosed. The common menstrually related conditions of this age group include the absence or loss of menses (amenorrhea), irregular menses (oligomenorrhea), painful menses (dysmenorrhea), and excessive menstrual bleeding (menorrhagia). Tumors and congenital abnormalities may also occur, though they are not common. Various problems may also arise involving the breasts.

OLIGOMENORRHEA AND AMENORRHEA

There are a number of reasons that menses fail to appear or become irregular. Some of these are simply the result of stresses of daily life, whereas others reflect serious pathology. Because of the complex nature of factors that control menstruation, consultation with a physician is always prudent when menses become irregular, cease, or fail to appear at the age-appropriate time. The discussion below speaks primarily of amenorrhea, but it generally applies to oligomenorrhea as well.

Primary amenorrhea refers to failure of menses to begin at the expected time. As discussed above, determination of the expected time is not as straightforward as it may seem. The relationship between the timing of a mother's menarche and that of her daughter's is so close that most physicians would diagnose primary amenorrhea in any girl who failed to menstruate within a year of her mother's age at menarche, even if she is younger than sixteen. Failure of menarche to occur within two years after initiation of breast development and within one year of the peak of the growth spurt may also warrant this diagnosis. Secondary amenorrhea refers to cessation of menses for at least three months.

Because interactions of hormones from the hypothalamus, pituitary, and ovaries are so critical in initiating and regulating menses, any disturbance in these organs or their interactions may result in amenorrhea. The most common cause of irregular or absent menses is immaturity of the regulatory system. The result is unpredictable ovulation. When ovulation does not occur, the ovary produces only estrogen. Without progesterone, the lining of the uterus builds up over the course of months before it is shed. This results in long intervals between menstrual periods. Some women, who are otherwise healthy and capable of reproduction, experience irregular menses throughout their premenopausal lives. Irregular menses is referred to as oligomenorrhea.

In addition to immaturity of the hormonal regulatory system, primary amenorrhea may be caused by genetic abnormalities (e.g., Turner syndrome) and birth defects of the reproductive tract. The most common and least serious of these is an imperforate hymen. This condition, in which there is blockage of the normal opening between the vagina and the exterior, is usually discovered when the young woman fails to menstruate at the age-appropriate time. In fact, she does menstruate, but the blood cannot exit the vagina. After a few months, the buildup of blood in the vagina behind the hymen results in pain and an enlarging lower abdominal mass. A similar scenario occurs with cervical stenosis, when the opening from the uterus to the vagina fails to develop. In this case, the enlarging "tumor" is the blood-filled uterus, rather than the vagina. The imperforate hymen is easily diagnosed by a physician's examination of the vagina, in which a bluish, bulging hymen is seen; the diagnosis of cervical stenosis typically requires a more extensive examination, including ultrasound study.

The most common explanation for secondary amenorrhea is pregnancy. Although this is the first thought that leaps to mind when the woman is an adult, it is surprising how often it is overlooked by physicians treating adolescents, as well as by the parents of adolescents. Secondary amenorrhea can also have many other causes, some of which (including immaturity of the hormonal system) may also result in primary amenorrhea. One of these causes is use of birth control pills; adolescent women are particularly susceptible to "post-Pill amenorrhea," which stems from the Pill's effects on the natural production of pituitary hormones (see Chapter 6).

Emotional and/or physical stress may interfere with menarche or menstrual regularity, sometimes to the extent of causing amenorrhea. The stress of going away to camp or college is a common reason for menses to cease. Strenuous athletic activity is becoming quite common as another reason for amenorrhea. It is still not entirely clear whether this results from the physical activity itself, the emotional stress associated with competition, or the lean body habitus of athletes. It is interesting that not all sports have the same impact on menstrual function. For example, it is rare that swimmers have amenorrhea, whereas runners commonly develop it, despite comparable training schedules. More research is clearly needed to better understand the physiologic effects of sports on women (see Chapter 10). Malnutrition, too, whether stemming from anorexia nervosa (see Chapter 7) or any other cause, commonly results in amenorrhea. Chronic illnesses such as inflammatory bowel disease cause cessation of menses through their impact on nutrition. Other chronic illnesses may adversely affect menstrual function by interfering with oxygenization (e.g., certain types of heart or lung diseases) or with hormonal balance (e.g., hyperthyroidism, adrenal hyperactivity, and certain ovarian tumors). Depression and drug use may also cause menstruation to stop (see Chapters 7 and 8).

Another pathologic condition that causes amenorrhea is polycystic ovary syndrome (PCO), also known as the Stein-Leventhal syndrome. This condition, which in its full-blown form consists of multiple small cysts in an enlarged ovary that is enveloped in a thick covering, has an interesting history. It was first discovered in infertile women who were in their thirties. These women tended to be obese, to have increased body and facial hair, and to have acne. Their hormones had a unique pattern: one of the two pituitary hormones that control ovulation (LH, or luteinizing hormone) was markedly elevated, and the other (FSH, or follicle-stimulating hormone) was normal. It was found that surgical removal of a wedge of tissue from the ovary often resulted in ovulation and enhanced the possibility of pregnancy. As time has passed, researchers have learned that the pituitary is the culprit and that the effects on the ovary are the result of the problem, not the cause.

Very importantly, it is now known that the condition begins in adolescence, before the physical appearance is affected. The usual features of this condition during adolescence are irregular menstrual periods for a longer time than usual (that is, for more than eighteen months following the first period), or absence or cessation of menses. The same abnormal hormone pattern previously identified in the older, infertile women is found in these young girls, most of whom are not overweight or hirsute and do not have excessive acne. It is important to make the diagnosis at the earliest possible age, because early initiation of treatment with birth control pills may prevent development of these unpleasant physical features. It is still uncertain whether this treatment can also prevent the infertility.

MENSTRUAL CRAMPS (DYSMENORRHEA) AND MENORRHAGIA

The leading cause of short-term school absence in girls is menstrual cramps. There have been numerous surveys to determine the prevalence of this problem, all of which come to similar conclusions: approximately one-third of adolescent girls have severe, disabling dysmenorrhea; one-third have mild or intermittent problems with menstrual cramps; and about one-third have no such problems.

Despite the fact that those in the first category often are bedridden and suffer significantly, only about 10 percent ever seek help from a physician (Klein and Litt 1981). The reasons for failure to seek medical treatment are many, including the fact that many teenagers (as well as their mothers) do not know that help is available. Another factor is that until recently the medical profession, as well as much of the lay public, erroneously considered menstrual cramps to be an emotional problem rather than a medical one. This position was bolstered by the anthropologic literature. Margaret Mead, for example, is widely quoted as having written that native Samoan girls did not suffer from menstrual cramps (Mead 1928). In my recent rereading of Mead's book, I interpreted her remarks as being consistent with the view that these girls had cramps but were not disabled by them. In addition, as recently as the 1960's, textbooks of gynecology and even popular books on childrearing described girls and women with menstrual cramps as neurotic, rejecting of their feminine roles, or worse. As is too often the case, when the medical profession didn't have a scientific explanation for a problem, it blamed the victim.

What has happened to change this attitude is the discovery that menstrual cramps are the result of contractions of the muscles of the uterus. The contractions are stimulated by substances called prostaglandins that are produced in the uterine lining. This is much the same phenomenon that occurs in labor, but obviously these contractions are not as strong. A variety of medications are now available to prevent or treat these cramps. They act by interfering with the production of the prostaglandins or by destroying them after they are formed. These medications are better known, through their wide use in the treatment of sports injuries, as the "nonsteroidal anti-inflammatory" drugs. Some of them, such as ibuprofen, are available without a prescription.

Another way to prevent cramps is through the use of birth control pills, which act in two ways. They limit the amount of uterine lining produced, which in turn decreases the amount of prostaglandins that can be made. They also prevent the ovaries from producing progesterone, which seems to make the uterine muscle more sensitive to the effects of the prostaglandins.

Rarely, these medications fail to cure the problem. For girls who do not get relief from them, it is important that the physician explore the possibility that the pain is the result of endometriosis. This results when tissue from the lining of the uterus forms in or extends to other parts of the abdominal cavity. Because this tissue responds to the effects of hormones in the same way as the uterine lining, it tends to cause pain at the time of menses. Endometriosis was, until recently, thought to occur only in adult women. With advances in the diagnostic technology, many women with chronic abdominal pain who, in the past, might have gone undiagnosed or been labeled as chronic complainers are often found to have endometriosis. The major tool for making the diagnosis is laparoscopy, which involves insertion of a tiny light and viewer through a small incision in the abdomen. Treatment of endometriosis may require surgery to remove an endometrial implant or, more commonly, the administration of medication that suppresses estrogens.

Despite these recent advances in both understanding of the causes of menstrual cramps and the technology for diagnosing and treating them, one "old wives' tale" continues to be valid. It has long been recognized that after childbirth, most women no longer experience menstrual cramps. The likely explanation is that childbirth causes a relaxation in the tone of the cervix and results in a decrease in the resistance offered to the contracting uterus during subsequent menstrual periods.

Excessive menstrual bleeding in the adult woman generally signifies serious pathology. In the adolescent, the causes of heavy bleeding are generally not as serious, but the impact of the experience can surely be major. Among the more serious, but rare, causes of this phenomenon in the teenage girl are clotting abnormalities and miscarriage. With adult women, cancer is often a worry when there is excessive bleeding, but this is not a consideration in the adolescent. More commonly, the cause in the teenager is hormonal. Although abnormalities in functioning of the thyroid gland may occasionally be responsible, the usual explanation is immaturity of the delicately balanced system that links the hypothalamus, the pituitary gland, and the ovaries. As discussed above under Oligomenorrhea and Amenorrhea, this immaturity may result in the uterine lining building up over several months. When it is finally shed, the bleeding is excessive. In more mature cycles, the presence of progesterone regulates the buildup of the uterine lining and, as a result, the amount of bleeding.

Most often, as long as the loss of blood is not so great as to cause anemia or light-headedness, a physician will not have to treat at all. When treatment is necessary, as is the case when bleeding is excessive, it is generally accomplished by giving the missing hormone, progesterone. Because we do not have to worry about uterine cancer as a cause of excessive bleeding in teenagers, a dilation and suction procedure is rarely, if ever, necessary.

TUMORS AND DEFORMITIES

Gynecologic tumors can occur during adolescence, although they are considerably more common in older women. Tumors of the ovary in adolescents, unlike those in adult women, are rarely cancerous. More typically, these are slow-growing tumors that have arisen from tissue of the embryo (dermoid cysts), from endometriosis, or as the result of ovulation (follicular cysts). Some ovarian tumors are discovered because their bulk causes pain or pressure on nearby structures. The most common cause of pain is endometriosis, when endometrial tissue has grown onto and into the ovary. This is called a "chocolate cyst" because of its appearance, resulting from monthly bleeding into the cyst at the time of a menstrual period. Because the blood is confined by the walls of the cyst, it cannot escape, and the cyst continues to grow. Other tumors of the ovary produce hormones that cause changes in the menstrual pattern or in the appearance (e.g., hirsutism, acne, enlarged clitoris). Cancer is rarely the cause.

Congenital abnormalities of the female genital tract other than those discussed above (e.g., imperforate hymen and cervical stenosis) are less common. They include structural deformities of the uterus, such as a double uterus or one divided by a partition ("bicornuate"), and ovarian malformations. Although the causes of most of these birth defects are unknown, some have resulted from exposure of the fetus to the effects of the hormone diethylstilbestrol (DES). From approximately the 1940's to the 1970's, this agent was often given to pregnant women with a history of prior miscarriage, in the belief that it would prevent a recurrence of this problem. Abnormalities of the reproductive organs of both male and female offspring, as well as some gynecologic tumors, were discovered during adolescence in many of the babies born following this maternal treatment. Accordingly, use of DES in pregnancy has been discontinued. Some of the defects it caused are correctable with surgery, but others may result in sterility. As discussed in Chapter 6, new technological advances now offer the possibility of reproduction for women with some of these abnormalities.

BREAST HEALTH PROBLEMS

Breast lumps are fairly common in young adolescent girls, but it is extremely rare to find breast cancer in this age group. The most common of their tumors are cysts that result from hormonal stimulation and typically regress within the next menstrual cycle. Cysts are usually painful and can be frightening to a young woman, but they are not dangerous. If they persist for more than three menstrual cycles, most doctors will insert a needle and remove the fluid, more to be sure that they are indeed cysts than for relief of symptoms.

The other common cause of a lump in the breast of an adolescent is a tumor called a fibroadenoma. This is quite firm and may grow to a large size. Because of the rare cancerous tumor in this age group, any tumor that lasts for more than three months will usually prompt a physician to recommend its removal. Mammograms are not generally useful in evaluating breast masses in adolescents because of the high density of the surrounding breast tissue at this age. Removal of a tumor will allow for its careful examination by a trained pathologist to be sure it isn't cancer. The technique for this surgery is much improved over past years, with only a small incisional scar remaining along the border of the areola, hardly noticeable as years go by.

Adolescents may also experience nipple discharge. Although the most common cause is pregnancy and subsequent lactation, it can also be caused by a number of other conditions. In adolescents, the most common of these is ingestion of some drug, prescribed or not, that stimulates the pituitary gland to produce an increased amount of the hormone prolactin. Drugs that may have this effect include oral contraceptives, some psychotropic drugs (such as phenothiazines), heroin, marijuana, some antihypertensive drugs, and antigastroplegics (e.g., metoclopramide). Rarely, and particularly if the discharge is accompanied by loss of menses and is not related to pregnancy, the cause may be found in the brain and its connection with the pituitary gland or the thyroid gland (particularly when the latter is less active than normal). Local effects on the breast from mechanical stimulation, infection, or trauma may also result in the production of a milky substance from the nipple.

It was once feared that injuries to the breasts of adolescent girls would result in the later development of breast cancer. There is absolutely no evidence that this is so, yet this belief was long used as medical justification for the exclusion of girls from sports. Now that legal protection has overruled these paternalistic restrictions, it is possible to gather data about sports injuries in girls. Interestingly, the risk of injuries is similar for the two sexes, the only difference relating to a slight increase in tendon and ligamentous injury in females. The breast is rarely involved in sports injuries, although irritation of the nipples as the result of jogging has become so common that it is now called "jogger's nipple." Some find petrolatum useful in preventing its occurrence.

Mortality

Adolescence is generally regarded as the healthiest time of life. Although the mortality rate for these years is lower than for other life stages, it is worrisome that adolescents are the only age group for whom this rate has increased in recent years. The manner in which vital statistics are reported in the United States cuts the adolescent age group between ages fourteen and fifteen and combines the younger half with children and the older with young adults. Therefore, mortality rates are reported for those 5 to 14 and those 15 to 24. In 1994, those rates were 22.7 per

100,000 for the younger age group (26.3 for males and 18.9 for females) and 99.6 per 100,000 for the older group (150.5 for males and 46.5 for females) (Singh et al. 1995). The higher mortality rate for males in both age groups is largely attributable to accidents, particularly motor vehicle accidents. In addition, the rates for homicide and suicide are far higher in males than females in the 15–24-year-old group.

The leading causes of death among adolescent and young adult females are listed in Appendix A.

CHAPTER TWO

Early Adulthood

This chapter addresses some of the health issues of greatest significance to women between the ages of 20 and 44. (The issues discussed in Chapters 5 through 10 are also, of course, highly relevant to women in this age group.) The major health issues for adult women relate to their social roles in relationships and careers. Those that are primarily determined by biologic factors are premenstrual syndrome, incontinence, high blood pressure, and immune system diseases. This chapter considers women's entry into the paid labor force and its consequences. In particular, it addresses the interface between work and pregnancy outcomes, heart disease, other causes of death, and nonfatal conditions such as repetitive motion syndrome.

Health Consequences of Entering the Paid Labor Force

The message has become more subtle, but it can still be heard all around us: "Venture into a man's world and you will be punished," or "Leave your children at home without you and they will suffer."

Welcomed into the paid labor force during wartime, women were promptly sent home when the last shot was fired. Or so it was before the 1960's. Since then, women have not only stayed in the country's work force, but have continued to join it in droves. As a result, over the last century, the percentage of women working outside the home has tripled (from 18 to over 50 percent). Women now are 45.6 percent of the work force, and this percentage is expected to rise to 47 by the year 2005 (Noble 1994). In 1960, only 17 percent of mothers returned to work within one year of a child's birth; in 1990, 53 percent did so (Carnegie Task Force 1994). By the time their children have reached three years of age, 54 percent of women are in the paid labor force, as are 57 percent with six-year-olds and 72 percent with children aged seventeen (Paula Reynolds, personal communication, 1990).

The kind of work women are doing has undergone a tremendous transformation. Aided considerably by the Equal Employment Opportunities Act of 1974, women have entered many professions in numbers equal to those of men. They have won the right to fly combat missions; 11 percent of American truck drivers are women; women are now "allowed" in the boardroom, albeit in token numbers; and women are now starting businesses at a rate five times faster than that of men.

Despite these considerable advances, rising unemployment and its emotional and economic threat to men in our country have once again brought pressure on these women to return to the home, as has been lucidly described by Faludi (1991). One strategy is to frighten women into thinking that competing in the highly stressful work world will have dire health consequences, either for them or for their children. The latter are targeted in newspaper headlines of the "Daycare Increases Infections in Toddlers" variety. The impact of these messages is reinforced by the difficulties encountered by women, many of them single parents, in securing child care. In fact, about half of women who return to work after maternity leave are no longer in the paid labor force one year later (Paula Reynolds, personal communication, 1991).

It is certainly true that women in the work force are exposed to many conditions that may have an adverse effect on their health. These include equipment designed for use by men, violence at the workplace, shift hours, extreme temperatures, and passive exposure to smoke. These realities lead to some special physical stresses for women in the workplace. But how true are the warnings women have received about workplace dangers? Let us look more closely at some of the health consequences often predicted for working women, and at some of those that have actually ensued.

FERTILITY AND PREGNANCY

It is shocking to find that there were almost no studies of the health of working women prior to the 1980's. Since then, a rash of reports have appeared in the occupational health literature to the effect that physical and chemical toxins in the workplace environment could be harmful to pregnant women or even those who might someday wish to have children. These reports stood in sharp contrast to several European studies that suggested that working women actually had better pregnancy outcomes than housewives—specifically, a lower rate of premature births (see Saurel-Cubizolles, Subtil, and Kaminski 1991; Ericson et al. 1987; Murphy et al. 1984).

It has been estimated that 80 percent of women pregnant with their first child are in the paid labor force. What is really known about the risk to unborn children from occupational exposures? The answer seems to vary with the type of factor to which women are exposed in the workplace.

The growing use of video display terminals (VDTs) raised concern that their electromagnetic radiation emissions might cause miscarriages. In a very detailed and careful study conducted over six years, researchers compared pregnancy outcome between hundreds of women who had been regularly exposed to VDTs during pregnancy and another group, similar in every way except for absence of such exposure. No differences in miscarriage rates were found (Schnorr et al. 1991).

On the other hand, a Swedish study found that passive exposure to smoke in the workplace increased the risk of miscarriage or stillbirth in the first trimester of pregnancy significantly among nonsmokers (Ahlborg and Bodin 1991). This finding, coupled with the knowledge that women exposed to cigarette smoke in the workplace have a 39 percent higher risk of developing lung cancer (Fontham et al. 1994), should prompt the banning of smoking, rather than of women, from the workplace.

Women in certain occupations in which they are exposed to chemical toxins have also been found to have an increased rate of miscarriages. For example, full-time workers in beauty salons, particularly those involved in perming, coloring, or bleaching hair or sculpting nails, are apparently at increased risk for this complication (John, Savitz, and Shy 1994).

Despite the absence of clear evidence of harm, a number of policies have been promulgated to "protect" women of all ages and their hypothetical unborn children from toxic exposures in the workplace. For example, one auto battery company required that women under the age of 70 (!) agree to sterilization or submit proof of infertility as a condition of employment, presumably to protect their unborn babies from exposure to lead. No similar policy existed to protect men. This policy was upheld by the U.S. Court of Appeals for the Seventh Circuit in 1989 as justified and nondiscriminatory under Title VII of the Civil Rights Act of 1964. However, it was reversed in 1991 by the U.S. Supreme Court.

There are data from experiments with rats showing that mating males exposed to low levels of lead with unexposed females resulted in offspring with brain defects. Among humans it has been found that children of *men* employed in jobs that expose them to lead had three times the rate of kidney tumors of those with nonexposed fathers. Significantly higher rates of brain cancer and leukemia have also been found among children with fathers exposed to paints, automobile exhaust, and solvents. Along the same lines, a recent report showed that more birth defects result from damage to sperm than to eggs. According to Davis (1991), "more than 50 therapeutic, occupational and environmental agents influence the ability of men to reproduce [and] . . . may irreversibly affect genetic material or temporarily affect the quality and quantity of sperm." The examples she cites include permanent sterilization among male agricultural and chemical production workers exposed to dibromochloropropane; twice the rate of premature babies born to wives of men who work in the glass, clay, stone, textile, and mining industries; and lower birth weight among babies of fathers who work with benzene and other solvents. These findings should not be surprising, given that rapidly growing and dividing cells are more vulnerable to the effects of toxins. Sperm cells divide extremely rapidly, especially in early adulthood, when a man produces 72 million sperm in each ejaculate. In comparison, a woman produces, on average, only 400 mature eggs in her lifetime from the two million immature eggs with which she is born.

Will we now see legislation barring men from work in high-risk environments? "Protective" legislation and company policies are more likely calculated to "protect" the male work force from female competition than actually to protect women or children. If the intent were truly to protect unborn children from the effects of occupational toxic exposure, the laws would apply equally to men and women. In the words of Davis (1991), "To protect the rights of workers, including their right to reproduce safely, workplace standards should protect the sperm, the egg and the embryo." Moreover, truly protective policies would cover the women working at hair salons who are at real risk from toxic exposure.

Existing discriminatory policies surely serve to frighten women and to make them feel guilty should they become ill or a baby be born with handicaps. A recent newspaper headline undoubtedly had that effect: "Chemical Plants Seen as a Factor in Breast Cancer" (Schemo 1994). The actual finding, though, related to living near, not working in, large plants producing chemical, rubber, or plastics.

The relationship between pregnancy outcome and physically stressful, though not necessarily toxic, working conditions has been examined in a number of studies. Saurel-Cubizolles, Subtil, and Kaminski (1991) found that occupation, rather than working conditions per se, affected the rate of prematurity. For example, women in manufacturing, sales, and service jobs had higher rates of premature births than those in managerial, clerical, teaching, and health jobs. Although working conditions as such were not found to affect outcome, it is important to note that more women who faced strenuous working conditions stopped working before the 28th week of pregnancy. Some earlier studies had, in fact, shown that pregnant women who worked standing at a conveyor belt, for example, or who lifted heavy weights in the course of their work had a higher rate of prematurity (Murphy et al. 1984).

The reasons that a number of more recent studies did not find this association are of interest. One theory is that over the last decade, working conditions have improved and industry has implemented preventive strategies. In support of this view are data from France indicating that the number of women reporting working while standing up during pregnancy decreased from 48 percent to 37 percent between 1972 and 1981 (Saurel-Cubizolles, Subtil, and Kaminski 1991). Working hours have generally decreased, as well. In evaluating all such studies, of course, one must also keep in mind the possibility of systematic bias in the reporting of adverse working conditions. For example, women with the fewest skills are more likely to have the most strenuous work conditions but also the greatest fear of job loss, should their complaints about these conditions to a researcher reach their employer.

The effect on pregnancy outcome of work-related psychologic stress was investigated by Homer, James, and Siegel (1990), who defined that stress as "work characterized by both high psychologic demands and limited control over the response to these demands" (p. 173). They found no association between job title, after accounting for physical exertion, and pregnancy outcome. However, for those women who did not want to remain in the work force, work-related stress did increase their risk of delivering a premature baby. This finding led these researchers to conclude, "Personal motivation toward work, as well as the physical effort of work, should be considered in evaluating the impact of a job's psychologic characteristics on pregnancy outcome" (p. 173).

Methodological concerns about the difficulty in separating the effects of socioeconomic status from those of work in earlier studies led to a well-controlled more recent study of female resident physicians. These women, who were working under conditions of both high physical and emotional stress, were compared with the wives of the male residents. This study found no difference in rates of miscarriage, stillbirth, delivery of premature or small babies, or ectopic pregnancy between the groups, despite the fact that the residents worked nearly twice as many hours (about 80 hours a week) during their pregnancies as did the male residents' wives. The only differences that were found were a higher rate of premature labor (but not birth) and of preeclampsia (pregnancy-induced high blood pressure) in the residents. Both of these findings may, alternatively, reflect increased vigilance among the residents. The authors concluded that "working long hours in a stressful occupation has little effect on the outcome of pregnancy in an otherwise healthy population of high socioeconomic status" (Klebanoff, Shiono, and Rhoads 1990: 1040).

CONSEQUENCES OF WORKPLACE STRESS

The growing literature on nonpregnant women in the paid labor force has focused on the health consequences of the emotional and physical stress generated by their work roles. The potential emotional stresses are many: low pay and status, shift work, sexual harassment, lack of professional and spouse support, and limited opportunities for advancement. These are often coupled with family responsibilities.

Emotional stress has been examined in studies of women's satisfaction with their major work roles (whether at home or on the job). This satisfaction has evolved as the most important predictor of health status and longevity: Women with multiple roles are found to be healthier. The healthiest women are actually those with "triple" roles (worker, spouse, and mother), whereas those women of comparable age with the poorest health are those who are unmarried and unemployed. This seems to be true regardless of race. These findings notwithstanding, the fact that married women who are employed full time outside the home work an average of 80 hours each week (counting housework and family-related activities), compared with 50 hours weekly for their employed husbands, surely has some adverse effects. These have primarily been seen in the higher incidence of both nervousness and anxiety in employed women (Zappert and Weinstein 1985).

One possible explanation for the finding of better health among women in the paid labor force is a self-selection bias. According to this interpretation, only the healthiest women can manage to work outside of the home, as well as fulfill their other role obligations. This has been labeled the "healthy worker" effect. In the best of the studies conducted, this possibility is considered and controlled for by matching the health conditions of the participants before and after they begin their employment. In the study by Kritz-Silverstein, Wingard, and Barrett-Connor (1992), for example, this was done by excluding women with known chronic illness from analyses at baseline. Parenthetically, the researchers found that the chronically ill working women excluded from analysis, the largest group of whom have diabetes, were still employed at the study's end, suggesting that it is not only healthy women who are in the work force.

Studies finding a positive association between satisfaction with employment and health for women may perhaps be explained by the presence of a third factor, rather than simply being attributable to cause and effect. Waldron and Herold (1986) suggest that certain personality factors may be responsible for both a positive job attitude and a healthier life-style. According to their interpretation, people with an "internal" locus of control, those who believe that what happens to them is the result of their own actions, are more likely to have a positive job attitude. Studies have also shown such personality types to have less physical and mental illness, to smoke less, and to exercise more than those with an "external" locus of control, who believe that they have little control over what happens to them (Waldron and Herold 1986). As a result, people with an internal locus of control may have both greater job satisfaction and a life-style that causes them to be healthier, independent of their employment status. Another study (Erdwins and Mellinger 1984) found that middle-aged women who were employed had more of a sense of personal control over their environment than women who were students or homemakers.

Just as these studies support a link between job satisfaction and good health, there is an apparent relationship between job dissatisfaction and poor health. One intriguing line of inquiry into this relationship is still in its infancy. This approach is based on findings that stress may lower immunity, thus increasing the risk of certain illnesses. One measure of immunity is the level of immunoglobulins in the blood. Research has shown a negative correlation between self-reported job stress and the level of immunoglobulins in samples of nurses and teachers (i.e., higher stress correlates with lower levels of immunoglobulins; Endresen et al. 1987; Ursin et al. 1984). Of the three types of immunoglobulin, immunoglobulin G is the longest lasting and most likely to reflect chronic stress. A more recent study (Theorell, Orth-Gomer, and Eneroth 1990) investigated levels of this factor, as well as subjects' ratings of job strain (defined by the ratio of demands to decision latitude) and of the amount of social support received, at four points in time over the course of a year. They found higher concentrations of immunoglobulin G with more job strain and with less social support. Immunoglobulin G increased more with increasing job strain in people who reported inadequate social support than in those with adequate support. The researchers found no difference in patterns between the men and women in their sample. Although it is too early to know all the implications of such a finding, it is interesting to note that immunoglobulin G may play a role in hardening of the arteries and heart disease as well as in protection against infections and possibly even cancer.

HEART DISEASE

Heart disease in women was generally predicted to increase as more women entered the work force because of the perception that they would experience additional stress in so doing. The first source of information on this subject is somewhat indirect, but intriguing. The World Health Organization examined the death rates from coronary artery disease in 30 industrialized countries between 1970 and 1985 (Uemurea and Pisa 1988). It found that the death rate for women fell more steeply than that for men in this period of time. This decline parallels the increase in numbers of women working outside of the home in these countries. This observation runs counter to the prediction that as women entered the paid labor force, their risk of heart disease would increase to approach that of men (LaRosa 1988; Passannante and Nathanson 1987).

In fact, more unemployed women of comparable age get fatal heart attacks than those in the workplace (Rosenberg et al. 1993). This is true even though there are more people with Type A personalities of both sexes (in the 30–35-year-old age group) in the workplace than out of it, and even though it has been demonstrated that having a Type A personality is a risk factor for getting a heart attack (Friedman and Rosenman 1974). One possible reason that employed women have fewer heart attacks is that, as discussed in Chapter 4, women's risk for heart attacks increases after the age of 65, which is often the age of retirement. In comparison, men's risk rises at an earlier age, when they are more likely to still be in the paid labor force.

If, apart from the age factor, there is a positive relationship between working outside of the home and a decrease in heart disease among women, what could explain it? One of the risk factors for heart disease is a high blood level of low density lipoproteins (LDLs) and a low level of high density lipoproteins (HDLs). A growing literature has developed on the association between women's work status and their levels of these cholesterols. One such study conducted in Germany (Haertel et al. 1992) initially looked at differences in cholesterol levels between women in the paid labor force and those at home, and subsequently followed these women for three years. These researchers found that employed women had significantly higher levels of HDLs than those who were full-time homemakers, even after they took into consideration all other factors that might affect these levels, such as diet, exercise, smoking, and alcohol consumption. Moreover, those women who, over the three years of follow-up, gave up their employment and became full-time homemakers experienced a significant drop in their HDL levels. Part of this decrease was associated with their increased alcohol consumption and pregnancies. The study concluded "that employment may exert a beneficial influence on coronary risk in women that is consistent with a positive association be-tween employment and HDL cholesterol" (p. 68).

A recent U.S. study (Kritz-Silverstein, Wingard, and Barrett-Connor 1992) examined the relationship between the employment status of 242 white, middle-class, middle-aged women and their risk factors for heart disease. The women who were employed outside the home had fewer risk factors, such as smoking and drinking alcohol, than unemployed women; they exercised more and had lower cholesterol, lower blood sugar levels, and a lower incidence of high blood pressure. The researchers concluded that "middle-aged women employed in managerial positions are healthier than unemployed women" (p. 215). This was also the con-clusion of another study (Hazuda et al. 1986) that was more racially di-verse in that it included Mexican-American women. On the other hand, the famous Framingham Heart Study (Hubert et al. 1987) found no dif-ference in health status based on women's employment status. This dis-crepancy among studies may actually reflect their different definitions of employment. The Framingham study, for example, classified a woman as "working" if she had worked outside her home for more than half her adult life, regardless of her current work status. The other studies, which used current employment as the basis for the classification, were the ones that found better health among employed women. If this is the explana-tion for the difference in results, it suggests that the life-style benefits of employment may be transient.

Those women who do get heart attacks while still employed are less often executives than clerical workers, particularly those who also have children. The recent revelation that heart attacks are the leading killer of women has been used as "evidence" that the workplace is dangerous to the women who dare to tread within it, particularly to those who aspire to executive positions. Despite such warnings to women that ascent of the corporate ladder might be harmful to their health, the research shows quite the opposite. A 1987 survey of 1,000 members of a national orga-nization of executive women found their scores on a health status ques-tionnaire to be very similar to those of women working in positions with lower status and pay. The executives were found to excel in measures of life satisfaction, social support, and health status. They were more likely than nonexecutive women to engage in health-promoting behaviors such as exercising and wearing seat belts, and were less likely to smoke. On the other hand, they were more likely to drink alcohol and less likely to know their blood pressure or cholesterol levels (LaRosa 1990). It would be of interest to compare these women to men in similar executive positions.

The observation that women executives are "heart-healthier" than their sisters in lower-paying and lower-status positions fits well with a study (Van Egeren 1992) that found that, for both men and women, working in a "high strain" job (one combining high psychologic work load and low worker control) was associated with increased blood pressure both at work and at home in the evening. Since elevated blood pressure is a risk factor for heart attacks, it follows that workers in these high strain / low control jobs are at higher risk for heart attacks. These conclusions, however, are somewhat inconsistent with another study, which found that people with Type A personalities are more likely to hold jobs high in both demand and personal control. In contrast, Type B's were found to be in jobs characterized by low demand and low control (Karasek and Theorell 1990).

The weight of the evidence is clearly that women in high-level professional and administrative positions have more favorable heart disease risk profiles than do unemployed women. The facts "do not support prior predictions that, as women attain male professional- or executive-level occupations, they will also acquire male coronary heart disease risk and mortality rates" (Kritz-Silverstein et al. 1992: 218).

The beneficial effects of employment on the health status of women are greater for unmarried than for married women, according to two studies (Waldron and Jacobs 1988; Repetti, Matthews, and Waldron 1989).

OTHER RISKS OF DEATH CORRELATED WITH EMPLOYMENT

For women, occupation is now the single most important determinant, after age, of their health status (Karasek, Gardell, and Lindell 1987). The leading cause of death for adult women (16 to 64 years old) in the labor force is breast cancer, and the second leading cause is heart disease. For those in this age group who are not employed outside of the home, this order is reversed. The third and fourth leading causes of death, lung cancer and cancer of the digestive tract, are the same for both groups. The fifth leading cause is motor vehicle accidents for those in the labor force and cirrhosis of the liver for those who are not. A California study (Doebbert, Riedmiller, and Kizer 1988) found that women who did not work outside the home were more likely to die from cirrhosis than women who did. The leading cause of cirrhosis currently is excessive alcohol consumption. It isn't at all clear from the way this study was done whether being at home all day led to more alcohol consumption or whether those who were already alcoholic were too ill to join the paid labor force.

The same study showed more suicide and homicide among women in the paid labor force. As with cirrhosis, the nature of the relationship in this finding is unclear, and there are a number of possible explanations. Does work outside the home lead to depression and suicide, or are the reasons for having to work the same as those that lead to depression?

Homicide is the third leading cause of death in young African-American adults. It is the third leading cause of workplace death in the United States. For all workers, nearly 13 percent of all occupational injury deaths from 1980 to 1985 in the United States were homicides. During that same period, 47 percent of the work force was female, but women suffered only 6 percent of all the fatal work-related injuries. It is astounding, therefore, that 41 percent of these women who died of work-related injuries were victims of homicide, making homicide the leading cause of traumatic death in the workplace for women in the United States (Bell 1991). Twice as many of these women were nonwhite as white, and their ages ranged from 16 to 93 years, with the highest homicide rate occurring in women over 65. Almost half of the victims were employed in retail trade, and most were killed by guns.

Mortality statistics for various occupations were examined in a 1993 report based on data from twelve states (*Monthly Vital Statistics Report* 1993). The report is of historical interest in that it is the first to include women since reporting began in 1890. The findings are not easy to interpret. For example, a reported association between cancer of the brain and nervous system and work in the transportation industry for women was not observed in men. The majority of female workers who died were employed in retail eating and drinking places. For them, a statistically significantly higher mortality resulted from cancers of the lip, mouth, throat, esophagus, and cervix, and from homicide than was found in homemakers or women employed in other areas. At least some of these deaths can be explained by increased exposure to alcohol and cigarette smoke in these settings. Although it will take time to fully understand the reasons for these findings, it is important that they be reported; it may be possible to analyze their origins and develop preventive measures.

The state of California found that the women at highest risk of early death were those who worked as waitresses, licensed vocational nurses and health aides, cosmetologists, telephone operators, housekeepers, janitors, launderers, and dry cleaners. Within each of these occupations there were few racial differences, and the risks were greater for women than for men (Doebbert, Riedmiller, and Kizer 1988). Within each job category, the causes of death are multiple, and deaths are not necessarily directly caused by the job. Here, again, there may be some element of self-selection. What these researchers found was that waitresses, at least in California, are at a high and previously unrecognized risk for heart attacks, suicide, lung disease, and homicide. Consistent with previous reports, they also ran a high risk of early death from cirrhosis, lung cancer, and motor vehicle and other accidents. The cirrhosis risk may relate to the higher intake of alcohol among workers in places where alcohol is sold. The high risk of lung cancer and other lung disease may result from passive smoking in restaurants prior to the recently imposed restrictions against smoking in most public places, as well as to a higher incidence of smoking among white waitresses, as observed in one study (Sterling and Weinkam 1976).

It has long been known that health workers, both male and female, in the United States as well as in Europe, have a higher risk of suicide than the general population or even other workers. Among physicians, the risk appears to be highest for pathologists and psychiatrists. Previous studies have documented that female doctors have suicide rates up to four times those of their age-mates in the general population, higher than those of female academics and higher than those of male doctors (Pitts, Winokur, and Stewart 1961). Apropos possible self-selection, studies of men and women at entry to medical school have not found any difference in the level of depression (Notman, Salt, and Nadelson 1984), suggesting that the higher rate of later depression and suicide must result from subsequent stress.

Indeed, female doctors face multiple sources of stress in addition to those generally experienced by male physicians, including conflict between family and career (Cartwright 1987; Notman and Nadelson 1973; Schermerhorn et al. 1986), prejudice (Franco et al. 1983), and paucity of role models. In surveys at a major medical center, the women residents consistently reported more feelings of isolation, depression, and job insecurity than the men (Koran and Litt 1988). Although most of these studies were done more than a decade ago and the numbers of women in medicine have increased tremendously in the interim, there is no indication that the stresses have abated. Sexual harassment, salary inequities (Kazis et al. 1993), and limitations on opportunities for advancement in academic medicine (American College of Physicians 1991; see also Chapter 12) continue to be sources of frustration and depression for female physicians even now. In addition, the lack of female role models is a continuing problem, because the increased numbers of female physicians are still at the lower levels of the occupational ladder (Bickel 1988).

In addition to the higher risk of suicide, female health workers were shown in the California study to be at increased risk for early death from high blood pressure, accidents, heart disease, strokes, and lung, breast, and digestive system cancers. The higher rate of smoking among female hospital workers (Sterling and Weinkam 1976) may account for these findings. If that is the case, the decrease in smoking over the last decade among health workers may improve these figures in the future—although studies documenting this decrease did not report gender differences, if any, and there has been a general increase in smoking among young women.

Another group found to be at high risk for early death in the California study, as well as in earlier studies in Washington State (Milham 1983) and Buffalo, New York (Decoufle and Stanislewczyk 1977), was cosmetologists. Their deaths resulted from accidents; cirrhosis; cancers of the lung, breast, and genitals; and heart disease. Among the possible causes are their exposure to dyes and other chemicals, as well as an increased rate of smoking.

The California and Washington studies found racial differences in the risk of women housekeepers and janitors for early death. For example, blacks in these occupations had a higher risk of dying from heart disease, high blood pressure, homicide, and liver disease. Similarly, among the female launderers and dry cleaners, the increased risk of death was found almost entirely in the blacks, who had three to six times the risk of early death owing to liver disease; cancers of the lung, digestive tract, and reproductive tract; heart disease; and high blood pressure.

These studies have probably raised more questions than they have answered. Nonetheless, their findings are critically important, especially for physicians, who must recognize the need to ask their female patients—as they have traditionally asked male patients—about occupation in order to better understand their health risks. These studies must also serve to alert governmental agencies charged with improvement in occupational safety to consider the possible gender differences in risk factors and prevention strategies, the better to educate and protect women workers from their special risks. This information must be used to rid the workplace of the dangers to women's health, rather than to rid the workplace of women.

REPETITIVE MOTION DISORDERS

Repetitive motion disorders reportedly occur more often in women than in men. Among these disorders, carpal tunnel syndrome has received the most attention. This condition is believed to be caused by compression of the median nerve between tendons of the wrist during flexion and extension of the wrist and by a resultant increase in pressure in the tunnel through which this nerve passes. One study showed that repetitive flexion or extension of the wrist and pinch grasping increase the risk of this disorder (Armstrong and Chaffin 1979). For people who engage in activities with either flexed or extended wrist for more than twenty hours each week, the risk is four- to fivefold greater than for people with a lower frequency of these movements (de Krom et al. 1990). Patients with carpal tunnel syndrome typically experience tingling, pain, and/or numbness in the thumb and first two fingers, which are served by the median nerve. The pain is often so severe as to awaken them from sleep. The formal criteria for the diagnosis include pain at least twice a week and physiologic testing that confirms nerve compression.

There is no clear biologic reason for this syndrome to occur more frequently in women. A study that examined possible effects of estrogens could find no association (Cannon, Bernack, and Walter 1981). It is of interest, however, that activities such as ironing and scrubbing are performed with the wrist extended, as is typing. Accordingly, the increased rate of carpal tunnel syndrome may reflect the increased exposure of women to the dangerous positions of the hand during the course of their paid work (in addition to their continuing work at home).

The higher incidence in women notwithstanding, more men are referred for surgical correction, at least in the Netherlands, the only place where gender-based referral patterns have been studied. The Dutch report explains it thus: "Regarding the sex ratios in the general population, which were different from those in the hospital cases, we hypothesize that most women in the Netherlands are housewives, who are able to avoid continuous wrist-burdening activities because they may vary their household activities. Men, however, have to perform their professional jobs continuously and therefore need to have their carpal tunnel syndrome treated" (de Krom et al. 1990: 1107–8). Perhaps someone should ask the women about this!

Other Health Issues in Early Adulthood

BREASTS

The mature female breast is made up of 15 to 25 lobes that radiate from the nipple. Each lobe is subdivided into many lobules that empty into ducts in the nipple. It is this system of lobes and ducts that produces milk and transports it to the nipple. The remainder of the breast is composed of fat tissue. With time, the fat tissue becomes more abundant and the functional tissue decreases in volume.

Contrary to images in the popular press, the typical adult breast does not resemble a grapefruit. According to Loren Eskenazi, a plastic surgeon at Stanford University who is creating the first database of normal breasts using computer imaging, the normal breast is likely to be "shaped like a teardrop, flatter on top and droopy below" (Raman 1995).

Many women have two breasts of unequal size; the difference is usually not noticeable when they are clothed. If further compensation is desired, padded bras often provide it, but some women still choose to have surgery to either reduce the larger breast or augment the smaller one.

Cosmetic breast surgery involving silicone-gel implants has been performed on more than two million women in the United States. Approximately 150,000 women have been receiving these implants yearly, and between one and two million women who had implants during the last 30 years still have them. Eighty percent of the implants have been for breast augmentation, the remainder for breast reconstruction following mastectomy. Concern has arisen about the safety of the implants following findings that between 4 and 6 percent of them have ruptured and that the urine of at least one patient who had a polyurethane sponge–covered implant contained a carcinogenic breakdown product of polyurethane. There have been allegations that the devices might be responsible for breast cancer (see also Chapter 3) and disorders of the immune system (see below). A number of studies have now been done to investigate this possibility.

The worry about implants and autoimmune diseases resulted from claims by thousands of women that they had developed these diseases after receiving the implants. So convincing were their experiences that the manufacturer recently agreed to settle their class action for $4.2 billion.

Studies are currently under way to evaluate the possible link between silicone-gel breast implants and immune diseases. It has been theorized that the immune system, stimulated by the silicone, produces antibodies against the foreign material that then attack the body's tissues. A recent report, as yet unpublished, describes antibodies to silicone that may potentially play a part in such an immune response. Dr. Nir Koosovsky of UCLA Medical School reported that his laboratory had found "that silicone . . . can bind to the patient's own molecules, damage them, and the body then produces antibodies. . . . These molecules are perceived as foreign bodies, and the body attacks itself." They found these antibodies in the blood of 9 of 250 women with implants (duration not given) and in none of the 89 women without implants. Until the study undergoes peer review for publication, the scientific merit of the research will not be known (Elias 1994).

Three large epidemiologic studies have, however, found no evidence to link silicone breast implants with immune disease. The most recent of these (Gabriel et al. 1995) found no increase in any disease or symptom in 749 women who had received the implants between 1964 and 1991.

In response to the concerns raised about silicone, the FDA, without scientific study, removed silicone-gel breast implants from the market in 1992, despite their provisional approval status since 1976. The effect of this action is that women who have chosen to alter their appearance, and with it their self-image, will be denied the option to do so. Women now may only receive breast implants if they are willing to become research subjects to evaluate their safety and if they meet one of the following two sets of conditions: (1) they have had mastectomies, or (2) they are over eighteen, are certified by physicians to have severe breast or chest deformity as a result of congenital or developmental problems, and have none of the following conditions: infection, pregnancy or lactation, immune disease, or any disease or skin problem that would affect healing or pose a surgical risk. In an excellent editorial in the *New England Journal of Medicine*, Dr. Marcia Angell (1992) raises a number of concerns about this action of the FDA's commissioner, Dr. David Kessler, with regard to its effect on women:

> It "has the effect of coercing women with breast cancer to become subjects" in research, despite federal regulations clearly mandating that such participation be voluntary.
>
> It has, without sufficient evidence, caused fear among those women who already have implants. Some have opted to have them removed, but others who wish to cannot afford to do so.
>
> It "ignores the social context. Targeting a device used only by women raises the specter of sexism."

Women contemplating reduction mammoplasty should be aware that this procedure, too, has risks. These include blood loss, possible loss of sensation, and possible interference with the ability to nurse.

Often the first hint of pregnancy is tenderness of the breasts. They increase in size, the areola darkens, and there may be some secretion from the nipple, all the result of rising levels of estrogen, progesterone, and prolactin. The production and secretion of milk from the breast result from the action of prolactin, which is produced in the pituitary gland.

For a detailed discussion of breast cancer, a disease more common among women over 50, see Chapter 3.

UROGENITAL PROBLEMS

Premenstrual Syndrome

In the second (luteal) phase of the menstrual cycle, levels of progesterone rise and those of estrogen fall. These hormonal changes often give rise to symptoms of fluid retention, decreased energy, acne, and/or headaches. For some women, these and other symptoms may be so severe and recurrent as to warrant the diagnosis of premenstrual syndrome (PMS), also called luteal phase defect. Common symptoms of PMS include dysphoria (depression, anxiety, nervousness, irritability, concentration difficulty, and tension); fluid retention (edema, bloating, and weight gain of up to ten pounds); breast tenderness; fatigue; food cravings (especially for chocolate, sugar, or salt); and headaches.

The cause or causes of PMS are not known, though there are many theories. The possibilities include excessive production of prostaglandins (which is the cause of menstrual cramps); nutritional deficiencies; progesterone deficiency; abnormalities of endorphin production; and imbalance of fluids. In the absence of a clear understanding of the cause of PMS, therapy has been largely unsatisfactory. Some women, however, claim to have been helped by some treatments, such as:

High doses of progesterone (Maxson 1987)

Vitamins (e.g., E, C). Although recommended by some, high doses of vitamin B_6 should be avoided because of the possibility of damage to the nerves (peripheral neuropathy) (Berger and Schaumberg 1984). Use of L-tryptophan may also be dangerous, having been implicated in the eosinophilia-myalgia syndrome (cough, joint pain, shortness of breath, fever, swelling).

Minerals (e.g., calcium)

Diets low in refined sugar, salt, and red meat and high in complex carbohydrates

Elimination of caffeine-containing beverages, smoking, alcohol, and chocolate

Aerobic exercise (for a minimum of 30 minutes three or four times
a week)

Prostaglandin inhibitors (Budoff 1987). These appear to be useful
when menstrual cramps accompany the PMS symptoms, as well as
when headaches are a prominent part of the picture.

Oral contraceptives (low-dose). The rationale for this approach is
to equalize hormonal levels across the menstrual cycle and
thereby eliminate the marked fluctuations in levels of estrogen
and progesterone.

Tranquilizers in the last week of the cycle (Smith et al. 1987)

Endometriosis, which can also cause pain at menstruation, frequently begins in adolescence but is not diagnosed until young adulthood. See
Chapter 1 for a discussion of endometriosis.

Incontinence

Urinary incontinence (involuntary leakage of urine) is generally
considered to be a problem of older women, many of whom wind up in
nursing homes because of it (see Chapter 4). The reality is, however, that
incontinence is a common problem for women throughout the life cycle. The underlying problem appears to be weakness of the pelvic (pubo-
coccygeal) muscles; anything that contributes to decreasing the strength
and endurance of these muscles will worsen the condition. Loss of tone
of the pelvic ligaments and urinary tract infections can also cause incontinence. One of the earliest students of the problem, Kegel (1951), believed that if women fail to develop what he called "a normal action pattern" when they are young, they will have problems of stress urinary incontinence for the rest of their lives.

It will come as a surprise to many women, and probably as a relief to
many more, that stress urinary incontinence is extremely common after
the age of 30. It affects about half of *all* women and worsens with advancing age, pregnancies, and menopause.

The first symptom is loss of a few drops of urine when laughing
(gelastic incontinence), sneezing, or coughing. The next symptom, the
need to get up in the middle of the night to urinate, is experienced by
71 percent of healthy women over the age of 45 (Cutler et al. 1992). With

time, the need to void during the night becomes more frequent. The muscle strength of the pelvis has been found to be lower in the afternoon.

Why don't we know more about this common problem? Probably because physicians are unaware of its ubiquity and don't inquire about its presence, and because women are too embarrassed to volunteer the information that they are affected. Cutler et al. (1992) recommend the inclusion of their simple questionnaire in routine health screening of female patients, especially those who are menopausal and/or have had more than two children. The entire questionnaire consists of just three questions: "Loss of urine sometimes occurs involuntarily. Does this ever happen to you? Under what situations? How often?" (Cutler et al. 1992: 260).

Most physicians are poorly trained to evaluate and treat this condition, and research is almost nonexistent, although nearly ten billion dollars are spent on this problem each year in the United States. When urinary incontinence does come to medical attention, most physicians will refer the patient to a urologist, who will likely perform a pelvis repair operation, with only limited success (Chalker and Whitmore 1990). Based on extensive study of Kegel's techniques for self-strengthening exercises, the current recommendation to physicians is to refer patients "to a biofeedback specialist for pelvic muscle training as a first step" (Cutler et al. 1992).

No studies have examined possible preventive strategies for this common problem. The limited data on the effect of estrogen replacement therapy on incontinence are inconclusive. It makes sense, however, to consider performance of some version of Kegel's exercises as a potential intervention (see Fig. 2.1). Surely it cannot be harmful, and it may just work. The following modification of these exercises is offered in *The New Our Bodies, Ourselves*:

> Begin exercising these [pelvic-floor] muscles by contracting hard for a second and then releasing completely. Repeat this ten times in a row to make up one group of exercises (this takes about twenty seconds). In a month's time, try to work up to twenty groups during one day (about seven minutes total). You can do this at any time—while sitting in a car or bus, while talking on the telephone, or even as a wake-up exercise. (Boston Women's Health Book Collective 1984: 333).

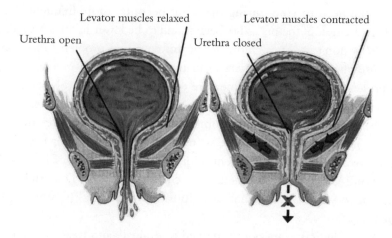

FIGURE 2.1.   Pelvic floor exercises. Sets of long and short contractions are done three times a day. Reproduced from Retzky and Rogers 1995, p. 28.

Other simple techniques, such as behavioral modification and regular voiding, may also help.

HIGH BLOOD PRESSURE

One factor that is only now being considered in studies of blood pressure in women is the effect of menstrual cycle phase. A recent study showed that blood pressure definitely varies throughout the cycle (in normal women, as well as in women with high blood pressure); it is highest at the beginning of menses and lowest during days 17–26 (Dunne et al. 1991). Lack of awareness of the influence of menstrual cycle phase until recently may have inadvertently confused previous studies of efficacy of drugs for the treatment of high blood pressure.

Although essential hypertension, the most common form of high blood pressure, has no known cause, there are other types of high blood pressure whose causes are known. One such cause is toxemia, which occurs during pregnancy and thus is obviously unique to women. Birth control pills, too, may raise blood pressure in some women (see Chapter 6). (For a more detailed discussion of high blood pressure, see Chapter 4.)

DISEASES OF THE IMMUNE SYSTEM

The immune system functions to fight invasion by germs (bacteria and viruses) and to resist the spread of cancer in the body by producing an inflammatory reaction. It does so through the manufacture of specialized cells (e.g., macrophages and lymphocytes) and chemical products (e.g., antibodies, complement, and cytokines). As a general rule, when the invading germ or other material is rapidly attacked and destroyed, the body is protected, whereas when the body is overwhelmed by the amount of foreign material or is slow in destroying it, the inflammatory reaction is more likely to damage the tissues of the host. Moreover, when the immunologic system is disarmed (for example, as eventually happens when the invader is the human immunodeficiency virus) or fails to develop normally (as is the case with certain genetic diseases), there is an inadequate or absent inflammatory response, the body is overwhelmed, and death often follows.

The same mechanisms that protect the body from foreign threats can, under certain circumstances, be directed against the body, as occurs in so-called autoimmune diseases, the most common of which are rheumatoid arthritis, lupus erythematosus, Sjogren syndrome, scleroderma, and mixed connective tissue disease.

For reasons that are not yet well understood, autoimmune diseases predominantly affect women. This fact has led researchers to implicate estrogens in their causation. However, the way in which estrogens may contribute is far from clear. The diseases are often worsened with hormonal changes such as those experienced during different phases of the menstrual cycle, the use of estrogen-containing oral contraceptives, and pregnancy. As discussed above, the role of silicone (such as that found in breast implants) in precipitating autoimmune disease is currently under investigation, with conflicting results. Genetic and viral factors are also being examined as possible causes.

Rheumatoid arthritis (RA) is a chronic disease in which the inflammatory process affects the entire body. Approximately 1 percent of all adults (about two million Americans) have RA. It is two to three times more common among females than males and affects all races and ethnic groups. It usually has its onset between the fourth and sixth decades but can appear as late as the seventh or as early as the first. It typically involves all of the body's connective tissue, including the bones, muscles, tendons, and ligaments, as well as many organs. Although in its mildest form RA may cause nonspecific problems such as fatigue and appetite loss, its diagnosis is predicated upon fulfillment of at least five of eleven criteria, including morning stiffness, pain when moving at least one joint or tenderness in at least one joint, swelling in at least one joint, X-ray findings typical of RA, and a positive laboratory test for rheumatoid factor.

The course of RA is quite variable. Some patients whose disease is diagnosed early may have it arrested by proper treatment. Others, however, progress to chronic disability despite vigorous treatment. The objectives of management include relief of pain, reduction of inflammation, minimization of side effects, preservation of muscle strength and joint mobility, and rapid return to a normal life-style. To achieve these goals, a number of modalities must be used, ranging from rest during the acute phases to supervised exercise; warmth; medication with salicylates or other anti-inflammatory agents; and, for those with irreversible joint damage, reconstructive surgery.

Lupus affects half a million Americans, the majority of whom are women of childbearing years. The female-to-male ratio is ten to one. African-Americans are affected three times as often as American Caucasians. It is estimated that a black American female has a 1-in-250 chance of developing lupus during her lifetime. The cause of lupus is not clear. Because of the finding that an identical twin has a 30 percent chance of developing the disease if her sister is affected, genetic, as well as hormonal, factors appear to play a role. Flare-ups can be triggered by a number of factors, including exposure to ultraviolet light, many drugs (e.g., a number of anticonvulsive drugs; some antibiotics, including tetracyclines and sulfas; and estrogen-containing oral contraceptives), some foods (e.g., alfalfa sprouts, figs, celery, and parsley), stress, surgery, infection, and injury. The symptoms can range from mild fatigue and fever to those resulting from severe damage to vital organs. The most common symptoms include a rash in the shape of a butterfly over the cheeks and nose, pain in joints and muscles, mouth sores, hair loss, pain of the fingers when exposed to cold, fevers, and loss of appetite. With rest and appropriate use of corticosteroid drugs, most patients can expect to live a normal life with occasional relapses. That notwithstanding, lupus can be fatal, causing approximately 5,000 deaths each year.

Sjogren syndrome results when the immune system attacks the salivary and lacrimal glands, resulting in decreased production of saliva and tears. It is ten times more common in women than in men and affects approximately two million people in the United States, half of whom also have RA. Its cause is not known, but the female preponderance implicates hormones such as estrogen. Symptoms include difficulty swallowing; dry eyes, mouth, nose, throat, tongue, skin, and vagina; swollen salivary glands; chronic constipation; recurrent bronchitis; pneumonia; deafness; and hoarseness. Approximately one-fifth of those affected will also experience pain in the fingers when they are exposed to cold. The diagnosis is usually made by careful examination of the eyes by a skilled ophthalmologist and/or specialized tests of the salivary gland function. Treatment is directed at the symptoms and includes use of artificial tears and salivary gland stimulants (e.g., chewing gum). Rarely, systemic treatment with corticosteroids is warranted.

"Scleroderma" literally means "hard skin," the major symptom of the disease. The great physician Osler described this hardening as restriction of movement "by an ever-tightening case of steel" (Wyngaarden and Smith 1988: 2018). Unfortunately, vital organs (e.g., lungs, circulatory system, kidneys, and gut) may be affected in the same way, and this involvement can result in death. Between 50,000 and 100,000 people in the United States are estimated to have scleroderma, 80 percent of whom are women between 25 and 55 years of age. The symptoms are like those of the other autoimmune diseases described, with the addition of skin thickening and discoloration and, often, difficulty swallowing. Ten percent of patients have joint changes indistinguishable from those of RA. Treatment is less than optimal, but glucocorticosteroids or D-penicillamine appear to be most useful. Successful management of high blood pressure has decreased the death rate from kidney disease. Now the leading cause of death is lung failure, a problem that is worsened by smoking, which should be avoided at all costs.

Mixed connective tissue disease (MCTD) is the name given to a combination of the symptoms of autoimmune disease. Patients with MCTD may have features of scleroderma, lupus, myositis, and other inflammatory diseases. There are no specific tests or features of this condition.

Mortality

The leading causes of death for women between 25 and 44 are listed in Appendix A. Of note is the fact that in just three years, AIDS has risen from sixth to third place (Singh et al. 1995). It is expected to rise to second place within the next few years. In just one year's time (from 1993 to 1994), for example, the rate of death from AIDS for women 25 to 44 years old increased from 9.1 per 100,000 to 11.6 per 100,000 population (Singh et al. 1995). In fifteen of the nation's largest cities, AIDS is already the leading cause of death for women. Consistent with the pattern in the rest of the world and in contrast with that for men, in 1992 the leading route of transmission of HIV in women became heterosexual activity (Altman 1995).

CHAPTER THREE

The Perimenopausal Years

The perimenopausal years are difficult to define precisely. We will define them as starting after age 44 (the official end of the "reproductive years") and extending to the middle of the seventh decade. Some of the most important issues for women's health at this stage of the life cycle relate to the gynecologic system, mainly to the effects of menopause, and to breast health.

In contrast with the earlier adult years, when issues of family and work tend to predominate, women at this stage of the life cycle often refocus on themselves. Stresses of divorce, retirement, partner retirement or death, financial issues, or care of elderly parents may cause pressure, but maturity and enhanced self-confidence, clarity of career or personal choices, and the support systems afforded by family and friends all contribute to enhanced ability to buffer the difficulties in a way that may not have been possible earlier.

Menopause

No women's health issue illustrates better than menopause the gap between the needs and expectations of the woman patient for information and what is provided by the physician. What women need to know (not necessarily in this order) are:

When will it happen?

How will I know when it is going to happen?

Is it going to change my mood and/or personality?

How will it affect my appearance?

How will it affect my ability to function (at work, sexually, etc.)?

How will it affect my health?

Should I take estrogens, and if so, when, how much, and
what type?

Frankly, physicians rarely have the time to address these critical questions during the course of a routine office visit. Patients, for their part, often feel pressured to focus on a physical complaint and rarely ask for this information. But they need to ask, because internists are not, as a rule, trained in the mode of "anticipatory guidance" that is the bedrock of pediatrics. Even when asked, however, physicians often lack the information necessary to answer these questions because of inadequate research and education on them. For example, the most comprehensive textbook of internal medicine (Wyngaarden and Smith 1988) devotes only one of its 2,404 pages to the subject of menopause. I will, therefore, attempt to fill the void by sharing the current information about menopause, with the understanding that we need to learn much more.

TIMING AND PREDICTORS

Some physicians define menopause in hormonal or symptomatic terms, but the generally accepted definition is that it is the end of menstruation (Lock 1991). The average age of menopause in the United States currently is 51, which means that the average woman will live more than one-third of her life in the postmenopausal state. However, the age range for onset is very broad, so it is difficult for an individual woman to predict when she will experience menopause. As with menarche, a useful but not perfect guideline is the time of menopause of close family members (mother and particularly sisters).

With a meticulous longitudinal study of characteristics of menstrual periods over the reproductive life of a large sample of women in Switzerland, Vollmann (1977) provided very useful information about indicators of approaching menopause. The most consistent finding was that in the year or so before actual cessation of menses, the length of the cycle decreased. A careful analysis revealed that this reflected a shortening of the phase between ovulation and bleeding, that is, the premenstrual or luteal phase of the cycle.

At the time of menopause, levels of estrogens in the blood are markedly decreased. Because of the finely tuned interaction between the ovaries, which produce estrogen, and the pituitary gland, which produces hormones (LH and FSH) that stimulate the ovaries, when levels of estrogen fall, those of LH and FSH rise. Therefore, at menopause and thereafter, levels of LH and FSH are quite high and are often measured to establish that menopause has occurred. But studies have also shown consistent increases in the levels of these pituitary hormones long before actual menopause. This has prompted the successful practice among some physicians of instituting estrogen replacement therapy at the time of elevation of LH and FSH and thereby eliminating symptoms of menopause.

SYMPTOMS

The symptoms of menopause are quite variable. Vasomotor effects or hot flashes are the most common symptoms, reported to occur in as many as 85 percent of postmenopausal women (Notelovitz 1989). A typical hot flash consists of reddening and warmth of the skin, especially that of the head and neck, lasting anywhere from a few seconds to two minutes. This is followed by cold chills. The precise mechanism of these changes is not known, but it is thought to involve that part of the hypothalamus that controls temperature regulation. Night sweats, palpitations, cold hands and feet, dizziness, headaches, anxiety, irritability, forgetfulness, inability to concentrate, vaginal dryness, insomnia, and depression are other symptoms reported with varying frequency.

Differences in frequency of these symptoms have been reported in different populations of women. For example, whereas approximately 65 percent of 45–55-year-old women studied in Manitoba, Canada, reported ever having a hot flash, a comparable group in Japan reported a 20 percent incidence of this symptom. This may reflect differences in biology, terminology, cultural meanings of biologic phenomena, or all of the above. Another factor to take into account is the source of the information. In many cultures, physicians are rarely consulted for symptoms of menopause, and physician reports of their prevalence may be accordingly biased. Now that there is more open discussion of menopause among women and in the media, it is to be hoped that a clearer view of its impact and symptomatology will emerge.

EFFECTS ON APPEARANCE

Menopause itself does little to the skin. With aging, however, the skin undergoes major changes that result in wrinkling, thinning, roughening, laxity, and uneven pigmentation (Wyngaarden and Smith 1988: 2306). And when estrogen levels fall, as they do following menopause, they cease to counteract the effect of androgens, hormones produced by the adrenal glands in both men and women. One result is slight growth of hair on the face.

The falling levels of both estrogen and progesterone with menopause result in declining stimulation of the ducts and glands of the breast. The end result is that breasts shrink and sag.

Menopause, itself, does not appear to cause weight gain. The best information on weight changes in this age group comes from a study of nearly 500 women who were evaluated first before menopause (at 42–50) and then again three years later. Some of the women experienced menopause in the interim; others did not. The average weight gain for all of the women was about five pounds, with no significant differences based on menstrual status. In other words, those who had experienced menopause gained, on average, the same amount as those who had not. The investigators found only three factors that appeared to be significant in predicting increased risk of weight gain: being black, living alone, and exercising less. They found a suggestion of more weight gain among the women taking estrogen replacement, but they did not have a large enough sample to prove this. The researchers were concerned that the weight gain was paralleled by increases in cholesterol and triglycerides as well as blood pressure, factors known to be associated with increased risk of heart disease and stroke. They suggested, but did not study, the possibility that attempts to prevent weight gain at this time in a woman's life might also prevent or reduce the likelihood of these serious threats to life (Wing et al. 1991).

The image of hunched-over older women is one that haunts many as they approach menopause. Curvature of the spine in old age results from at least two factors. One is loss of elasticity and resulting compression of the collagen "cushions" between the vertebrae that support and protect the spinal column. This is what causes women to gradually become shorter in their later years. The other is loss of bone and resulting compression of the vertebrae themselves as a result of osteoporosis, which is discussed below.

EFFECTS ON SEXUALITY

In our fitfully puritanical society, sex is rarely discussed openly, and its portrayal in the mass media suggests that it falls within the exclusive domain of those too young to act responsibly or too physically attractive to be real. Our youth-worshiping society ignores, denies, or rejects the possibility that sex is enjoyable for women in the second half-century of life. Yet, whenever this question is raised in surveys of women in this age group, it is clear that for many, sex is in many ways even more enjoyable than it was earlier. Gone is the threat of pregnancy, as well as the possibility that lovemaking will be interrupted by a wandering child. Improved self-confidence and self-image and comfortable communication with a familiar partner all combine to make sex more enjoyable.

Libido appears to be more related to the body's level of androgens than to that of estrogen. Menopause is not associated with a decrease in androgens, so there is no reason to think that libido will decrease at this time of life. It is also possible that the lower levels of estrogen after menopause allow the androgens to exert an even greater effect in this regard. In Britain, physicians make available an office procedure that involves inserting under a woman's skin every six months a pellet that slowly releases testosterone (an androgen hormone) in order to restore sexual response (Thom and Studd 1980).

On the other hand, physical changes associated with menopause may interfere with some of the newly gained psychologic and situational liberation. Lower estrogen levels may make the walls of the vagina thinner, less elastic, and drier. Intercourse under such conditions may lead to irritation, itching, and even increased susceptibility to infections. Estrogen replacement therapy usually prevents or reverses these changes. Alternatively, lubricating agents (e.g., K-Y jelly or saliva) can help the problem of dryness, and Kegel exercises (see Chapter 2) can improve vaginal tone.

Moreover, certain medications may decrease libido, although most of the information on this topic comes from studies of men. (The major textbook of internal medicine [Wyngaarden and Smith 1988] devotes two pages to the subject of reduction of libido and impotence in men without mentioning the subject in women.) Among the drugs shown to be capable of decreasing libido and erections in men are some of the antihypertensive drugs, some sedatives, antiulcer medications, tranquilizers, and alcohol. Taking synthetic progesterone as part of hormone replacement following menopause may decrease libido in some women. Some chronic physical diseases and depression may also cause lowered sexual interest. L–dopa, a drug used to treat Parkinson disease, may have the opposite effect.

ESTROGEN REPLACEMENT THERAPY

The issue of estrogen replacement therapy (ERT) is complex. When the use of estrogens in menopause is discussed, I often hear criticism of "the medicalization of aging" or attacks on efforts by the male-dominated medical profession to "control women's bodies" by prescribing estrogens. Such charges and concerns are understandable, given the history of the treatment of women patients by the medical establishment, but we must take care not to let such emotionally charged rhetoric further harm the health of women by discouraging application of new information that may actually prolong life and improve its quality. To the charge that prescription of estrogens in menopause is yet another way in which the male-dominated medical profession is attempting to control our bodies, I would offer the opposite argument: This may be one of the few instances when the medical profession has acknowledged that women have roles and needs other than those related to their reproductive function. Moreover, as the number of women physicians increases, "they" are becoming "we." In fact, recent information indicates that female doctors were twenty times more likely than male physicians to prescribe ERT for their postmenopausal patients (Angier 1992).

In trying to sort out the relevant information on ERT, I will first discuss its advantages, then review its known disadvantages, and finally address questions of the best way to implement it. But first, a caveat: As we review the research on ERT, it is critical to be aware of the many limitations on that research. First of all, thus far studies have been done primarily on white women. It is unclear which, if any, of their findings apply to women of other races, particularly since minorities often have poorer health than whites in this country. Also, these studies have been mainly retrospective, evaluating the effects of estrogens on women who have independently decided to take them, rather than assigning women systematically to groups that do and do not get estrogens. This self-selection bias means that it may be some other characteristic of women who choose to take estrogens that is responsible for the effect that is being attributed to the estrogens. For example, perhaps the type of woman who is more careful in general about her health and diet is more likely to choose this therapy. Thus, studies may unwittingly be measuring the effect of good living and good health care, rather than estrogens. The studies that are now being undertaken under the NIH Women's Health Initiative will attempt to correct this possible bias by randomly assigning women to different therapy groups and following them up for ten years. In the shorter term, there remains a need for more research and for research that includes women of all ethnic groups.

Advantages

It is clear that most of the bothersome effects of menopause, such as hot flashes, vaginal dryness, and mild depression (when it is not caused by other factors), can all be dramatically improved by taking estrogens (Premarin) in the proper dose. However, from a health perspective, the other benefits of estrogen are more significant.

Studies have unanimously found that estrogen replacement will prevent the progression of osteoporosis and will thereby decrease a postmenopausal woman's chance of having a hip fracture by 50 percent (Melton 1990). However, it will not reverse osteoporosis or loss of bone density that has already occurred. (For more on osteoporosis, see Chapter 4.)

The risk of coronary artery disease dramatically increases after menopause. This has been suspected to result from loss of the protective effect of estrogen. Knowledge of the factors that contribute to heart disease in animals suggests that estrogens protect by reducing the blood level of "bad" cholesterol, LDLs, and increasing the level of "good" cholesterol, HDLs. It now appears that this mechanism exists for humans as well and provides the basis for the practice of replacing estrogens after menopause.

Although the cholesterol-lowering effects of estrogens are the most likely reason for the improved cardiovascular status of women on ERT, it is important to mention some other possible factors. For example, one study showed that estrogen users weighed less than nonusers and had lower levels of total cholesterol, lower blood pressure, and lower fasting blood sugar levels (Barrett-Connor et al. 1979). Because this was a study of women who had self-selected to take estrogens and had not been evaluated before they started taking them, it is impossible to know if these findings were themselves the result of the estrogens or were unrelated to them and independently caused other beneficial health effects.

After reviewing nineteen studies on the effect of ERT on coronary artery disease, including that of Sullivan et al. (1988), which showed that estrogen users had a significantly lower risk of coronary artery constriction than nonusers, Barrett-Connor and Bush (1989) concluded that by taking estrogens, a postmenopausal woman decreases her risk of heart disease by 30–50 percent. This appears to be true regardless of whether menopause occurred naturally or was the result of surgical removal of the ovaries (Gruchow et al. 1988). Estrogen has been shown to have a beneficial effect in preventing strokes, especially for women over the age of 75.

Recent research suggests that ERT may also help prevent colon cancer. Using a case-control study design, Newcomb and Storer (1995) showed a reduction in risk of colon cancer of one-half among postmenopausal women using either estrogen or estrogen with progestin. ERT apparently also reduces the chance of developing Alzheimer disease and may have other positive effects on mental state. See Chapter 7 for more information on this.

Disadvantages

There is some concern that ERT may increase the risk of certain cancers. It does not, however, appear that taking 0.625 mg of estrogen for the short term will increase the risk of getting breast cancer for women in low-risk categories. Taking estrogen for ten or more years, however, appears to increase the risk by 10 percent.

In a major prospective study of 121,700 female nurses who were between 30 and 55 at its commencement and who were followed for ten years, it was found that past use of any estrogens (which meant birth control pills for most), even use for more than ten years, was not associated with an increased risk of breast cancer. Current use did, however, significantly increase the risk, particularly with increasing age—but only in women who consumed alcohol (Colditz et al. 1990). (As discussed in Chapter 14, alcohol use may affect estrogen levels, and vice versa.) Interestingly, this risk did not increase further with increasing dose of estrogen or with longer duration of use, the latter in contrast with studies mentioned above. The difference between past and current use may reflect an early effect, reversible upon discontinuation of the estrogen. The study did not have enough subjects to evaluate the possible protective effect on the breast of simultaneous use of progestins postulated by some. One possible interpretation of the finding of more breast cancer in long-term estrogen users is that they are under better surveillance by physicians and therefore more likely to have mammograms. This possibility was, however, investigated and rejected by Colditz et al. (1990).

Interestingly, however, another important study showed that women who were receiving replacement estrogens and developed breast cancer had a lower risk of dying from it (Bergkvist et al. 1989). The reasons for this are not yet certain. It may be that there is a biologic difference in the tumor when estrogen is being administered and that this results in a better outcome. More likely, women who are taking replacement estrogens are being watched more closely by their doctors. If they develop breast cancer, it is more likely to be detected earlier because of regular checkups, including mammograms, and therefore caught in time to prevent death.

At this point in time, the recommendation is that women who are at high risk for breast cancer, either because they have already had it in one breast or because a close biologically related family member has had it, should not take replacement estrogens.

Concern still exists about whether estrogens may contribute to cancer of the uterus. This risk appears to be small, however, and is significantly reduced by the coincident administration of progesterone (Provera). Sadly, there has been no research on the effects of exogenous estrogen on the metabolism of drugs often prescribed simultaneously for postmenopausal women, including psychotropics (see Chapter 7).

Implementation

In implementing ERT, there are questions about when to begin it, how long to continue it, what dose of estrogen to use, how to administer it, and whether to administer progesterone as well. The weight of the present evidence is that estrogen replacement should begin as soon as there is evidence of rising levels of LH and FSH. However, even for women who are already years past menopause and have not been taking estrogens, it appears that there is an advantage to starting. Among women who, based on findings of coronary angiography, already have coronary artery disease, the ten-year survival rate is better for those who have ever used ERT than for those who have never used it (Sullivan et al. 1990). This means that the beneficial effects of ERT on heart disease exist regardless of how long it is started after menopause. This advantage is not so obvious regarding osteoporosis; if more than ten years have passed since menopause, osteoporosis has likely already taken its toll.

Most physicians now believe that ERT should continue indefinitely. This has certainly been shown to be the case for the effect on preventing heart disease (Barrett-Connor and Bush 1989).

The dose of Premarin necessary to avert hot flashes and other irritating symptoms is obviously not the same for all women, but it is generally in the range of 0.3 to 1.2 mg. The optimal dose is one that is high enough to suppress menopausal symptoms and below that which causes tenderness of the breasts. According to Barrett-Connor and Bush (1989), a dose of 0.625 mg daily is adequate to reduce the risk of heart disease.

Estrogen may be supplied through a pill, a patch, or an implant. The patch and implant have the obvious advantage of avoiding the need to remember to take a pill each day, but there is concern that they may not be as effective as the orally administered form in preventing heart disease. There is little research comparing animal and vegetable sources of estrogen.

If progesterone is taken along with estrogen, however, the beneficial effect of the estrogen on cholesterol appears to be lost. The way in which taking progesterone along with estrogen changes the odds of getting breast cancer is still not certain. Progesterone further reduces the already small risk that estrogens will increase the rate of uterine cancer. In the NIH's multicenter study, the Women's Health Initiative, a number of different combinations and routes of administration of hormones will be studied to gather more accurate information on these issues, but, unfortunately, we will have to wait a decade or more for results.

Breast Cancer

Breast cancer can occur at any age, but most of its victims are over 50; about one-quarter of cases occur in women between 40 and 60. It has been estimated that one in nine American women will get breast cancer if she lives long enough. It is the most commonly diagnosed cancer in women (striking about 180,000 women each year) and the second leading cause of cancer death in women in the United States after lung cancer; it was the leading cause until lung cancer rates began to rise in the early 1980's. The current reported incidence rate in the United States is about 113 cases per 100,000 women (1991 figures; Devesa et al. 1995). This is one of the highest rates in the world, on a par with that in Wales. The incidence is lower in Brazil, Greece, and the former Yugoslavia, and lowest in Japan and Taiwan.

In 1991, about 44,000 women died from breast cancer, giving a death rate of 27 per 100,000 women in the population. Age has a profound effect here, with a fifteenfold higher death rate for women over the age of 50 than for those under 50. Between 1950 and 1990, there was a 52 percent increase in the annual incidence of breast cancer, with a 4 percent increase in the death rate (Hankey et al. 1991). Thirty percent of the increase in incidence occurred over the last fifteen years, during which time the death rate decreased by about 2 percent (Devesa et al. 1995). There is controversy about whether these numbers indicate an actual increase in the incidence of breast cancer, as is clearly the case with lung cancer, or reflect improved detection. Some point to the news of a falling rate of diagnosis of new cases from 1991 to 1993 as evidence that improved detection was responsible for the increase in cases reported in the 1980's.

RISK FACTORS

Much epidemiologic research has focused on determining the risk factors for developing breast cancer, the first step in efforts to prevent it. Thus far, a number of possible risk factors have been studied.

1. Family history: There is good evidence of a genetic basis for at least one type of breast cancer, that affecting women under the age of 50. Dr. Mary-Claire King at the University of California at Berkeley has been searching for the responsible mutant gene for seventeen years. She

estimates that 600,000 women in the United States are carriers of the gene and therefore at risk for the disease (Friedman et al. 1994). A Harvard study of genetic risk among 117,000 women, followed prospectively, concluded that 6 percent of the 2,389 cases of breast cancer that developed in the group could be attributed to a family history (Colditz et al. 1993). It is good news that the incidence of breast cancer found in this group is significantly lower than those reported by earlier, less well designed studies. Nonetheless, it implies that a woman whose mother or sister had breast cancer has twice as great a risk of contracting the disease as a woman without such a history.

2. History of other types of breast disease: It appears that having fibrocystic disease of the breast may increase risk of later breast cancer slightly. This observation may simply reflect the high incidence of fibrocystic disease, rather than a true risk factor.

3. Age at menarche: The average age for onset of menses is currently twelve and a half years in women in industrialized societies. The earlier menses begin, the longer a women is exposed to elevated levels of both estrogen and progesterone. The duration of exposure obviously also relates to other life events that affect estrogen levels, such as pregnancy, use of birth control pills, vigorous exercise, malnutrition, and age at menopause. Epidemiologic studies (Bernstein, Ross, and Henderson 1992) have found that the risk of breast cancer is decreased by 5 to 15 percent for each year that menarche is delayed after the age of twelve. In countries with lower rates of breast cancer, the age of menarche is later than that in the United States. Furthermore, in Japan, for example, not only is menarche later, but women have longer menstrual cycles, both factors reflective of lower estrogen exposure.

Even if there is a population-based relationship between earlier menarche and higher breast cancer risk, it is not certain that it is one of cause and effect for an individual woman. Other, independent factors may cause both phenomena. For example, the leaner the woman, the later her menarche, and likely the lower her intake of fat (see below).

4. History of pregnancy: Whether and when a women has her first child is considered one of the most important factors, next to genetics. There have been consistent findings of a decreased lifetime risk of breast cancer with early birth of the first child. The mechanism for this protection has been suggested by animal experiments showing that breast cells

become less susceptible to carcinogens at the first birth (Russo and Russo 1987). It has, however, also been found that there is an immediate, though possibly transient, increase in risk of breast cancer immediately following the birth of the first child. This is presumed to result from estrogen stimulation of hyperplastic cells (Pathak and Whittemore 1992).

5. Use of birth control pills: Current evidence suggests that use of the Pill does not increase the risk of breast cancer, although women with a family history of breast cancer should be careful about using the Pill. (See Chapter 6 for more information.)

6. Age at menopause: For the same reasons that relate to age of menarche, having fewer years of exposure to estrogens as a result of early menopause appears to confer some protection against breast cancer. Pathak and Whittemore (1992) conclude that "each year of delayed menopause confers about a 4 percent increase in risk" (p. 165). Women with nonsurgical menopause before the age of 45 have been found to have only half the risk of breast cancer of women with menopause after the age of 55 (Trichopoulos, MacMahon, and Cole 1972). Surgical menopause seems to be even more protective than natural menopause (Bernstein, Ross, and Henderson 1992), probably because it tends to occur at an earlier age.

7. Estrogen replacement therapy: As discussed above, there are many reasons to be concerned about possible harmful effects of estrogen in promoting breast cancer. As we have seen, earlier menarche and later menopause, both of which expose women to estrogen for a longer time, are associated with an increased risk of the disease. In addition, other studies have shown higher estrogen levels among women with breast cancer (Key and Pike 1988). There are also animal studies showing that estrogens promote breast cancer. Moreover, the way that tamoxifen (the drug now under study as a possible inhibitor of breast cancer) works is to compete with estrogen at cell-binding sites (Early Breast Cancer Trialists' Collaborative Group 1988).

8. Race: The incidence of breast cancer is higher in white women than in women of other ethnic groups. This may reflect more effective detection; white women are more likely to have mammograms, owing to their generally higher socioeconomic status and the link between ability to pay and utilization of this critical breast cancer screening mechanism. Although the incidence rate is higher in white women, the death rate is lower. For example, the death rate for black women with breast

cancer is now twice as high as that for white women. This rate is higher for black women regardless of age (CDC 1994c). The greater survival rate of white women, too, has been attributed to the earlier detection of their tumors and the better outcome related to that fact.

There is more to the story, however. It is true that white women are more likely than blacks to have their breast cancer diagnosed at an earlier stage (Hankey et al. 1991). A recent study found that 40 percent of the higher death rate in black women was the result of the cancer having been more advanced at the time of diagnosis (Eley et al. 1994). But even controlling for the stage at diagnosis, whites appear to survive longer than blacks after the diagnosis is made (CDC 1994c).

Moreover, at least in California, African-American women have a much higher rate of mammograms than white women (61 percent versus 56 percent) (CEWAER 1993), yet their death rate from the disease is considerably higher than that of any other ethnic group. It may be that African-American women start getting mammograms later than white women. This possibility is supported by California data from 1988–89 that show that more African-American (and Latina) women were diagnosed at a late stage of the disease than white women (42 percent, 43 percent, and 32 percent, respectively) (CEWAER 1993). This may reflect the fact that Medi-Cal (California Medicaid) was not required to cover the cost of mammograms until 1991, so poorer women did not start getting them until that year. Moreover, federally funded screening programs for poor women do not generally pay for the follow-up care after a breast tumor is diagnosed.

Other possible explanations for the racial differences in death rates include ethnic differences in risk factors, in the cell type of the cancer, and in survival rates. Analysis of risk factors is complicated by the fact that in the United States, many women from ethnic minority groups are in the lower socioeconomic strata, itself a risk factor for poor health.

9. Socioeconomic status: The rationale and findings are similar to those discussed under the category of race, because the two are commonly linked in the United States. Moreover, poor people, because of problems of access to proper nutrition and health care, as well as increased stress, often have more illness and poorer outcomes than whites, who are more often in the higher socioeconomic strata. Statistics comparing ethnic minority women living in the United States to those living

in their country of origin may, therefore, be helpful in examining the role of ethnic differences. For example, Asian women in the United States have a higher rate of breast cancer than those living in Asia. This difference may reflect lower socioeconomic status in the United States and/or differences in customs.

10. Body weight: Before menopause, there is some variation in the findings with regard to weight and its relationship to breast cancer risk. In high-risk countries such as the United States, it has been found that the more obese a premenopausal woman is, the lower her risk of breast cancer (Pathak and Whittemore 1992). The reasons for this are not clear. One theory is that it is harder to detect a breast tumor in an obese person, so the reported lower rate is an artifact. This is not, however, consistent with some of the data, specifically, the lack of finding of a protective effect of adiposity in "moderate-risk countries" (Pathak and Whittemore 1992). All studies seem to agree that following menopause, the higher the body mass, the greater the risk for this cancer.

11. Fat intake: Some studies have suggested that fat plays a role in producing breast tumors, perhaps by increasing estrogen or growth hormone levels. A recent study, however, examined nearly 5,000 cases of breast cancer and found no evidence of an association between total dietary intake of fat and the risk of breast cancer (Hunter et al. 1996).

12. Smoking: An epidemiologist, Dr. Eugenia Calle, and her associates followed 600,000 initially cancer-free women for six years and found that smokers had a 25 percent greater likelihood of dying from breast cancer than nonsmokers and former smokers. The risk was proportional to the number of cigarettes smoked, with those smoking two or more packs each day having a 75 percent greater chance of developing fatal breast cancer than nonsmokers. The mechanism of this increased risk is not at all clear from the study (Calle et al. 1994). It is possible that smokers have a different life-style—for example, one that does not include mammograms—or that smoking somehow affects immunity to breast cancer. The finding of a lower risk of breast cancer in smokers who had had breast cysts than smokers who had not may support the former theory because this group would have been more likely to have mammograms. The study also debunks the common myth that because smoking decreases estrogen levels in the body, it might protect against breast cancer.

13. Silicone breast implants: These implants (which are discussed more fully in Chapter 2) have recently been the subject of concern with regard to their possible role in causing breast cancer. A 1992 study that evaluated women who had had the procedure from 1973 to 1986, with an average time interval of 10.2 years, was reassuring. It found a lower risk of breast cancer in these women than in the general population, despite their higher-risk demographic profile (Berkel, Birdsell, and Jenkins 1992). The recipients of implants were predominantly white and of higher than average socioeconomic status. There are a number of possible explanations for this finding unrelated to the implants themselves. For example, the women most likely to have the implants were those at biologically lower risk for the disease (such as those who were slim and small-breasted). In addition, there is the possibility that tumors may be more difficult to detect in such women.

14. Exposure to ionizing radiation (Kelsey 1993).

15. Toxic exposure: A recent study by the health department in Nassau County, Long Island, gave credence to concerns of environmentalists about the risks of industrial pollution. This study found a 62 percent higher incidence of breast cancer in postmenopausal women who had, between 1965 and 1975, lived within five-eighths of a mile of plants that produced plastics, rubber, or chemicals. The difference was felt to be statistically significant, but obviously more research needs to be done using prospective studies. Dr. G. Iris Obrams is beginning a five-year prospective study of the higher breast cancer incidence on Long Island for the National Cancer Institute (*New York Times*, Apr. 13, 1994).

PREVENTION AND DETECTION

In the absence of a known clear cause of breast cancer, researchers have based their studies of prevention on the well-recognized association between estrogen and increased risk for developing this tumor. Preventive approaches have aimed to decrease the exposure to estrogen of those considered to be at increased risk because of family history of breast cancer. These approaches are currently being tested; it is too soon to know if they will prove effective. Some side effects of estrogen reduction, such as diminished protection against heart disease and osteoporosis, must also be considered in evaluating the usefulness of these agents.

Different specific preventive strategies are being tested in a variety of experiments for different age groups of women considered to be at increased risk for breast cancer because of family history or history of previous breast cancer. Premenopausal women are being treated with a chemical that blocks release of the hypothalamic hormone (luteinizing hormone-releasing hormone, or LHRH) that stimulates the pituitary hormone responsible for causing ovulation. Postmenopausal women are being treated with tamoxifen. This chemical, an "antiestrogen," blocks the receptors in the breast that bind to estrogen. It also appears to have a blunting effect on the production of growth hormone in the brain and may inhibit tumor growth as a result (Bernstein, Ross, and Henderson 1992). A large study (at the University of Pittsburgh, financed by the National Cancer Institute) of use of tamoxifen by 11,000 women at high risk for breast cancer because of family history was recently suspended before all 16,000 women were enrolled when it was found that the drug was associated with an increased risk of cancer of the uterus (*New York Times*, natl. ed., May 22, 1994). Concern has also been expressed that tamoxifen has other serious side effects.

A novel approach to reduction in exposure to estrogen has been suggested. Its appeal lies in the fact that it does not depend on the administration of drugs or hormones, but follows from the observation that vigorous exercise inhibits ovulation and decreases estrogen levels. The idea is that engaging in vigorous exercise in early adolescence will delay the onset of menses and, according to some studies, may lower estrogen levels and sex hormone–binding globulins for the rest of a woman's life (Bernstein et al. 1992). Again, the possibility of placing women at later risk for osteoporosis and heart disease must first be evaluated before any such intervention can be justified.

Another line of research in primary prevention of breast cancer has focused on dietary manipulation. Most dietary research has examined the possible effect of reduction in dietary fat (Prentice et al. 1988). This will be extensively evaluated in the NIH's Women's Health Initiative Study. Other nutritional interventions studied in this connection include increasing consumption of vitamin C, carotenoids, and the phytoestrogens in soybean products and olive oil (LaVecchia et al. 1995). Studies of vitamin C have mainly been done on mice and in tissue culture. In the mouse studies, researchers from the Linus Pauling Institute gave large quantities of ascorbic acid to a strain susceptible to spontaneous development of breast tumors. This was associated with delay in appearance of the tumors. In the test tube, large amounts of ascorbic acid were shown to kill breast cancer cells. In the Canadian National Breast Screening Study, there was no statistically significant reduction in the risk of breast cancer associated with vitamin C intake (Rohan et al. 1993). This study did, however, show a beneficial effect of dietary fiber on reduction of breast cancer risk. Much work remains to be done to evaluate any possible role of vitamins and other dietary factors in prevention of breast cancer.

If it is not possible to prevent this disease, it may still be possible to reduce its mortality rate. Of the three most common cancers in women, only breast cancer is amenable to early detection when it is still at a curable stage. When it is diagnosed before it has spread, the survival rate is 75 percent better than when it is discovered after it has spread (CDC 1994c).

Women's knowledge of the procedure for self-examination of the breast has been shown to vary by ethnicity. One study (CEWAER 1993) found that, whereas only 5 percent of white and African-American women reported that they did not know how to perform breast self-examination, the proportions among Latinas and Asian/Other women were 14 percent and 19 percent, respectively. Unfortunately, efforts directed at teaching self-examination of the breast are largely ineffective. Women generally do not comply, out of embarrassment (in certain ethnic and cultural groups, in adolescents [Cromer et al. 1992], and in the elderly) or even fear of finding a lump. Furthermore, even performance of self-examination is an insufficient detection mechanism, because by the time a breast cancer is palpable, it is usually far advanced. Nevertheless, women should be taught how to perform this examination, which is far better than using no screening mechanism at all. Women should also be on the lookout for changes in the skin of the breast (particularly if it takes on the appearance and feel of the skin of an orange) or a discharge from the nipple, either of which may be a sign of cancer. Nipple discharge can obviously be caused by a number of other factors, including pregnancy, lactation, certain drugs (such as some psychotropics, antigastroplegics, and blood pressure medications that stimulate the production of prolactin), pituitary or thyroid problems, and local infection or injury. However, because a discharge may also occasionally indicate breast cancer or certain other cancers elsewhere in the body, any such discharge should be checked by a doctor.

It is generally agreed that mammography is the most effective tool for early detection to improve outcome. Through mammography, the death rate for breast cancer has been reduced 30 percent for women between the ages of 50 and 69; that is, women between 50 and 69 who get mammograms have a 30 percent lower death rate than women in that age group who do not. Such a reduction has yet to be shown for younger women, however (Fletcher et al. 1993). The lack of data on younger women has, unfortunately, been used by insurance companies, health maintenance organizations, and the federal government as an excuse for not covering the cost of routine mammograms in women between 40 and 49. Although the cost of an individual mammogram is only about $100, the direct cost of having covered the five million women in their forties who got mammograms in 1990 would have been half a billion dollars. An estimated 6 out of every 100 of those mammograms in 40–49-year-olds were abnormal, requiring repeated mammograms or other tests, at an additional estimated cost of $31 million, and biopsies, at a cost of $120 million. On the other side of the argument, however, 13,500 young women were found to have breast cancer that would not have been discovered early if they had not had mammograms. The cost of the mammograms and other tests and treatment works out to about $48,000 for each of these women, a small price to pay for saving a young life. Further, as the American Medical Women's Association points out, the decision not to cover mammograms for women between 40 and 49 is premature and is based on studies that were not optimal for a number of reasons (Freedman 1994).

In 1997, the National Cancer Institute and the American Cancer Society finally recommended mammograms for all women over 40. Prior to that, the policy was for women over 49 to get a screening mammogram and clinical breast examination every one to two years. Yet only 57.8 percent (median) of women in this age group appear to be in compliance with even this recommendation (CDC 1993a). It has been estimated that less than one-third of physicians advise their female patients over 50 to get annual mammograms (Centers for Disease Control 1990). As mentioned above, there are major ethnic and other factors associated with lack of utilization of mammography, which may be responsible for some of the differences in outcome. Lack of access because of inadequate health insurance coverage is a major barrier to receiving regular mammograms. Low-income women had a compliance rate more than 15 percent lower than that of middle-class women. Also, Hispanic women are less likely to get mammograms than white women (43 percent versus 56 percent in California from 1989 to 1991 [CEWAER 1993]). Within this group, acculturation appears to be an important contributing factor. One study found that only 13.8 percent of Hispanic women over the age of 35 living in Los Angeles who spoke Spanish exclusively had ever had a mammogram, compared to 47.1 percent of those from the same communities who also spoke English (Stein and Fox 1990).

This study also discussed ways in which cancer prevention and screening efforts might be made more accessible and relevant to women of different cultural backgrounds. For example, the women who were interviewed in Spanish preferred television to either Spanish-language newspapers or radio as a means of receiving such messages. The study also stressed the importance of going beyond mere translation of health-promotion messages into other languages. Cultural relevance and reading level also need to be taken into account if we are going to meet the year 2000 health objective of clinical breast examination and mammogram for 60 percent or more of Hispanic women over 40. Studies to improve the likelihood of women obtaining mammograms are under way.

It is astounding and frightening that with the decisions (to say nothing of lives) dependent on mammograms, there were prior to 1993 no federal standards for mammography screening. This was finally recognized and rectified by the Breast Cancer Screening Safety Act, which became part of the Women's Health Equity Act introduced by Senators Brock Adams and Barbara Mikulski and Representatives Patricia Schroeder and Marilyn Lloyd. This legislation, which was enacted in 1993, established long-overdue national standards for mammography and a process for mandatory accreditation of mammographers by an approved body.

TREATMENT AND RESEARCH

Throughout recorded medical history, breast cancer has been treated with radical mastectomy. This approach was institutionalized by the father of modern surgery, William Halsted, almost a hundred years ago and was unchallenged until very recently. Radical mastectomy involves the removal of the breast and surrounding lymph nodes and tissue. Reexamination of the appropriateness of this procedure was prompted by the recognition that tumors are now diagnosed at earlier stages and when they are smaller than was the case in Halsted's day, thanks to the advent of mammography. In addition, we now know that even when a tumor is found early, it is likely that cancer cells have already entered the bloodstream and been carried away from the tumor itself, regardless of the extent of the local surgery. Because of this new information, surgeons in the early 1980's began evaluating the possibility that comparable survival rates could be achieved by more limited local removal of the tumor and surrounding tissue and lymph nodes (lumpectomy), accompanied by irradiation to kill cells that had reached more distant sites. Indeed, in a number of prospective trials in which patients were randomly assigned to receive either radical mastectomy alone or lumpectomy followed by radiation, survival has been found to be comparable. This prompted the NIH Consensus Development Conference in 1990 to conclude that breast conservation was preferable to radical mastectomy for most women with early (Stage I or II) breast cancer. For these women, the rate of recurrence eight to ten years later was the same (2–10 percent, varying with the amount of time after surgery) for both methods.

It appears that the application of this recommendation varies for a number of reasons. For example, breast-conserving lumpectomy is more likely to be performed on women who are younger, married, living in urban areas, better educated, and more affluent. Most women with early breast cancer seem still to be treated with radical mastectomy, at least as of 1990 in Washington State, where an extensive study was undertaken (Lazovich et al. 1991).

After years of relative neglect, breast cancer research support has been substantially increased in recent years. In 1994, the budget of the National Cancer Institute of the NIH for this research was estimated at more than $260 million, an increase of about $70 million from the previous year.

Through a strange series of events, the Pentagon's so-called peace dividend resulted in millions for the study of breast cancer.

The focus of this research ranges from the biomolecular to the behavioral. For example, studies of genes are ongoing in order to understand which women might be at risk for breast cancer, why the cancer spreads in some and not others, and what factors influence repair of DNA after X-ray and chemical treatment. The value and cost-effectiveness of screening mammograms for women under 50 continues to be a focus of research. As mentioned above, others are studying the possibility of prevention through the use of the controversial drug tamoxifen. This study is part of the Breast Cancer Prevention Trial, a five-year national collaborative study that planned to enroll 16,000 women. A major study to evaluate the difference in outcome of lumpectomy versus extensive, radical mastectomy continues. Different approaches to treatment of breast cancer are being studied by other researchers. These include refinements of bone marrow transplantation and a number of immune therapies, in addition to studies of RU-486, the antiprogesterone drug.

Recently, concern has arisen about some treatment research results following the finding that one of the surgeons in a study done at the University of Pittsburgh and financed by the National Cancer Institute falsified data (Altman 1994). The entire study is now being reevaluated without the data from that physician. Preliminary findings are reassuring but not yet conclusive (Altman 1994).

Ovarian Cancer

Currently, about 13,000 women die from ovarian cancer each year in the United States, making this the fourth leading cause of cancer death among women in the nation. (The first three, in decreasing order of prevalence, are lung cancer, breast cancer, and cancer of the colon or rectum.) Ovarian cancer strikes 1–2 percent of women, with about 20,000 cases diagnosed each year. The causes of this deadly disease are currently under intense study. The one definite risk factor is family history. Women who have a sister, mother, grandmother, daughter, or aunt with the disease have a 5 percent risk of contracting it. Women who have never borne children are also at increased risk. Other associations have been reported with talc, milk, and tamoxifen (the drug being tested for the prevention of breast cancer).

Some degree of protection against ovarian cancer appears to result from using birth control pills. Some studies estimate the risk reduction to be 40–50 percent in women who have used the Pill for a minimal period of three years. Protection increases with longer periods of use. At ten years of use, the risk is reduced by 80 percent, according to the Cancer and Steroid Hormone Study of the Centers for Disease Control and the National Institute of Child Health and Human Development (1987). This protection appears to continue for at least fifteen years after the Pill is discontinued. It is particularly heartening that a recent study reports the protective effect of the Pill to extend to women who are at increased risk for ovarian cancer by virtue of family or pregnancy history. Five years of continuous birth control pill use by women who had never given birth reduced their risk to a level equal to that of non-Pill-using women who have had children. Among women with a family history of ovarian cancer, Pill use for ten years appeared to reduce their risk so significantly that it fell below that of non-Pill-using women without a family history of the disease (Gross and Schlesselman 1994).

Protection also appears to follow tubal ligation. A study of 78,000 premenopausal women followed from 1976 to 1988 found that those who had this procedure reduced their chance of getting ovarian cancer by one-third (Hankinson et al. 1993). The explanation for this observation is not at all clear. Although the possibility of hormonal changes following this procedure had been suggested, studies of hormone levels have had different findings. Nor could this finding be attributed, as originally thought, simply to earlier discovery of problems in the ovaries when they were seen at the time of the procedure.

There is presently no noninvasive or inexpensive screening test for ovarian cancer. Although ultrasound examination of the ovaries can detect malignancies, it has a high rate of false positives. That is, ultrasonography may suggest that a woman has a cancerous tumor when she does not. The growths seen on ultrasound may in fact be cysts or noncancerous tumors. Opponents of general use of ultrasound for ovarian cancer screening argue that it would lead to many unnecessary operations. Use of this procedure for screening is currently reserved for women with a family history of the disease. Similarly, the blood level of the tumor marker CA-125 is elevated in women with ovarian cancer, but it is also elevated by other conditions; thus, using it as a method of ovarian cancer screening also results in many false positives.

Because there is no good screening test, and because the ovaries are well hidden from view, cancer of the ovary is generally discovered after it has advanced. It isn't surprising, therefore, that the survival rate is relatively low. The overall survival rate following diagnosis is given as 39 percent, but only 19 percent survive for over five years (American Cancer Society 1992).

Treatment for ovarian cancer currently includes surgery followed by chemotherapy with the platinum-containing drug cisplatin. A new, experimental drug currently under investigation is taxol. This drug has received a lot of publicity recently because its only known source is the endangered Pacific yew tree.

Endometrial (Uterine) Cancer

Cancer of the endometrium, the lining of the uterus, typically occurs in women over the age of 50. It affects approximately 12,000 women each year, and incidence has been fairly constant over the past decade. The rate is higher in white than in black women, although the death rate is approximately twice as high for blacks as for whites. The reasons for this racial difference in death rates are not clear, but likely relate to detection at a later stage of the disease in women with more difficulty accessing the health care system.

The risk of developing this cancer is higher in women who are obese, who have been infertile and/or had irregular or absent menstrual periods, and, to a lesser extent, who have taken estrogen treatment. Despite this last factor, it appears that birth control pills, which also contain estrogen, offer some protection against this disease (see Chapter 6). Recent drug trials with tamoxifen for the prevention of breast cancer have reported an increase in the incidence of cancer of the uterus, a finding that will be examined carefully in future research.

The typical symptoms of uterine cancer include heavy and/or frequent menstrual bleeding or any vaginal bleeding occurring after menopause. Of course, the same symptoms can occur in women with other sorts of problems, including "fibroids" and hormonal imbalance. It is important, therefore, that any woman with such symptoms be examined by a physician. If there is any question about the diagnosis, the physician will perform an endometrial biopsy and have the tissue examined by a trained pathologist. Treatment usually consists of surgery alone; in some cases radiation treatment is also necessary. The survival rate for endometrial cancer is relatively high if the cancer is discovered early. About 85 percent of women are alive five years after diagnosis and treatment.

Hysterectomy

In a hysterectomy, the uterus is removed, and usually, though not always, the ovaries as well. Much has already been written about hysterectomies, most of it worrisome. During the nineteenth century, many women were subjected to unnecessary and dangerous hysterectomies out of the misguided but widely held belief among physicians of the time that most of women's ailments were the result of dysfunction of the uterus or ovaries (hence, the word "hysterical," from the Greek word for uterus). Among other benign conditions, menstrual cramps in young girls were often treated in this grossly inappropriate and cruel manner.

Even more recently, some find the high percentage of hysterectomies suspicious. *The New Our Bodies, Ourselves* (Boston Women's Health Book Collective 1984: 440, 511) records the following statistics about the incidence of hysterectomies: 40 percent of women will have had one by the age of 40, 50 percent by the age of 65, and 62 percent by the age of 70. The rate in the United States is twice that in England and Sweden. Women of color have hysterectomies at twice the rate of white women, and doctors' wives have proportionately more than any other group.

It is, therefore, understandable that with the rise in women's consciousness in the 1960's and 1970's, the medical profession was targeted for criticism of its poor treatment of women. Out of this collective indignation, women were encouraged and empowered to cure themselves, particularly in the area of gynecologic problems. As an alternative to hysterectomy, for example, some publications advocated exercise, vitamins, and avoidance of certain foods. The details may have changed in the ensuing thirty years, but the message continues.

Gail Sheehy in her recent best-selling book about menopause, *The Silent Passage*, warns women against "passive surrender of organs." Others warn of the "medicalization of aging." It is not surprising, therefore, that an intelligent and articulate woman like Jane Gross (1994) might write that her decision to undergo a hysterectomy "leaves me feeling guilty for selling out the sisterhood." Along the same lines, *The New Our Bodies, Ourselves* (Boston Women's Health Book Collective 1984), long a bible for feminists, includes a cartoon by Bülbül picturing a woman being wheeled into surgery with the caption: "I hope you can justify this hysterectomy to my women's health group" (p. 513).

Although it is true that even today some of these operations are unnecessary, it is important also to recognize that in many cases a hysterectomy can be life-saving. To condemn every physician for suggesting it and stigmatize every women who agrees to it is irresponsible. Some of the conditions for which a hysterectomy is necessary include advanced cancer of the uterus, cervix, or vagina; cancer of the fallopian tubes and/or ovaries; large or bleeding "fibroids"; uterine bleeding that is uncontrollable by hormonal treatment or curettage (scraping); some complications of pregnancy, including rupture of the uterus; incapacitating pain from endometriosis (see Menstrual Cramps and Menorrhagia, in Chapter 1); and prolapse (dropping) of the uterus. Failure to have a hysterectomy when indicated can result in death, a fact that is often overlooked by critics of the procedure.

Mortality

The leading causes of death of 45–65-year-old women are listed in Appendix A. They resemble closely the leading causes of death for older women.

CHAPTER FOUR

The Older Years

The "graying" of America is dramatically illustrated by the fact that since the turn of the century, there has been a tenfold increase in the number of people over the age of 65. The elderly make up about 15 percent of the population of the United States. It is estimated that by the year 2030, there will be more than 66 million "older" Americans (the term preferred by the American Association of Retired Persons) and that they will make up almost 22 percent of the population.

Among the approximately 31 million Americans in this category in 1989, more than half (18.3 million) were women, a ratio of 145 older women for every 100 older men. This ratio increases with age. Within the 65–69-year-old group, it stands at 120 to 100, but for those 85 or older, it is 258 to 100, almost three women for every man. As of 1992, women are expected to outlive men by an average of 6.8 years (Kochanek and Hudson 1994).

So much for the "female advantage." On the other side of the coin, older men are twice as likely as women to be married. Half of all older women in 1989 were widows (five times the number of widowers). In 1992, 57 percent of women who died had been widowed, compared with only 18 percent of men (Kochanek and Hudson 1994). As a result of this difference, as well as the fact that more older women than men are divorced (there has been a 2.9-fold increase since 1980 in the number of older women who are divorced, compared to a 1.9-fold increase for older men), more than 40 percent of older women who are not institutionalized live alone or with nonrelatives. Five percent of older women lived in nursing homes in 1985; the numbers increased with age, from 1 percent at the lower end of the older age group to 22 percent of those over 85 (the age group largely composed of women). Finally, the poverty rate among older women was almost twice that among older men. Against this background of longer life expectancy and higher rates of isolation and poverty, we can now examine the health status of older women. Not surprisingly, the major health concerns of these women relate to their fear of dependency and loss of mobility.

More than one-third of the nation's personal health care costs are expended on those over the age of 65, a group that in 1984 constituted only 12 percent of the population. This reflects the higher incidence among older people of chronic illness and functional disability, as well as advances in technology that have prolonged the lives of people who in previous eras would likely have died of their illnesses. Approximately 20 percent of people over 65 years of age have multiple disease processes that cause functional limitation on their normal activity. This is the group referred to by geriatricians as the "frail elderly." After the age of 85, the percentage of frail elderly rises to 46 percent. Viewed in a slightly different way, the elderly are 4.5 times more likely to experience limitation on their activity than younger people (American Medical Association Council on Scientific Affairs 1990).

In 1988, older women averaged 34 days of restriction of usual activities because of illness or injury, compared with 26 days for older men. On average, women spent sixteen of these days in bed, and men spent twelve. In 1984, 25 percent of older women (compared with 19 percent of older men) reported having difficulty with one or more personal care activities (such as bathing, dressing, eating, or transferring from bed to chair) as a result of a health problem (American Medical Association Council on Scientific Affairs 1990).

Although women have a longer life expectancy than men, their "active" life expectancy (the ability to perform basic activities of daily living unassisted) has stayed the same. The net effect is that women spend more of their life in a dependent state (Katz et al. 1983). For example, in the early 1980's it was estimated that women between 65 and 69 would live 54 percent of their remaining years in a dependent state, compared with 46 percent for men of the same age. This discrepancy persists for every age group over 65. It is projected that by the turn of the century, among those over the age of 75 experiencing limitations in their daily activities, three-quarters of a million will be men and one and one-quarter million will be women (Rice and Feldman 1983).

Despite the higher incidence of health problems in women in this age group, in 1990 men over the age of 65 made more visits to the doctor than did women. In fact, the highest per-person rate of doctor visits in any gender/age group was seen in males over the age of 75, who averaged 5.4 visits that year. This may be less a reflection of health status than of men's greater likelihood of having health insurance coverage that allows for such visits.

Gerontologists have now begun to think about the health problems of the elderly in a more functional way rather than in the traditional organ system–based way. As a result, they now discuss practical problems that have a profound effect on the well-being of the elderly in terms of "syndromes." These syndromes include falling, instability, functional impairment, deconditioning, incontinence, delirium, constipation, fecal impaction, dehydration, nutritional deprivation, sleep disorders, sexual dysfunction, family stress, and adult abuse (Ham 1988). Unfortunately, most physicians are trained to think in terms of organ systems and discrete entities and are challenged more by making the rare and exotic diagnosis than by making a constipated older person comfortable.

Physicians, as a group, have been criticized by their own colleagues for their poor management of the frail elderly, including "(1) inappropriate institutionalization, (2) incomplete medical diagnosis, (3) poor coordination of community support services, (4) overprescription of medications, and (5) underutilization of rehabilitation" (American Medical Association Council on Scientific Affairs 1990: 2460). This same report suggests the use of a "comprehensive geriatric assessment" that is "multidimensional and interdisciplinary and seeks to define and quantify biomedical, functional, psychological, and social variables" (ibid.: 2461; see Appendix B). This kind of comprehensive approach has been shown to increase the number of new diagnoses while decreasing the number of prescriptions given, the use of acute care hospitals, the number of nursing home placements, and overall health care costs over time. Nevertheless, few physicians use this type of evaluation, either because of lack of familiarity with it, lack of time to do it, or lack of resources to follow up on the identified problems.

There is some hope that this may change. The American Medical Association's Council on Scientific Affairs (1990) describes recent research into one syndrome that will have a far-reaching impact on the quality, and possibly the quantity, of life of the elderly. In investigating the reason for frequent falls after meals among nursing home residents (a topic that, in the past, would not have attracted much interest among medical researchers or funding agencies), Lipsitz et al. (1983) discovered that eating may cause a fall in blood pressure in elderly patients. This finding has stimulated further research into possible preventive treatment, but in the meantime it has alerted nursing home personnel to the need to alter staffing and procedures in order to prevent problems at and after meals. This research may also help prevent the need for nursing home placement; instead, in-home assistance might be scheduled to provide assistance to the elderly around mealtimes.

Medical science has made considerable progress in the technology that allows people with chronic debilitating illness and even those with some illnesses previously considered fatal to live longer and more functionally satisfying lives. For example, with hip-replacement surgery, thousands of people with degenerative joint diseases are now mobile and pain-free. It even appears that retinoic acid may be able to reverse or prevent skin wrinkles.

All this leads to the possibility that some of the aging process may be slowed, prevented, or reversed. With such possibilities comes the challenge to better understand the process of aging. We know very little about how much of the body's deterioration with age is inevitable and whether or not, with more research, we may be able to prevent some illnesses from occurring.

Health Problems of Older Women

The ten most common chronic conditions in the elderly are arthritis, high blood pressure, hearing impairment, heart disease, deformity or orthopedic impairment, chronic sinusitis, visual impairment, diabetes, varicose veins, and abdominal hernia (National Center for Health Statistics 1985).

Although most older Americans suffer from at least one chronic illness, many have more than one (American Association of Retired Persons n.d.). Most of these conditions are more serious and/or more common in older women than in older men. Women are more likely to develop neurologic illnesses such as Alzheimer disease, parkinsonism, blindness, or deafness. The risk for muscular-skeletal diseases such as arthritis and osteoporosis is not only greater in older women but a major cause of limitation of mobility. This places them at increased risk not only for compromising their quality of life by becoming dependent, but also for developing fatal complications such as pneumonia.

Moreover, the older woman has a greater chance than a man of the same age of developing congestive heart failure, stroke, heart attack, high blood pressure, and chronic obstructive lung disease (e.g., emphysema). These chronic diseases are responsible for higher out-of-pocket health care expenses for older women; the acute illnesses more common in older men are less expensive (Clancy and Massion 1992).

The most common causes of poor quality of life for women in their later years are conditions or syndromes that increase their dependency, limit their mobility, and cause social isolation. Among these, the most common are impairment of vision and hearing. Others include incontinence, osteoporosis, osteoarthritis, and complications resulting from hospitalization and long-term care. Older women also face changes affecting their appearance, as well as the more serious dangers of breast cancer, high blood pressure, and stroke. But perhaps the deadliest threat to this age group is heart disease.

VISUAL IMPAIRMENT

Visual impairment is defined as having difficulty seeing with one or both eyes when wearing corrective glasses. About 11 million Americans fit this description, and almost half of them are 65 or older. Legal blindness is defined as having corrected vision in the better eye of 20/200 or less or having a restricted visual field of 20 degrees or less in the better eye. More than 50 percent of all legally blind persons in the United States are 65 or older. The leading causes of blindness in this age group include cataracts, glaucoma, diabetes, and degeneration of the macula. Cataracts are curable with surgery or possibly newer nonoperative techniques; glaucoma is usually treatable with medication if detected early; and the visual complications of diabetes may be prevented with good control of the diabetes itself. For all of these reasons, it is critical that the elderly have regular vision evaluations and not assume that their failing vision is just the result of aging.

HEARING IMPAIRMENT

Between one-quarter and one-half of individuals above the age of 65 have impaired hearing. Aging may cause problems in the part of the inner ear responsible for hearing pure tones and discriminating nuances of speech, as well as the part that maintains balance. In addition to the obvious decrease in functional capacity resulting from these problems, hearing impairment often leads to psychologic difficulties. It is not uncommon, for example, for the hearing-impaired elderly to become angry, fearful, depressed, frustrated, and anxious. In some cases, an erroneous diagnosis of dementia or a determination of incompetence has resulted when the possibility of hearing loss has not been considered. Early identification of hearing problems and individualized treatment, often including hearing aids, lipreading, and other rehabilitative measures, can make the difference between dependence and independence in elderly women.

INCONTINENCE

Incontinence is another common chronic syndrome in women, often beginning in the early adult years (see Chapter 2). We are now all familiar with radio and television ads by the likes of June Allyson and other popular and wholesome movie stars of the past inviting women to "come back into life again" despite their incontinence. Besides increasing sales of the advertised products designed to provide protection against embarrassing accidents, these ads have really served as public service messages. Women now know that they are not alone in having this problem and may develop the courage to discuss it with their physicians, which it has been estimated that only one in twelve women with the problem does (Older Women's League 1991).

Because of widespread reluctance to report incontinence, it's difficult to know how common it really is. The medical literature estimates that it affects between 10 and 20 percent of community-dwelling people over the age of 65; about one-third of those in this age group who are in acute care hospitals; and almost 50 percent of those in nursing homes (Solomon 1988). The Older Women's League (1991) provides a prevalence estimate of about one-third of all women over the age of 50. Another report shows that 80 percent of all people with incontinence are women, constituting nearly 10 million women in all (Pharmaceutical Manufacturers Association 1991). The problem takes an inestimable toll in terms of human suffering, as incontinence, especially fecal incontinence, is often the precipitating factor in the decision to place an elderly person in a nursing home.

Despite its high incidence, incontinence is not simply a consequence of aging. As discussed in Chapter 2, it usually has a specific cause, which may be treatable. Therefore, it is important for women with this problem to be evaluated by a physician.

OSTEOPOROSIS

Osteoporosis poses a significant threat to women's lives and well-being. It affects about half of women over the age of 45 and nine out of ten of those over 75. At greater risk of developing osteoporosis are white women, those who are thin with small musculature, smokers, those who drink a lot of alcohol, and perhaps those with premature graying (Rosen, Holick, and Millard 1994). Conversely, it is less common in blacks and in the obese. Despite considerable media attention to studies reporting a decreased risk in athletes, the jury is still out on that question. It does, however, seem to be true that weight-bearing exercise is beneficial in this regard (see below).

Osteoporosis is a condition of decreased bone density and strength. The bones become more fragile and may be more easily broken. Certain bones, like those of the wrist, the vertebral column, and the hip, are most likely to break. This probably reflects a combination of fragility at those sites and their particular vulnerability during falls, an increasingly common problem as aging robs the body of defenses such as vision and balance. Falls account for almost 90 percent of all fractures among the elderly.

Fifteen percent of women with osteoporosis will experience a hip fracture. Each year, nearly 200,000 elderly people fracture a hip in a fall. Almost 10 percent will die within six months; of the survivors, 20 percent will spend more than a year in a nursing home or other long-term care facility. Fifty percent of those who suffer a hip fracture will die within the next five years. This death rate is higher than those for many types of cancer (AMA Council on Scientific Affairs 1990).

Ten percent of women with osteoporosis will fracture their vertebrae. Like a hip fracture, fracture of vertebrae is extremely painful and can result in limitation to bed rest. It may also lead to serious deformities as well as to life-threatening pneumonia.

Although the end result of osteoporosis, namely fractures, occurs in the later years, the process of bone thinning has been shown to begin in the twenties. Women seem to lose bone density at a rate of about one-half percent each year during the twenties, thirties, and forties. After menopause, this rate increases for approximately ten years, such that 15 percent of bone loss occurs during this time. The rate of loss, fortunately, then falls to zero, so the older woman with strong bones is likely to keep them. This information was not known until recently; as a result, all the studies of osteoporosis have been done on the elderly, with frustrating results.

Prevention is obviously the best way to improve outcome. The time to prevent osteoporosis is adolescence. Bones achieve their lifelong supply of substance and strength (60 percent) during puberty and go downhill from then on. Studies are now ongoing to learn how to maximize bone strength during the pubertal years. It appears that having regular menstrual periods, being of normal or above average weight, exercising, and consuming adequate calcium (about six servings of dairy products or supplements to achieve about 2 g of elemental calcium each day) are important factors. The specific role of exercise in prevention of osteoporosis is being carefully evaluated; one recent study of women over the age of 62 showed that women who walked about one mile each day delayed the onset of osteoporosis by four to seven years in later life. It appears that swimming does not benefit bone density, whereas gymnastics does. Additional research is obviously needed to help us learn more.

What about those of us well beyond the adolescent years? What can be done to help? Treatment can prevent further loss of bone strength and substance, although it cannot reverse any of the losses that have already occurred. Research has shown that taking estrogens to replace those no longer produced by the ovaries after menopause, taking calcium to supplement that in the diet, engaging in moderate, weight-bearing exercise, and not smoking all help to prevent further postmenopausal loss of bone density and decrease the risks from osteoporosis. Estrogen replacement therapy is associated with a 50 percent reduction in future hip fractures and a 70 percent decrease in spine fractures resulting from loss of bone density (Melton 1990).

A study by Agriculture Department scientists and the Jean Meyer Human Nutrition Research Center on Aging at Tufts University recently found that women who walked more than 7.5 miles each week reduced their risk of loss of bone density. These walkers were found to have the equivalent of up to seven years' more reserve bone than the nonwalkers. They had 7 percent more density in the bones of their legs and 4 percent more over their entire skeleton than women who did not walk. Of interest was that the walking did not have to be done as exercise per se; it was equally effective if done in the course of daily activities (*New York Times*, natl. ed., Dec. 7, 1994, p. B9). Recent studies by Robert Marcus of Stanford University School of Medicine showed that even very elderly women can benefit from a program of weight-bearing exercise, but its value is mainly to improve muscle strength and thus to prevent falls, rather than to prevent progression of osteoporosis (Marcus et al. 1992).

Why don't we hear anything about osteoporosis in men? It does occur, but it is much more rare. This is because men don't start to experience bone loss until they are over 40, and the loss rate of about one-half percent each year is constant for the rest of their lives. At that rate, they would have to live to the age of about 120 to reach the level of bone thinning of the average woman half that age, assuming she had menopause at 50. There are, of course, certain disease states and medications that accelerate bone loss in men and that can cause osteoporosis at earlier ages.

OSTEOARTHRITIS

Osteoarthritis of the knees, hips, hands, and feet is a condition characterized by degeneration of cartilage and overgrowth and remodeling of bone at the joints. It rarely occurs in people under the age of 55 and is the leading cause of joint pain and disability in middle-aged and elderly patients (Wyngaarden and Smith 1988). It is more common in women after menopause, particularly women who are obese. It has long been considered a disease of aging, but recent research suggests otherwise. One of the currently active areas of investigation seems to point to estrogen itself, rather than its decrease after menopause, as the cause of degenerative changes in the cartilage of the joints during earlier adulthood. It is possible that progesterone protects the joints from these effects of estrogen and that the loss of progesterone after menopause contributes to the damage (Tsai and Liu 1992). Some forms of osteoarthritis may be prevented by avoidance of prolonged immobilization and repeated trauma. Treatment is initially focused on pain relief using nonsteroidal antiinflammatory drugs (NSAIs), joint rest and protection, relief of associated muscle spasm, and weight reduction when appropriate. After pain and muscle spasm are relieved, prolonged home exercise, often involving hydrotherapy, is beneficial in maintaining function.

CONSEQUENCES OF HOSPITALIZATION AND LONG-TERM CARE

In many cultures, it is well known that you go to the hospital to die. Although modern scientific advances and technology have changed that for most people in industrialized societies, for the elderly the hospital remains a dangerous place and one that should be avoided whenever possible. For example, one study (Reichel 1965) of 500 hospitalized patients over the age of 65 showed that there were 237 complications (47 percent); this figure compares with a rate of 36 percent for hospitalized patients of all ages, including the elderly, in another study done 26 years later (Steel et al. 1981).

Older patients not only appear more vulnerable to typical complications of hospitalization, such as reactions to medications or transfusions and procedure mishaps, but are at greater risk of contracting serious infections while in the hospital. In addition, they are at high risk for becoming confused, falling, not eating, and losing control of their urinary or bowel function. These problems were reported to have occurred in 40 percent of the elderly in one study, compared with 9 percent of patients under 70 (Gillick, Serrell, and Gillick 1982). They often lead to complications: A patient who stops eating often requires tube feeding, which increases the risk of puncture of the esophagus; one who loses bladder control typically has a catheter inserted, which increases the risk of urinary tract infection; falling leads to restriction to bed, or, worse, to physical or pharmacologic restraints, both of which increase the risk of developing blood clots in the legs and possibly fatal clots in the lungs, as well as pneumonia.

To these well-described risks of hospitalization, one might add ageism. It is obviously difficult to assess the extent to which negative attitudes of young, inexperienced doctors toward their elderly patients might contribute to a lower quality of care. This was pointed out to me not by my medical training but by my aunt. At the age of nearly 80, this remarkably energetic, youthful-thinking, and astute woman was admitted to the hospital for a coronary bypass operation (after convincing her physician to allow her first to walk the Great Wall of China). When she realized that the nameplate on the door to her hospital room included her birth date, she instructed me to cross it out, stating that if she had a cardiac arrest, she didn't want any young intern to see her age, rationalize that she had already lived a long life, and be less than vigorous in attempting resuscitation. She is still going strong ten years later, and I continue to learn from her.

CHANGES TO SKIN AND HAIR

With age, in both men and women, the skin roughens, thins, dries, wrinkles, becomes less elastic, and develops uneven pigmentation and a variety of lumps and bumps (most, but not all, benign). Although most of these are viewed negatively, there is one positive aspect of aging skin: a decrease in its responsiveness to immunologic challenges, which translates into a decrease in contact dermatitis.

Graying of the hair results from a gradual loss of enzymatically active melanocytes in the skin. The rate of loss is about 10 to 20 percent each year (Wyngaarden and Smith 1988: 2306). The decrease in production of androgens in both sexes is responsible for a gradual decrease and thinning of body hair, on the head as well as in the axillae and pubic regions.

BREAST CANCER

About three-quarters of all cases of breast cancer (see Chapter 3) occur in women over the age of 60. Mammography rates among poor women and women over 65 are even lower than those among women in general (see Chapter 3), resulting in an unacceptably high rate of disseminated breast cancer owing to delay in its detection in these groups. One of the major reasons for this problem has been the lack of Medicare reimbursement for screening mammography prior to January 1991. Many women with private health insurance similarly are denied coverage.

Treatment of breast cancer seems to differ according to the age of the patient (and possibly that of the physician). A study was done to see how doctors treated early breast cancer prior to the development of recommendations by the NIH Consensus Development Conference in 1990. It found that the recommended approach of breast-conserving lumpectomy followed by radiation therapy was less likely to be used for older women than for those who were younger. Of even greater concern was the finding that women older than 70 were "at significantly increased risk of not receiving postoperative radiation therapy; fully 56 percent of women aged 80 years or older who had conservative surgery were not treated with radiation. Widows were more likely not to receive radiation therapy than married women, even after adjustment for age" (Lazovich et al. 1991: 3,436). This is particularly worrisome, given recent findings of increased risk of recurrence of breast cancer in women who undergo lumpectomy without subsequent radiation (Kolata 1994).

There are many possible explanations for these findings. Is it the physicians' choice or bias, or the patients'? The answer is probably both. In a number of studies (Liberati et al. 1987), when doctors were given vignettes describing different clinical situations, they more frequently recommended radical mastectomy for older women than for younger women with the same stage of breast disease.

Older women themselves are also more likely to choose mastectomy when given a choice (Ward, Heidric, and Wolberg 1989), but it is possible that they do so because of physician biases in providing information to them. When this issue was explored in another study, it was found that older women were less satisfied than younger women with the information they received from their doctors. Among those 60 to 70 years of age, only 61 percent were satisfied, compared with 85 percent of women younger than 50 (Cawley, Kostic, and Cappello 1990).

HIGH BLOOD PRESSURE AND STROKE

High blood pressure is the leading cause of visits to internists in the United States and the most common reason for prescription medications (Anastos et al. 1991). It is more common in blacks than in whites. Among blacks, it is more common in women than in men. Although in whites the reverse is true, in absolute numbers there are more women than men with this disease because of the greater number of women in the overall population. It has been estimated that sixteen million (58 percent) of all people with high blood pressure are women (Pharmaceutical Manufacturers Association 1991).

The incidence of complications of high blood pressure increases steadily with age. In the 65-to-74-year-old group, there are more women than men with high blood pressure and its complications, the most serious of which are heart disease and stroke. It is unclear why postmenopausal women have a higher incidence of high blood pressure than either men or younger women.

High blood pressure is the major risk factor in two of the leading causes of death, strokes and heart disease. (For a discussion of heart disease, see below.) Strokes are the third leading cause of death among older women, after heart disease and cancer. There are two types of deadly stroke. One is caused by blockage of a blood vessel in the brain, the other by a hemorrhage in the brain. Although both men and women are at risk for both types of strokes, women tend to have more of the second kind and to have them earlier in their lives. Women who smoke increase their risk for stroke, as do women who take birth control pills that contain estrogen after the age of 35. Women who both smoke and take birth control pills have a tremendously increased risk of stroke.

The treatment of high blood pressure significantly reduces the risk of fatal heart disease and stroke in men, but not in women. In 1991 treatment of high blood pressure in women was estimated to cost $13.7 billion in the United States (Pharmaceutical Manufacturers Association 1991).

There is a difference of opinion as to what constitutes high blood pressure. For adult women, there is agreement that the upper safe levels are 140 mmHg (systolic, the upper number) and 90 mmHg (diastolic, the lower number). For adolescents, however, these levels are determined by the average range of blood pressure for sex and age. Therefore, high blood pressure is defined as a level greater than that of 97 percent of others of the same age and sex, though it is not certain that exceeding these ranges is dangerous at all ages.

The effect of treatment with antihypertensive drugs on risk reduction in women is as yet unclear. According to Anastos et al. (1991: 287), "current recommendations concerning the treatment of hypertension do not differentiate between women and men: Both sexes are encompassed in a single set of guidelines. . . . A similar gender blindness exists with respect to the adverse effects of antihypertensive medications. It is not clear that this universal approach is warranted."

These authors reviewed available medical literature to determine if the present gender-blind treatment of high blood pressure is justified. They found that medication trials that included women showed benefit to black women, but not white women. In fact, there was a suggestion that treatment for high blood pressure might actually be harmful to white women. Most important, they found that no studies examined the effect in women of antihypertensive drugs on levels of cholesterol and lipids, factors known to affect the risk for heart disease and stroke. They also noted that although studies of these drugs had evaluated their effect on sexual functioning in men, "few data have been published on the frequency of sexual dysfunction in treated hypertensive women" (Anastos et al. 1991: 287). Furthermore, as discussed in Chapter 3, there is currently no information about whether postmenopausal ERT increases the risk of high blood pressure.

Thus far, we have focused attention on "essential hypertension," the most common form of high blood pressure, which has no apparent cause. However, some factors are known to cause other types of high blood pressure. Among them is kidney disease, particularly what is called "renal vascular hypertension from fibrous dysplasia." The kind of high blood pressure caused by this disease is more common and more serious in women than in men (Becker 1990).

HEART DISEASE

Coronary heart disease has long been considered a male problem. Although its tremendous toll among women has only recently been recognized, it is not a new phenomenon. It was previously unappreciated for two main reasons. First, heart disease occurs later in women than in men (about ten years later, in general), largely because of the protective effects of estrogen for premenopausal women. In the most influential study about heart disease, the Framingham study, the majority of women were premenopausal. Not surprisingly, few developed heart disease, reinforcing the conventional wisdom among physicians. The second reason is that physicians have diagnosed heart disease much less often in women.

However, as discussed below, this does not necessarily mean their female patients have not had the disease.

The reality is that almost one-third of all deaths of women in the United States (more than one-quarter of a million per year) result from cardiovascular disease. Half the people who die of heart attacks are women. By the age of 60, one in five men suffers a heart attack, compared with one in seventeen women. Ten years after menopause, this gap is almost nonexistent; after the age of 65, the heart attack rates between the sexes are comparable. By the age of 67, "heart disease becomes the most common cause of death among women" (Altman 1991). Moreover, many more women than men are incapacitated by their heart disease. In 1987, it was estimated that the direct cost for care of coronary artery disease in women was $14 billion (Pharmaceutical Manufacturers Association 1991).

Causes

The paucity of research on coronary artery disease in women means that there is still much we do not know about its causes. Some of the risk factors identified for the well-studied male population, however, appear to hold true for women as well. Cigarette smoking, which has unfortunately been increasing among women, is a known predisposing cause of this type of heart disease. High blood pressure and elevated plasma cholesterol levels are independent risk factors. It is not simply high cholesterol, but the relative amounts of the so-called "good" and "bad" cholesterols (HDLs and LDLs) that is significant. The higher the HDL and the lower the LDL, the lower the risk for a myocardial infarction (MI). In general, women have higher HDL levels than men, a factor presumed to explain the gender difference in incidence of MIs. Studies in men have demonstrated the benefit of reduction in total cholesterol in lowering their risk of MIs. Overweight is clearly a risk factor in men, independent of its association with high cholesterol levels, and recent reports link certain body shapes (specifically, an "apple" shape, or truncal obesity) to risk in males as well. Diabetes mellitus increases the risk for coronary artery disease in both sexes, but it is associated with a greater risk of death from heart disease in women than in men for uncertain reasons (Corrao et al. 1990).

Age, too, is important. In women, it is unclear whether this is solely because of the reduction of estrogen levels that takes place at menopause, or whether age is an independent risk factor, as it is in men. Birth control pills containing estrogen increase the risk of heart attacks, presumably by increasing the levels of LDLs and of blood-clotting factors when taken by women over the age of 35. The combination of smoking and use of birth control pills increases this risk still further (Hatcher et al. 1990). One caveat about this information: It is based on long-term follow-up studies of women who took the original Pill, which contained a hundred times as much estrogen as the pills that are currently being used (Hatcher et al. 1990).

It may be confusing that estrogens used after menopause appear to *decrease* the risk of heart disease, when estrogen-containing birth control pills *increase* this risk. One possible explanation is that the estrogens used postmenopausally are conjugated estrogens, while those in birth control pills are synthetic estrogens. There is evidence that conjugated estrogens increase HDL levels and lower LDL levels, which may explain their pro-tective effect. Another possibility is that birth control pills may have an effect opposite to that of estrogen taken alone because they also contain progesterone, which has been shown to increase the risk of heart disease by changing blood cholesterol and lipid levels. It is also possible that women who self-select to take birth control pills have different health characteristics than those who self-select to take ERT. However, this last possibility was refuted by one of the largest studies of women using ERT, the Nurses' Health Study (Stampfer et al. 1991), which found that nurses who were taking postmenopausal estrogens were actually more likely to have used oral contraceptives in the past.

Diagnosis

One of the most important revelations in the medical literature in the past few years is that serious heart disease has been underdiagnosed in women patients. The most common symptom of coronary artery disease in both men and women is chest pain. Diagnosis of this disease is ini-tially based on performance of an electrocardiogram (ECG) followed by a stress ECG. The latter involves having the patient exercise on a treadmill while cardiac activity is monitored; it is often supplemented by an injec-tion of a radioactive isotope of thallium, which enables visualization of the blood flow through the arteries (a "nuclear" exercise test). If one or more of these test results are abnormal, referral is made for cardiac catheterization and coronary angiography. In cardiac catheterization, a tube is introduced into an artery in the groin and passed into the heart, where dye is released. The lumen of the coronary arteries can be seen by X ray (angiography) as the dye passes through them. Obstructions will prevent the passage of the dye, and narrowing of the artery because of buildup of plaque on its walls can commonly be seen. The stress tests are considered noninvasive and catheterization invasive, because of the need for a surgical procedure to insert the catheter.

Treadmill testing is considered reliable in men, but there is some confusion about its value for women. One of the few studies to include women reported that this test was misleading in 35 percent of them. Twenty-two percent of the tests produced false positives, suggesting heart disease that was not confirmed by subsequent angiography, and 13 percent produced false negatives, that is, failed to show heart disease that later invasive testing found to be present. Although the false negative rate was the same as that for males, women had a much higher rate of false positives (Barolsky et al. 1979).

The explanation for this difference is not clear. Two studies have suggested that it is related to the phase of the menstrual cycle (Clark et al. 1988) or to use of contraceptives (Barrett-Connor et al. 1986), suggesting that female sex hormones may play a role. Other explanations that do not involve hormones have also been suggested, however. It is also said that treadmill testing is less reliable for women because they "seem to have a different physiologic response to exercise than do men" (Altman 1991). Because of these concerns about treadmill testing in women, attention has been focused on a different kind of test, nuclear imaging. This test appears to have similar results in men and women when interpreted by experienced personnel, but those who are less experienced were found in one study to be confused by the artifact produced by breast tissue (Desmarais et al. 1993).

A 1987 study reported that men were ten times more likely than women to have cardiac catheterization after a positive nuclear exercise test, all other things being equal (Tobin et al. 1987). And a recent study of patients admitted to hospitals for possible coronary heart disease in two different East Coast cities showed that men are more likely to undergo coronary angiography than women with the same health and demographic characteristics (Ayanian and Epstein 1991). The authors of this study suggested four possible explanations for their findings. Physicians may view coronary heart disease as more severe among men because they believe a greater number of men develop the disease; physicians may view the coronary procedures as more risky or less effective in women than in men; women may decline coronary procedures more often than men; and/or the differences in use of coronary procedures may represent a sex bias in the delivery of medical care (Ayanian and Epstein 1991).

The first explanation is likely correct, given the paucity of information about this disease among women. The second explanation is also correct. But although many physicians do believe that coronary procedures are less effective for women (e.g., Becker 1990: 2 recommends against noninvasive diagnostic testing in women), this belief is based on inadequate data. The impression exists among physicians that breast tissue may obscure portions of the heart on X rays (e.g., Altman 1991, quoting Dr. Robert Bonow of the National Heart, Lung and Blood Institute of the NIH). These beliefs have not been carefully studied, but they obviously influence the practice of medicine to the detriment of women patients, often with fatal outcomes.

The third explanation has not yet been studied. If it is true that women are more likely than men to refuse these diagnostic studies, one must consider the possibility that they do so on the advice of their physicians, advice that is likely to be different from that given to male patients, given the long-standing gender biases among physicians about heart disease. This brings us to the fourth explanation, which is the one most in need of study: that there is gender bias in the delivery of care to women with heart disease. This bias may operate in a number of ways. Women may have been socialized by the medical profession not to worry about or even consider heart disease as a possibility, so that they would be less likely to seek medical attention when chest pain or excessive fatigue occurs. Alternatively, women may be more stoical than men and tolerate chest pain. Most likely is that physicians are more apt to attribute women's somatic complaints, particularly fatigue, to depression, rather than consider heart disease. They are more likely, therefore, to prescribe antidepressant medication, rather than to refer for diagnostic tests for heart disease. This response prolongs the delay until the correct diagnosis is made, if indeed it is ever made. In turn, this delay contributes to the poor outcome of corrective procedures in women, which completes the circle by reinforcing physicians' bias against referring women for diagnostic tests.

Treatment

Surgery to bypass obstruction of one or more coronary arteries to improve blood flow to the heart muscle and thus prevent heart attacks (myocardial infarction) has become one of the most commonly performed operative procedures in the United States. In 1988, for example, there were 175,000 such procedures performed (Sabiston 1988). More than three-quarters of these were in men, for whom the outcome is generally good. As early as 1975, reports in the medical literature (Loop et al. 1983; Fisher et al. 1982) showed a worse outcome, including many more deaths, among women than men undergoing the procedure. This finding was not only used as an excuse for recommending that women not be operated upon, but also explained away as being caused by the smaller size of their blood vessels and the resulting greater technical difficulty in achieving a satisfactory surgical result (Fisher et al. 1982).

This explanation was critically examined and challenged by Khan et al. (1990), who found that the lower surgical success rate was not caused by the smaller size of women's blood vessels but by the fact that women had been referred for the operation much later in the course of their disease, when they were in poor shape already. The women were older and more likely than the men to have already had a heart attack, to be in congestive heart failure, and to have the highest grade (that is, the most severe form) of heart symptoms (New York Heart Association Class IV). Conversely, the men were more likely than the women to have been referred quickly, after their abnormal exercise test, and therefore to be significantly earlier in the course of their illness.

When the researchers compared men and women on their functional status (that is, their ability to perform activities of daily living at the time of surgery) alone, they found no sex difference in the outcome of the surgery. Surgery after later referral increases the chances of operative death. They found their results to be in agreement with Taylor's hypothesis that "the severity of disease is greater in the gender that less often presents with a disorder" and that "treatment outcomes may also be influenced by disease prevalence" (Taylor and Ounsted 1989). Taylor's hypothesis by implication was confirmed in a study of over 2,000 subjects with a history of recent heart attacks. It found that women were more apt to have had disabling symptoms before their attack and less likely to have been referred for angiography or bypass surgery (Pfeffer et al. 1992).

Cardiac Rehabilitation Following Myocardial Infarction / Bypass

There also appear to be gender differences in the process of rehabilitative treatment after a heart attack. "Overall, a scarcity of research has been devoted toward women recovering from [MI]. However, clinical investigations have determined the following: 1) women enter cardiac rehabilitation programs less frequently than men; 2) women enrolled in rehabilitation programs are more likely to drop out than men; 3) women return to work less frequently than men and require a longer duration of sick leave; 4) women resume sexual activity later and less frequently than men, and more frequently experience anxiety and clinical symptoms" (Becker 1990: 3).

Of even greater concern is the finding that women are more likely than men to die following a heart attack. This was originally attributed to the fact that women are generally older than men when they have their attacks (Hsia 1993). However, when these findings were more closely analyzed in a large Israeli study in which the risk of dying after a heart attack was 1.7 times greater for women than men, it was found that even after accounting for age and other potentially important factors, being female remained the most important predictor of death (Greenland et al. 1991).

Mortality

The ten leading causes of death for older women are listed in Appendix A.

Although the death rate for all causes, adjusted for age, decreased by about 6 percent for women between 1985 and 1994, it fell 9 percent for men (Singh et al. 1995). During that time, there were increases in the rates of three of the ten leading causes of death for women of all ages. These included blood and lymphatic cancers, chronic obstructive lung diseases (e.g., emphysema), and diabetes. The increase in deaths from diabetes was 12 percent for the year 1988–89 alone (Advance Report 1992).

PART TWO

Special Health Issues for Women

CHAPTER FIVE

Sexually Transmitted Diseases

Over the past decade, the subject of sexually transmitted disease (STD) has emerged from the shadows into our daily consciousness, largely owing to the specter of AIDS. As a result, what was once considered a problem of "others" has, by now, touched everybody in some way. Although infection by the human immunodeficiency virus (HIV) has received most attention, knowledge about other STDs has also increased dramatically in recent years. In medical schools 30 years ago, there were thought to be just two STDs (which, in those days, were called venereal diseases), syphilis and gonorrhea. We now recognize the existence of at least 25 infections that can be spread through sexual contact.

Women are disproportionately impacted by these infections by virtue of their biologic, social, and economic vulnerability. Although women obviously share the life-threatening consequences of infections such as HIV, they are at unique risk for other problems involving pregnancy, family planning, and fertility. For example, gonorrhea or chlamydia can jeopardize a woman's fertility and increase her risk of ectopic pregnancy. In addition, infection with herpes, syphilis, chlamydia, or HIV may place the life of her newborn infant at risk. Affluence affords no protection against these infections or their sequelae, but poverty increases the likelihood of high-risk sexual encounters for women. Social inexperience and poor self-image also increase the risk of contracting such infections, particularly for young women unable to communicate their wish for "safe sex." Victimization, whether it be within the family setting or on the street when an abused girl becomes a runaway, is another factor contributing to women's increased vulnerability.

This chapter discusses the STDs (and other infections and infestations involving the female genitalia) that are common or serious, with emphasis on their effects and consequences for women. It first reviews the major STDs (in alphabetical order), then discusses their unique features in preadult stages of the life span.

STDs and Similar Diseases

BACTERIAL VAGINOSIS

Bacterial vaginosis is a common condition that may be transmitted either sexually or nonsexually. The usual symptom is a foul-smelling vaginal discharge, sometimes described as "fishy." It is thought to result when the normal bacteria of the vagina (the *Lactobacillus* species) are replaced by anaerobic bacteria. These bacteria are also found in cultures of women who have no symptoms, so there is controversy about their relationship to producing disease. As a result, the common practice is to treat only if there are symptoms of a discharge, and if no other cause is found. It is not necessary to treat sexual partners.

The standard treatment has been with metronidazole, given twice a day for one week. This medication cannot be used in the first three months of pregnancy, because it may cause birth defects, and patients cannot take alcohol the day of treatment, and probably not for a few days afterward, without risking stomach pain. Even without alcohol use, some patients experience nausea and abdominal pain and develop a metallic taste in their mouths when they take this drug.

Recently, the FDA has approved two new forms of treatment of bacterial vaginosis. The first is a gel containing metronidazole, the second a cream containing another antibiotic, clindamycin. Both are applied directly to the vagina (*Medical Letter* 1992). Although the gel form is better tolerated than metronidazole taken by mouth, it still has possible side effects because of the small amount absorbed through the wall of the vagina. Though to a lesser extent than the oral form of the drug, the gel may cause some abdominal discomfort and a metallic taste in the mouth.

As with the oral preparation, the woman should not drink alcohol within 24 hours of its use and should not use the gel during the first three months of pregnancy. It is not necessary to treat sexual partners. The clindamycin cream may cause yeast infection and should not be taken by people with a history of bowel disease. In addition, the mineral oil in this cream may damage latex or rubber condoms or diaphragms.

Use of yogurt may be considered for prevention if there is recurrence. However, this has not been specifically studied for this condition, as it has for yeast infections (see below).

CHANCROID

Chancroid is caused by a bacterium called *Hemophilus ducreyi*. It is becoming more common, but because doctors are not required to report this disease to health departments, we do not know its precise incidence rate. The infection is characterized by painful ulcers in the vagina and enlarged and tender lymph nodes in the groin. These lymph nodes may go on to ooze pus if not treated correctly. Because a woman with chancroid has open sores, there is a high likelihood that she also has syphilis or herpes, and she is more susceptible to HIV.

Treatment is with a cephalosporin antibiotic given by injection. As with any of the STDs, the sexual partner should be promptly treated, even if he has no symptoms.

CHLAMYDIA

Many consider chlamydia to be the most prevalent STD in the United States. It is not currently required that chlamydia infections be reported to health departments, so there are not good data about the extent of this infection. However, it is estimated that there are four million new chlamydia infections each year, with the highest rate among adolescent females. Figure 5.1 shows chlamydia rates by gender for the years 1984 to 1992. The causative organism, an obligate intracellular parasite, is in the same family as *Chlamydia trachomatis*, which causes most of the world's blindness. In the United States, the sexually transmitted species of *Chlamydia* can affect the eyes of newborn babies. Its most common

rate (per 100,000 population)

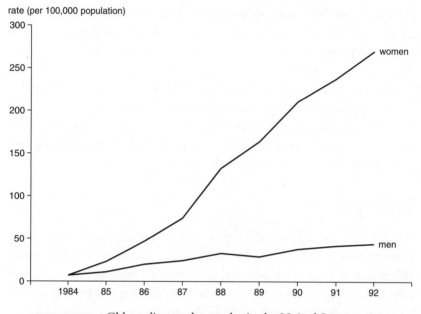

FIGURE 5.1.   Chlamydia rates by gender in the United States, 1984–92

symptom in males is penile discharge. In the female, chlamydia often has no symptoms. It causes infection of the vagina or fallopian tubes similar to that caused by gonorrhea. It is usually effectively treated with a form of tetracycline called doxycycline. No tetracycline should be given directly to a child or to a pregnant woman because of the danger to the child of bone and tooth damage. In these cases, erythromycin is often prescribed, but this tends to be less effective and may also cause nausea and vomiting. All patients with chlamydia should be tested for other STDs and treated for gonorrhea, because it is often difficult to tell these infections apart. Sexual partners must be treated.

GONORRHEA

Gonorrhea is caused by a bacterium called *Neisseria gonorrhoeae*. It continues to be mandatory for doctors to report gonorrhea cases to health departments, so the data are better for this infection than for chlamydia, with which it often coexists. There are an estimated one million new infections in the United States each year. The rate of reported cases of gonorrhea is higher for females than males, particularly in the younger age groups.

Infections in males generally cause symptoms of penile discharge within a few days of contact. As a cause of penile discharge it is as common as chlamydia, and treatment should always be designed for both infections, because it isn't always possible to know which is the cause.

For females, gonorrhea may cause a vaginal discharge, anal pain or discharge, or sore throat, depending on the entry point to the body. At this stage, gonorrhea can be treated with penicillin, although some strains of the gonococcus have become resistant to penicillin and some other antibiotics, which is making it increasingly difficult to treat these infections. Culture results can be inaccurate. If a woman has symptoms, even if her cultures are negative, both she and her partner should be treated.

More often, however, gonorrhea causes no symptoms at all until it has spread to the fallopian tubes (see below under Pelvic Inflammatory Disease) or into the bloodstream. The bloodstream infection can be life-threatening. It is typically characterized by high fever and pain and swelling in the joints of the legs and hips, sometimes with a skin rash. This infection is generally treated with intravenous penicillins and cephalosporin antibiotics.

HEPATITIS B

Hepatitis B is a viral infection of the liver that causes approximately 5,000 deaths each year in the United States. Anywhere between one-third and two-thirds of the approximately 250,000 new cases that occur in the country each year are caused by sexual transmission (CDC 1993c). Almost 10 percent of those who are infected become carriers, capable of infecting others even if they themselves have no symptoms.

There is no effective treatment, so the most prudent approach to this disease is prevention. A safe and effective vaccine has been widely used in the United States for more than ten years. All newborns and previously unvaccinated children over the age of twelve should receive three doses of this vaccine following a standard schedule. In addition, it is especially important that people with multiple sex partners (or more than one sex partner in the preceding six months), those with any other STD, partners of known carriers of the virus, and intravenous drug users and their

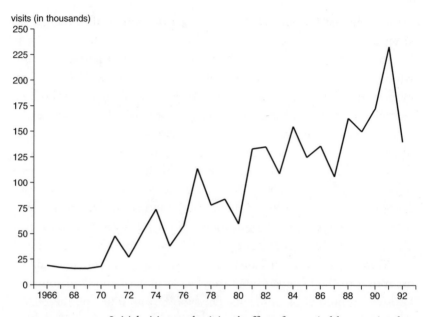

visits (in thousands)

FIGURE 5.2.   Initial visits to physicians' offices for genital herpes simplex
virus infections, United States, 1966–92

partners be vaccinated against this virus. Other preventive measures
should include condom use, as well as exclusivity in sexual relationships.

HERPES SIMPLEX 2

Herpes type 2 is caused by a virus that is in the same family as the one
that produces "cold sores" in the mouth (which may, rarely, be transmitted to the genitals) and a cousin of the one that causes chicken pox and
shingles. This type of herpes virus is transmitted by sexual contact and
lives within the body, presumably for life. Approximately 30 million people in the United States are thought to have this infection, and its rate
has increased significantly over the last three decades (see Fig. 5.2).

Some people have only one episode, others recurrent bouts. The virus
is activated at times of stress and hormonal change and under a variety of
other conditions. It causes small, fluid-filled, extremely painful blisters in
the vagina and/or the anus and the surrounding skin. The vaginal swelling

may become so severe as to make urination difficult. The sores then typically break, leaving small, raw craters in their wake. Before the blisters appear, there can be increased sensitivity and pain in the region of the nerves that extend from the spine to the inner aspects of the thighs. The chance of transmitting the virus to a sexual partner is greatest during the time that sores are visible, although the desire for sexual contact under these painful circumstances is significantly diminished. Condoms should be used in the unlikely event of intercourse during this time.

Treatment for the first infection with herpes should be with acyclovir, an expensive antiviral agent, which must be taken by mouth five times daily for ten days or until symptoms disappear. This treatment decreases symptoms and the period of time that the virus is shed, but it does not cure the infection or prevent its recurrence. There is a difference of opinion as to whether it is of value for treatment during recurrences. My patients vote yes. Women who have six or more recurrences in a one-year period may benefit from daily prophylactic therapy with this drug.

The herpes virus has been implicated as a cause of later cancer of the cervix. Women with herpes must, therefore, get yearly Papanicoulou (Pap) smears to detect this condition early.

HUMAN IMMUNODEFICIENCY VIRUS (HIV)

The human immunodeficiency virus produces AIDS, which may take anywhere from months to more than twelve years to develop, with a median time of ten years for adults, with or without therapy. AIDS is the most rapidly increasing cause of death among adult women. Worldwide, it is now the leading reason that young women die. In nine major cities in the United States, it is the leading cause of death of women aged 25–44. Throughout the country, it is the sixth leading cause of death for black women aged 25–34.

Approximately one-third of female cases of AIDS result from intravenous drug use, another third from heterosexual contact, one-fifth from transfusions with blood products, and the remainder from a variety of unspecified causes. The greatest recent increase has been in the proportion of women with heterosexually acquired infection. The risk of contracting HIV from an infected heterosexual partner is greater for a woman than for a man. This risk is further increased in women who have other STDs that cause ulcers in the vagina or rectum. These include syphilis, herpes, and chancroid.

According to Gena Corea (1992), a man is at least ten times as likely to transmit HIV to a woman during sex as he is to get the virus from her. Yet many men refuse to wear condoms, and many women become infected because they do not suspect that their partners in heterosexual, monogamous relationships have HIV. Furthermore, Corea points out, prostitutes have been criticized for transmitting the disease, but society has ignored the real scandal, which is their own risk of contracting it.

The diagnosis of HIV is based on blood tests for the antibody against the virus. This test becomes positive within six months of contracting the virus in more than 95 percent of people. The initial screening test must be confirmed by a more specific test (e.g., the Western blot assay) because of the rare possibility of false positive antibody tests. The tests in the United States are for the HIV-1 strain. People who have been exposed to HIV-2 through contact with infected partners from West Africa, Angola, Mozambique, Portugal, or France should also be tested for this strain. Currently, specific and informed consent must be given before the test for HIV can be performed. This is best done after counseling.

The spectrum of symptoms caused by HIV is very broad, ranging from no symptoms to death. Symptoms appear at variable times, typically as the result of suppression of the immune system and the acquisition of infections such as tuberculosis and PCP, a special kind of pneumonia caused by the organism *Pneumocystis carinii*. Women may get severe and persistent vaginal yeast infections, although these may certainly occur also in otherwise healthy women and should not be a cause for alarm if all else is normal.

Cervical cancer is a common complication in women with the disease. Because AIDS was first discovered in males, its case definition was based on the way the disease appeared in males. In 1993, more than ten years after the epidemic began, cervical cancer was finally added to the criteria for making a diagnosis of AIDS, and a number of very sick women were given the diagnosis overnight. These women had previously been kept from receiving services and benefits available to AIDS patients. Their official invisibility distorted our knowledge about the disease in women, as well as the statistics. The reported 151 percent increase in cases of AIDS in women between 1992 and 1993 clearly resulted largely from the expansion of the case definition of AIDS that year (CDC 1994a).

There is no curative treatment for AIDS at this time, but therapies for a variety of symptoms, including AZT (azidothymidine) and newer drugs such as protease inhibitors, have been useful in prolonging life. However, another complication of women's long exclusion from the category of confirmed AIDS cases has been their exclusion from the major drug trials for treatment of this disease. We find ourselves in the dangerous position of having to extrapolate from studies done on men to treatment for women without knowing how hormonal changes or other biologic differences might affect the metabolism of the drugs.

At one time, it was thought that pregnancy would hasten the demise of a woman with AIDS, but this no longer appears to be of concern. AIDS can, however, be transmitted from a pregnant woman to her fetus. In fact, for many women who do not realize they have been infected with HIV, the tragedy is that the diagnosis is made with the birth of an infected, and thus doomed, infant. It has recently been learned that administration of AZT to an HIV-infected pregnant woman can decrease the risk of its transmission to the unborn baby. This finding underscores the importance of testing the blood of pregnant women for this infection, so that they will know their status early enough to take steps to protect their babies. Ironically, another reason that women have been banned from drug trials is the concern that they may be pregnant and that the drug may harm their unborn babies. We are now in the position of having to try to treat these very babies.

Women with AIDS receive fewer services than men with the disease. A woman with AIDS is 20 percent less likely to be hospitalized than a similarly diagnosed male, and her asymptomatic counterpart is 20 percent less likely to receive AZT than an asymptomatic HIV-infected male (Hellinger 1993). Even when both genders have health insurance, as in the case of recipients of Medicaid, HIV-infected women use medical services less than HIV-infected men (Hogan et al. 1991). My colleague Dr. Bonnie Maldonado, who runs a program for HIV-infected children at the Packard Children's Hospital at Stanford, has been heartbroken to find that there are many resources for these children, but that their mothers are rarely provided with the services and supports that they need to survive, let alone care for their sick children.

There are several possible reasons for the disparity in medical services received by women and men with HIV. Delay in diagnosis and treatment for women was associated with their being less likely than men to have private health insurance and more likely to be covered by Medicaid, to be admitted as emergency cases, and to receive their care in hospitals with less experience in treating this infection (Bastian, Bennett, and Adams 1993). The need of these sick women to care for their children has been cited as another reason that they are less likely than men to be hospitalized during the course of their illness. According to Dr. Fred J. Hellinger, "discrimination against women with HIV could be another factor" (Hellinger 1993: 1). And J. L. Mitchell et al. (1992: 38) offer this perspective: "The poor and minorities, regardless of gender, tend to be crisis-oriented in their 'health seeking behaviors,' primarily due to the need to survive and to prioritize one's responsibilities. Health, even if one is HIV-infected, finds itself far down the list behind food, shelter, personal safety, caretaking, etc."

Regardless of the reason for their receiving fewer services, the result is that women with AIDS have a lower rate of survival than men, even after controlling for differences in the severity of the disease. One study found that among women hospitalized for their first episode of HIV-related *Pneumocystis carinii* pneumonia, a common and serious complication of AIDS, one-third died in the hospital, compared to only one-quarter of the men admitted for this condition (Bastian, Bennett, and Adams 1993).

HUMAN PAPILLOMA VIRUS

Annoying and unsightly, warts in the area of the vagina and anus were largely ignored by researchers until recently. What sparked renewed interest was the finding that some strains of the virus that causes these warts (Human papilloma virus, or HPV) can also cause cancer of the cervix in later years. There has been a marked increase in the incidence of these warts over the past three decades (see Fig. 5.3). Teenaged women have the highest incidence of this STD.

Men typically have no symptoms, though they may occasionally have warts on the penis. Diagnosis in women depends on seeing a characteristic pattern of cells in the lining of the vagina and cervix through the colposcope after a vinegar-like solution has been applied to these areas. The

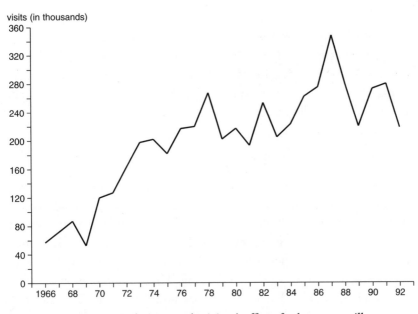

FIGURE 5.3. Initial visits to physicians' offices for human papilloma virus infections, United States, 1966-92

strain of the virus is determined through DNA typing tests available in special laboratories.

Research is under way to find the best treatment for this condition. Treatment methods have traditionally been crude and painful, involving painting the affected area with chemicals that burned the warts (and the adjacent skin). Newer techniques being evaluated now include the use of lasers and interferon. Any woman who has had these genital warts must have yearly Pap smears for the rest of her life to be sure to identify cancer of the cervix early if it develops.

LICE

Lice (pediculosis pubis) are not transmitted sexually, but by close bodily contact or contact with the bedclothes of an infected person. Therefore, they can be transmitted to and by children through nonsexual means. Infection typically causes intense itching in the pubic area, and lice may be found attached to the pubic hair. Treatment with lindane shampoo

(1 percent) is preferred, although neither pregnant or lactating women nor children under the age of two should be treated with this chemical. Bedding and clothing should be dry-cleaned or washed in a washing machine and machine-dried on heat cycle. It is not necessary to fumigate living areas, as was once recommended. Sexual partners, if any, should be treated at the same time.

LYMPHOGRANULOMA VENEREUM

Lymphogranuloma venereum, caused by a relative of the organism that causes chlamydia, is rarer than the other STDs we have discussed. Women may first notice a small ulcer in the vagina; they then typically develop infection in the rectum and even the bowel. In some, the disease progresses to the point where fistulae are established between the bowel and the area between the vagina and the anus. The lymph nodes in the groin become large and tender, and may ooze pus if not treated. Treatment is with a tetracycline antibiotic, doxycycline, taken twice each day for three weeks. Sexual partners should also be treated.

PELVIC INFLAMMATORY DISEASE

Pelvic inflammatory disease (PID) is caused by the spread of the gonococcus or the chlamydia trachomatis (see above) from the cervix into the fallopian tubes. This usually occurs at the time of a menstrual period, so that the pain is often confused with that of menstrual cramps. Once in the fallopian tubes, the organism causes pain and fever. If it is not treated promptly and vigorously, it can cause permanent damage to the tubes and sterility or ectopic pregnancy. Again, because of the similarity between chlamydial and gonococcal infections, treatment must be effective against both (see above under Chlamydia and Gonorrhea). This usually requires hospitalization with intravenous administration of antibiotics.

It is worrisome that there has been a marked decrease in the rate of hospitalization of women for treatment of PID over the last decade although there has been no significant change in its rate of occurrence (see Fig. 5.4). This suggests that physicians are hospitalizing women less often. This translates into poorer care and increased risk of developing infertility and other complications. The trend is partly the result of pressures

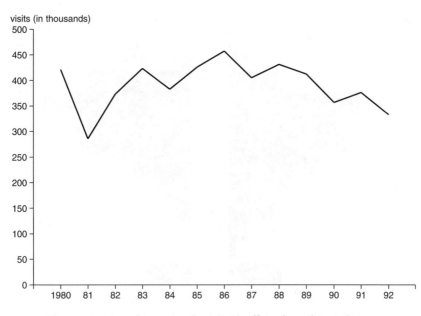

visits (in thousands)

FIGURE 5.4.   Initial visits to physicians' offices for pelvic inflammatory disease by women ages 15-44, United States, 1980-92

from managed care systems and others to decrease health care costs. In the case of PID, however, this approach is clearly not cost-effective. The cost of treatment of infertility and chronic pelvic pain far outweighs any short-term savings from withholding necessary hospital care for PID. It has been estimated that the financial burden of caring for infertility and ectopic pregnancy approached $3 billion in 1990, one-third of which came from public sources (CEWAER 1993). The emotional toll is impossible to measure.

SCABIES

Scabies is also called "crabs," because the insect that causes it looks very much like a crab when viewed under the microscope. Although scabies may be sexually transmitted among adults, children often get it without evidence of sexual abuse. It typically produces severe itching and little bumps on the skin. The location may vary, but the classical picture is an itchy rash between the fingers and on the buttocks. Treatment is with

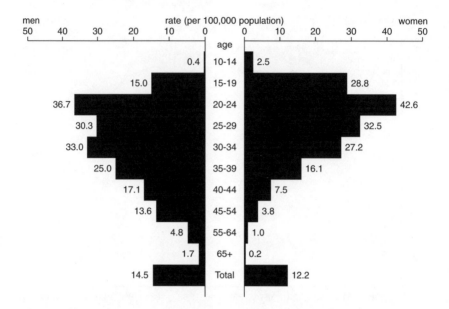

FIGURE 5.5.   Age- and gender-specific rates of primary and secondary syphilis, United States, 1992

permethrin cream (5 percent) applied to affected areas and washed off within eight to fourteen hours. Other control measures are the same as those for lice (see above).

SYPHILIS

Syphilis, whose history has been written into that of civilization, is caused by the cork-shaped microscopic creature (spirochete) called *Treponema pallidum*. Although syphilis is relatively easy to cure with penicillin, it has become much more common over the last twenty years in the United States. (Fig. 5.5 shows the rates for 1992 by age and gender.) Syphilis occurs in three stages, the first consisting of a nonpainful ulcer on the penis, vagina, or cervix (or even the skin elsewhere on the body if infected body fluid comes in contact with a cut). If this chancre is not diagnosed and treated with penicillin, it will still disappear. Some weeks later, however, the disease will emerge anew with an entirely different and extremely variable range of possible symptoms: fever, rash, enlarged lymph nodes, bumps in the vagina or anus, or even a rash on the palms and soles. Sometimes there are no symptoms. It can be diagnosed with a blood test (e.g., Venereal Disease Reference Laboratory, the one required for obtaining a marriage certificate in some states). Its treatment is relatively simple, consisting of a single injection of penicillin. The sexual partner should, of course, be treated as well. If it is not properly diagnosed and treated at this stage, it enters a chronic and debilitating form that affects the heart, spinal cord, eyes, and ears, and is very difficult to treat. This is termed tertiary syphilis.

TRICHOMONIASIS

Trichomoniasis is quite common as a cause of a foul-smelling yellow-green vaginal discharge and irritation. Men rarely have any symptoms and are not routinely tested for the protozoan (*Trichomonas vaginalis*) that causes it, so they can spread the infection without ever knowing that they have it. Until recently this condition was thought to be merely an annoyance. Now, however, there is concern that it may be associated with complications of pregnancy, such as premature rupture of membranes and premature births.

Diagnosis depends on finding the causative organism in fluid from the vagina viewed under a microscope or by culture. Treatment is quite effective with metronidazole, taken by mouth. The same precautions discussed above under bacterial vaginosis apply. Both sexual partners must be treated simultaneously to prevent reinfection.

YEAST INFECTION

Yeast infection (vulvovaginal candidiasis) is not an STD, but it is discussed here because it causes a vaginal discharge and thus is considered in the physician's evaluation of a woman with this symptom. It is undoubtedly the most common cause of vaginal discharge and may occur in girls and women who are not sexually active. It has been estimated that 75 percent of women will have at least one yeast infection during their lifetime and that 40–45 percent will experience two or more such infections (Sexually transmitted diseases treatment guidelines 1993). Fewer than 5 percent will be plagued with recurrent infections, which are more of a risk in women who are immunocompromised (e.g., from AIDS), who take certain medications for long periods of time (e.g., tetracyclines, corticosteroids), or who have diabetes mellitus.

The symptoms of yeast infection include a vaginal discharge that resembles cottage cheese; itching; and burning, especially with urination. A culture can confirm the presence of yeast. Many women have yeast in their vaginas without ever having symptoms. Therefore, most physicians prefer not to treat unless symptoms appear.

Treatment with vaginal cream containing antifungal medication is effective. These creams are now available over the counter, but it is advisable to consult a physician if the symptoms do not abate with this treatment or if they later recur. Because this is not a sexually transmitted infection, there is no need to treat sexual partners. Women with recurrent infection may benefit from daily administration of an antifungal medication, but this is not without side effects. Some women have been able to prevent recurrences (if there is no underlying medical condition) by eating yogurt cultures. These can restore the normal flora of the gastrointestinal tract that may have been changed by antibiotics or other factors.

Special Issues at Early Life Stages

SEXUALLY TRANSMITTED DISEASES IN INFANCY

Newborn infants may contract an STD from their mothers through the placenta, during passage through the birth canal, or from nursing. Different infections are passed along in different ways. Syphilis, hepatitis B, and possibly herpes may be transmitted through the placenta, HIV through the placenta or through breast milk, and herpes, chlamydia, and gonorrhea during passage through the birth canal. Both chlamydia and gonorrhea can cause serious eye infections in babies, and chlamydia may cause pneumonia as well.

The risk of transmission of hepatitis B to the unborn infant ranges from 10 to 85 percent. These babies typically become carriers of the virus and run a high risk of developing serious, often fatal, chronic liver disease. The infection of an infant can be prevented by vaccination of the mother, even if she is already infected. In the case of syphilis, treatment with penicillin during pregnancy can cure both the mother and the fetus.

A pregnant woman with active herpes sores in the vagina will usually be delivered by cesarean section. Recent studies have, however, questioned this practice on the basis of data showing less than a 1 percent rate of transmission to infants born to women with recurrent genital infection. For women with a first infection causing sores in the genital area at the time of labor, the risk of transmission to the infant is between 35 and 80 percent. In these cases, cesarean delivery is critically important. Even this practice will not, however, prevent infection of the infant in every case. Studies show that about 20 to 30 percent of infants with the infection at delivery are born by cesarean delivery (Randolph, Washington, and Prober 1993).

It appears that between 15 and 39 percent of infants born to women infected with HIV are themselves infected. We know very little about HIV during pregnancy, but, as discussed above, giving the drug AZT to pregnant women has been demonstrated to help prevent the transmission of this deadly disease to their unborn babies. Of course, this approach presupposes that an infected woman knows she has the virus. Very often, however, this is not the case, because she is unaware that her partner has been infected.

SEXUALLY TRANSMITTED DISEASES IN CHILDHOOD

Sexual abuse of girls (see Chapter 9) may result in their contracting STDs. Some of these infections (e.g., chlamydia, gonorrhea, hepatitis B, and syphilis) are preventable if a child is treated within a day or two of her attack. Unfortunately, many cases of abuse are not reported, and the opportunity to prevent infection is thus lost. Other infections, such as herpes and HIV, cannot be prevented at this point in time.

When gonorrhea occurs in a child, its clinical course is somewhat different from that in an older woman. The child's vaginal wall is thin and quite susceptible to infection. With puberty, the wall thickens and becomes more resistant to infection, and the fluid in the vagina becomes more acid, which adds protection. Therefore, when gonorrhea strikes a child, it most often causes an infection in the vagina itself, whereas in a girl who has gone through puberty, it usually infects the cervix, which makes it more likely to ascend to the fallopian tubes.

Children may contract lice or scabies from close, but not necessarily sexual, contact. Caution is urged in treating children (under two years of age) for these infestations, because lindane can be absorbed through the skin and cause damage to the central nervous system, particularly if it is applied after a hot bath. Other agents are preferred for this reason.

The typical symptoms of a yeast infection in a young girl are vaginal burning and itching, and occasionally a white discharge. Treatment is as described above under Yeast Infection. The possibility that bubble bath or washing detergent has caused this problem should be explored.

SEXUALLY TRANSMITTED DISEASES IN ADOLESCENCE

Because adolescence is often a time of heterosexual exploration, many adolescent women are at risk for sexually transmitted infections. "Women and girls ages 15 to 25 are at the leading edge of an epidemic of over 30 STDs that infect 12 million Americans each year," according to a recent report of the American School Health Association (1989). Adolescents have the highest rates of all STDs except AIDS.

Within this age group, females have higher reported rates of STDs than males (Office of Technology Assessment 1991: II-268). Some of this reported gender difference may result from the fact that adolescent females are more likely than males to see physicians, often in the course of obtaining family planning care, and to be screened for STDs. On the other hand, males are more likely to have symptoms with their STDs than are females, and they are apt to seek medical care when symptoms occur. How these factors balance out is not clear. Because girls may have no outward symptoms of an STD, or may confuse the discharge caused by an STD with a physiologic discharge, its discovery and treatment may be delayed. In addition, even those girls who are aware of the possibility of such an infection are often reluctant to seek treatment out of embarrassment or inability to access services for financial or other reasons. Perhaps for both of these reasons, infections typically result in more severe complications in girls than in boys.

The percentage of U.S. adolescent females who reported having had sexual intercourse in 1970 was 28.6; in 1975, 36.4; in 1980, 42; in 1985,

44.1; and by 1988, 51.5 (Office of Technology Assessment 1991: II-326). Within this age range and time period, the greatest increase occurred among fifteen-year-old girls (from 4.6 percent in 1970 to 25.6 percent in 1988). There are no good sources of national data for girls under the age of fifteen, but these data on fifteen-year-olds, pregnancy data, and isolated smaller studies suggest that there has been an increase among younger girls as well.

Often the first episode of intercourse, and undoubtedly many thereafter, takes place without the benefit of any protection. Although the AIDS epidemic has caused an increase in use of condoms, this has mainly been on the part of older adolescents and adults. Young adolescent females often lack the communication skills and self-confidence to raise the issue of protection with a prospective sexual partner. They fear that they will sound sexually experienced or that the boyfriend will be offended. Moreover, one study found that adolescent girls were sure that no boy with whom they considered having sex could possibly have an infection (Sorensen 1973). Another problem is that adolescents, as a group, tend to feel invulnerable. "It can't (or won't) happen to me" is a common attitude. In one study, teenagers from a rural environment were found to have more information about HIV and its transmission, but to be less likely to use protection against the virus, than teens from an urban area (DiClemente et al. 1993). This attitude, fostered by much of the publicity about AIDS being a problem for poor, minority, and urban people, has created a false sense of security among other groups of adolescents.

With new advances in birth control, protection against STDs is increasingly becoming uncoupled from contraception. Whereas older methods such as latex condoms and spermicidal foam provided some protection against both STDs and pregnancy, methods such as birth control pills, Depo-Provera, and Norplant prevent only pregnancy. The idea of using latex condoms for STD protection along with one of these excellent birth control methods (the "belt and suspenders" approach) typically falls on deaf ears in young adolescents. The female condom has not yet been tested in adolescents.

Not only are heterosexual adolescent females at increased risk of these infections, but so are young lesbians. At a time in their lives when they are dealing with the stress of self-identity and fear of disclosure, some throw themselves into a sexual relationship with a male, often with the dire consequence of pregnancy or STD.

Chlamydia is the most common STD among adolescents, and adolescent females are the age and sex group with the highest prevalence of this infection. The disease appears to be more common in urban areas and among blacks, but this may be an artifact of the location of STD clinics and of reporting biases. Because chlamydia often causes no symptoms, adolescent females are at high risk for infertility as a result of PID resulting from this infection.

Gonorrhea is the second most common STD among adolescents, with findings of infection rates among females ranging from 3 percent in whites to 18 percent in ethnic minorities screened in a variety of studies (Office of Technology Assessment 1991). In 1989, the rate for ten-to-fourteen-year-old girls was more than three times that for males of the same age, and for those fifteen to nineteen years old, the female rate was 1.5 times the male rate (Office of Technology Assessment 1991: II-269). The cervix during puberty undergoes a transformation from one cell type to another. During this transition, it appears that there is a greater chance of developing gonorrheal infection at the cervix.

Little is known about the incidence of herpes infection in adolescent females. An unpublished study done by the author over twenty years ago found that more than 10 percent of sexually active females (average age: fourteen) in a juvenile detention facility in a major East Coast city had positive cultures for this virus, although they denied any symptoms. Because the virus is associated with later development of cancer of the cervix, it is critically important that young women at risk for herpes receive yearly Pap smears.

The absolute number of cases of AIDS in adolescents is still low relative to that of other STDs (568 cases as of August 1990; Office of Technology Assessment 1991: II-263). Compared with a ten-to-one male-female ratio in adults, that of four to one in adolescents is noteworthy. There were 200 deaths among women in this age group in 1994 (Singh et al. 1995). However, 70 percent of new AIDS infections in women are occurring in those under the age of 25. This fact, coupled with the known incubation period of more than five years between the time of infection with HIV and that of developing symptoms of AIDS, suggests that many of these women are getting infected during adolescence.

Moreover, the largest increases in reported cases in 1993 were in heterosexual women between the ages of thirteen and nineteen (35 percent of cases in this age group were women), particularly blacks and Hispanics (CDC 1994a). There are, in fact, more black female victims of AIDS among adolescents than in older age groups. Fifty-eight percent of adolescent females with AIDS are black, compared with 30 percent of adolescent males (Office of Technology Assessment 1991: II-262).

Most important, in the United States the percentage of women who have become infected with HIV through heterosexual contact is higher among adolescents (12 percent) than among older women (5 percent) (Office of Technology Assessment 1991: II-261). Another way of looking at this problem is that 45 percent of thirteen-to-eighteen-year-old females with AIDS contracted the disease through heterosexual intercourse. Nationally, the male to female ratio for AIDS is ten to one for adults over the age of 25; for adolescents, it is four to one, closer to the adult ratio in Africa, where most of the cases result from heterosexual contact. The risk is especially high in adolescents with multiple sex partners and those with other STDs. Although there are still more urban than rural cases, the numbers are growing in rural and midwestern areas among adolescents.

Despite their increasing infection rate, a recent study found that "women and adolescent girls infected with [HIV] receive fewer medical services, such as medications, hospital admissions, and outpatient visits, than similarly diagnosed men. . . . In particular, an asymptomatic, HIV-infected female is 20 percent less likely to receive azidothymidine (AZT) than an asymptomatic, HIV-infected male" (U.S. Department of Health and Human Services 1993: 1).

Human papilloma virus is now considered the most common STD, "affecting 20–50% of adolescent females," according to Mary-Ann Shafer (1994: 1). Cases of HPV are not required to be reported, so its true prevalence is impossible to know. One study of inner-city, predominantly black, teenaged females found that 13 percent were positive for HPV (Office of Technology Assessment 1991: II-269).

The first two stages of syphilis may occur during adolescence. The third stage requires many years to develop, so it is a problem only for adults. The 1987 infection rate was the highest reported up to that time for adolescents, almost entirely because of its increase among adolescent

females. For example, between 1977 and 1987, the rate for females between the ages of ten and fourteen and those between fifteen and nineteen increased about 120 percent, while that for ten-to-fourteen-year-
old males was unchanged and that for fifteen-to-nineteen-year-old males
increased only 33 percent (Office of Technology Assessment 1991: II–
270). The rate for adolescent women in 1992 was 28.8 per 100,000 population (CDC 1992b: 10). If the denominator had been the number of
sexually active females in this age group, the prevalence obviously would
have been much higher and more reflective of true risk.

Prevention of STDs

For the foreseeable future, our only hope of dealing with AIDS is to try
to prevent it. One of the greatest barriers to prevention is psychologic.
Women must force themselves to consider the possibility that their
prospective sex partners, including their husbands, may be infected with
AIDS. You can't tell by looking! You may not even be able to tell by asking, for your partner may not know that he is infected. Many people have
become infected after a single episode of unprotected sex or a one-time
experience with a contaminated needle during a dare as an adolescent. It
happens to rich people, rural people, and white people, although most of
the publicity has been about groups with the highest incidence, namely
the urban, the poor, and minorities.

J. L. Mitchell et al. (1992: 38) caution against the view that all women
are alike or that they should be seen simply as victims:

> The initial focus on women as vectors or vessels of the infection
> negated the worth of women as persons. Because the majority of
> women infected were poor, either African-American or Hispanic/
> Latina, and drug users, characterizing them as infection bearers or vec-
> tors was easy. The spread of this disease to a more "acceptable" group
> of women, often times portrayed as "unsuspecting partners of (devi-
> ous) men" has allowed issues related to women to be embraced by a
> larger community. This tactic is as destructive as the initial approach.
> While the demographics of the infection in women may be growing
> in terms of heterosexual spread, the ethnicities and the cultures of the
> women remain the same. Although they may not be drug users, they

know and have come to accept the fact that many of their partners are users. Why they then continue to put themselves at risk is difficult for many to comprehend. Comprehension will come only when one realizes that with cultural diversity come many norms. What may be unacceptable to some is perfectly acceptable to others.

In addressing issues of cultural diversity, one must be aware not only of differences in norms, perceptions, and behaviors among the diverse ethnicities of women, but of the effects of acculturation and context on some of these. These issues were underscored in a survey of more than 1,000 adult women of color interviewed in homeless shelters and drug recovery programs. The study found that Latinas who were less acculturated were least likely to engage in behaviors considered high risk for contracting HIV, compared to the "high-acculturated" Latinas, who had a higher prevalence of intravenous drug use. In comparison, African-American women in this sample had less risk from intravenous drug use, but higher risk from their sexual activity (Nyamathi et al. 1993).

Much has been written about the use of latex condoms as the only effective form of protection against STDs (other than abstinence). Whenever one partner has been diagnosed with an STD, latex condoms should be used in subsequent intercourse to prevent recurrence. Indeed, under laboratory circumstances, latex condoms are virtually impermeable to all STDs studied. In practice, however, the picture is not as optimistic. Laboratory studies of spermicidal foams and jellies have shown them, too, to be effective in killing some of the major organisms that cause STDs, including HIV (Hicks et al. 1985). In a study involving more than 4,000 women, it was reported that women using the contraceptive sponge (which contains the spermicidal chemical nonoxynol-9) or diaphragm (which is used with a spermicidal jelly containing this chemical) had more than a one-third lower rate of infection with gonorrhea or trichomoniasis than women using no contraception (including those who had had tubal ligations). This compared favorably to the rates in women using condoms, who had a 34 percent lower rate of gonorrhea and a 30 percent lower rate of trichomoniasis than the group using no contraception. The study concluded that users of "female-dependent" methods had significantly lower rates of both gonorrhea and trichomoniasis, and a somewhat lower rate of chlamydia, than women who had used no contraception. Those who used condoms substantially reduced their risk of these STDs, but not to the same extent, which suggests that condoms are often used inconsistently or improperly (Rosenberg et al. 1992). This study underscores the importance not only of providing women with the skills to communicate their desire that protection be used, but of educating them about measures they themselves can take to ensure that they are protected. The contraceptive sponge had been particularly attractive in that regard because it could be purchased without a prescription or health care worker involvement, in contrast with the diaphragm, which requires initial fitting by a skilled practitioner. Unfortunately, the sponge has now become unavailable.

The challenge for the coming years is both technical and behavioral. To better protect themselves against the threat of STDs, women need both improved prophylactic methods and the means for exercising their right to that protection.

CHAPTER SIX

Pregnancy and Its Prevention

Although the medical establishment has focused too narrowly on women's reproductive health, it is nevertheless true that many women's health issues relate to pregnancy—facilitating it, ensuring its positive outcome, preventing it, or terminating it. Regarding normal pregnancy in adult women, this chapter touches on a few issues that deserve more attention than they commonly receive. It then addresses facilitating pregnancy via assisted reproductive technologies, preventing it via contraception, and terminating it via abortion. Finally, it discusses issues of pregnancy and contraception unique to one life stage, adolescence.

Pregnancy

MATERNAL HEALTH

There are about three million spontaneous vaginal births each year in the United States. The number of women giving birth out of wedlock has grown tremendously and includes women of all ages and races. (The meaning of this finding is uncertain, particularly since it has recently been found that many states record as unmarried any couple who have different surnames.)

Although intrauterine pregnancy poses no special risks to a healthy young adult, there are 14 deaths annually per 100,000 women from pregnancy complications in the United States. The death rates from complications of pregnancy and childbirth are 3.5 times greater for black women than for white women. One major complication is ectopic (tubal) pregnancy, which occurs in approximately 0.5 to 1 percent of all pregnancies. Ectopic pregnancies are the leading cause of pregnancy-related death for black women. These pregnancies result when the egg is fertilized while still in the fallopian tube and divides and grows in this space, which is not equipped to handle it. As a consequence, the growing mass eventually causes the tube to rupture, causing extreme pain and the risk of death from blood loss.

Ectopic pregnancy typically is caused by blockage of the fallopian tube or other structural damage that results in loss of its ability to contract and relax. This movement is necessary to propel the egg along into the uterus where it is normally fertilized. The most common cause of these problems is an inadequately treated STD, typically gonorrhea or chlamydia (see Chapter 5). Use of an intrauterine device (IUD) can also be a factor, although, as discussed below, the risk of pregnancy is quite low among IUD users. Other pregnancy-related causes of death include toxemia, postpartum hemorrhage, and uterine infection.

Little has been written about the non–life-threatening effect of pregnancy and delivery on the health of the mother in industrialized societies. In the first study of its kind, a group of researchers followed up nearly 12,000 women who had delivered in the same hospital over a seven-year period (MacArthur, Lewis, and Knox 1991). They found that 47 percent of these women had had at least one new health problem that lasted more than six weeks and began within the three months after delivery. One of the most common was backache, which was more of a problem for women who had had spinal anesthesia. Almost 10 percent had other musculoskeletal symptoms, with more problems reported by women who had undergone cesarean deliveries. More than 10 percent of women experienced stress incontinence, especially those who had had difficult labors, large babies, and forceps deliveries. The onset of hemorrhoids was common and they were persistent, with the same risk factors as for stress incontinence. Almost 10 percent reported depression (see Chapter 7) and about 12 percent extreme tiredness, with more than half improving within a year's time. Depression was more common among young, unmarried mothers and those who were breast-feeding. Fatigue, not surprisingly, was more common in older mothers and those with twins or small babies.

Fewer than half of those with any of these problems consulted a doctor, with the others perhaps being resigned to their fate. One result of this, the authors stress, is "that the full extent of post-partum morbidity is not recognised by the medical profession" (MacArthur, Lewis, and Knox 1991: 1195). These findings suggest that women should be advised to see their physicians regularly after the traditional six-week postpartum checkup and that these physicians should be educated to probe beyond the narrowly defined perimeter of reproductive health.

These findings also raise concern about the absence of a secure governmental policy of adequate paid maternity leave in this country. Mothers need not only safe and affordable care for their young children, but more support and health care for themselves during the year following delivery. The fact that more than 50 percent of new mothers now return to their workplace makes this need more acute (see Chapter 2).

INFANT HEALTH

Although it fell 4 percent from 1993 to 1994, the infant mortality rate (the number of babies per 1,000 live births who die within their first year) remains unacceptably high in the United States (7.9 in 1994). The mortality rate for African-American babies in 1992 (14.4) was more than double that for white infants (6.9).

Prenatal Care

Although smoking is an important contributor to poor pregnancy outcome (including spontaneous abortion, premature birth, and low birth weight; see Chapter 8), the major determinant of that outcome appears to be prenatal care. When it is absent or inadequate, the risk to the fetus is enormous and the incidence of complications high.

The infant mortality rate is significantly impacted by prenatal care. Among infants whose mothers began prenatal care in the first trimester of pregnancy, this rate was 9.7 per 1,000 live births. With care initiated later in pregnancy, the rate rose to 12.5 per 1,000; with no prenatal care, it leaped to 48.7 per 1,000 (Alan Guttmacher Institute 1993a). The benefits of prenatal care are reflected in the health of surviving babies as well. They have a lower incidence of learning disabilities, respiratory infections, congenital anomalies, and hospitalization during the first year of life (Carnegie Task Force 1994). These differences likely represent the impact of the care itself as well as a certain amount of self-selection bias; women at the highest risk for poor pregnancy outcomes (e.g., adolescents and drug abusers) would be the least likely to receive prenatal care. These confounding factors notwithstanding, it has been clearly demonstrated that even the highest-risk patients derive health benefits for themselves and their fetuses when they receive prenatal care.

Care at Delivery

Another factor that influences pregnancy outcome relates to the resources and facilities available for the management of complicated pregnancies and deliveries. Studies have shown that when women and their physicians who anticipate problems choose to deliver at teaching hospitals with high-level, sophisticated newborn intensive care units, there are lower rates of infant deaths. The problem here is that many women who are at high risk for problems at delivery do not have this choice. Some of the same factors that place them at increased risk for dangerous pregnancies and deliveries also cause them to have no health insurance or to be covered by Medicaid, which limits their access to many hospitals. A study that analyzed 61,436 deliveries in the San Francisco Bay area in 1985 found that high-risk women with Medicaid coverage were more likely to deliver at hospitals that had no newborn intensive care units (and had records of worse infant mortality rates) than high-risk women who had private insurance (Phibbs et al. 1993).

Most vaginal births in the United States are attended by physicians, primarily obstetricians and family practitioners, but this is likely to change dramatically. The rising numbers of malpractice suits against physicians when there are birth defects and complications of pregnancy and delivery, and the resulting increase in rates for malpractice insurance, have driven many physicians out of the practice of obstetrics. Midwives are, for the most part, filling the void. For example, between 1975 and 1989, their proportion has increased 40-fold, from 1 to 4.6 percent of all births (Baldwin, Hutchinson, and Rosenblatt 1992).

Midwives and nurse practitioners are increasingly providing family planning services to women as well. A study of family planning clinics found that 72 percent of patient visits were to such practitioners, with only 28 percent to physicians. In general, these providers spend more time with patients and are more likely to provide needed counseling (Alan Guttmacher Institute 1993b). Not surprisingly, there is a higher degree of patient satisfaction with this type of care.

CESAREAN DELIVERY

About one-quarter of the approximately four million deliveries in the United States each year are by cesarean section (CS). The rate of 25 percent in 1987 was the highest recorded, and it has decreased to about 23 percent since 1990. This rate places the United States third highest among countries reporting CS rates, following Brazil and Puerto Rico. CS is now the most common surgical procedure performed in the United States.

There are significant regional and demographic differences in the number of CSs performed. For example, many more are done in the South than anywhere else in this country. Women over the age of 30 have a higher rate than younger women. The rates among different health care delivery systems vary widely and are largely reflective of patients' payment status. The chance of having a cesarean delivery is higher among women in proprietary and smaller hospitals and women who have private health insurance (CDC 1993d). The observed link between CS and ability to pay exists in other countries as well. A recent study in the Lazio region of Italy, for example, showed the highest rate in private hospitals (almost 35 percent) and a correlation between the rate of its use and mode of hospital care payment (Bertollini et al. 1992).

Does this mean that because some women can and do pay, they get better care, or are they being exploited? Should there be more CSs for poorer women or fewer for the rich? The answer is not simple. It depends on the indications for the procedure and its risks and benefits.

CS is necessary when labor fails to progress normally and/or when the health of the baby or mother is jeopardized by waiting for spontaneous vaginal delivery. One long-standing indication for CS has recently been questioned, however. It has been standard medical practice to perform a CS for any woman with active herpes infection of the genitalia in an effort to prevent transmission of what is often a fatal infection for the newborn. A recent study (Randolph and Prober 1993) has shown that this is necessary for women with first-time infections but is probably unwarranted for women with recurrent infections (see Chapter 5). Eliminating this common indication would reduce the yearly total of CSs by 1,600 at a saving of $2.5 million per case of neonatal herpes prevented (Randolph and Prober 1993). Another time-honored indication for CS recently challenged by new data relates to deliveries among women who have previously had a CS. Repeat CSs have now been shown to be unnecessary in most of these cases (American College of Obstetricians and Gynecologists 1988).

The only way to answer the question about the correlation of ability to pay with CS rate is to examine some complication of pregnancy that is universally judged to be an indication for CS. The Italian study did this by examining the CS rate when the baby was in the breech position (with its feet rather than its head down). They found that more CSs were done for breech presentation in private than in public hospitals, tending to confirm the existence of two classes of care.

CS is often necessary, but it carries an increased rate of complications, primarily infections of the site of incision and of the urinary tract. Even when there are no complications, it doubles the length of hospital stay and cost of hospitalization. Accordingly, one of the national U.S. health objectives for the year 2000 is reduction of the overall cesarean rate to 15 or fewer per 100 deliveries. If this had been the rate in 1991, the savings would have been more than $1 billion.

There is a delicate line between the need to decrease the number of CSs performed for economic reasons and the need to retain the health benefits of the procedure in well-chosen, selected cases. The only acceptable reasons for CS are to save lives and improve the health of mother and baby. Profit motives and fear of malpractice suits have too often tipped the balance toward performance of this procedure, as has the convenience of the patient and/or the physician. None of these has a place in medical decision making.

Assisted Reproductive Technologies

An exciting and critically important aspect of reproductive medicine is that of assisting women previously unable to bear children. "Artificial" insemination has been performed for many years and has, for example, recently been increasingly used by lesbian couples desirous of bearing children. In addition, since the birth of Louise Brown, the first "test-tube" baby, in 1978 in England, the field of assisted reproductive technologies (ART) has flourished. It is estimated that between 1985 and 1990, there have been 12,181 deliveries as a result of ART in the United States alone (Medical Research International and SART 1992).

There are three main approaches to improving the chance that an egg will meet a sperm so that fertilization will take place: gamete intrafallopian transfer (GIFT); in vitro fertilization with embryo transfer to the uterus through the cervix (IVF-ET); and zygote intrafallopian transfer, or in vitro fertilization with tubal embryo transfer (ZIFT). (See Appendix C for further definitions.) These approaches share the need to stimulate production of multiple eggs in each cycle and to retrieve them from the ovary at the optimal time.

In GIFT, after eggs are retrieved, they are mixed with sperm and returned immediately into the fallopian tubes. This is the only technique among the three in which fertilization takes place within the body. Accordingly, it requires at least one healthy fallopian tube. This is generally the first procedure performed for women with unexplained infertility or those whose partners have moderate decrease in sperm production.

In IVF-ET, eggs are fertilized with the partner's sperm in a petri dish. The resulting embryo is placed in the uterus through the cervix about two days later. This technique is most suitable for women whose tubes have been damaged by previous STDs, ectopic pregnancy, or endometriosis. It is also a recommended technique for couples whose problem is male factor infertility (suboptimal sperm production) or immunologic infertility, in which a woman's antibodies attack certain antigens on the partner's sperm, resulting in its death. With IVF-ET, it is postulated that her antibodies may not recognize and attack these antigens in the embryo, and pregnancy may ensue (Milki et al. 1992).

In ZIFT, the fertilized embryos are placed in the fallopian tube, rather than the uterus. This is an appropriate approach for women who have at least one healthy fallopian tube and who are experiencing male factor, immunologic, or unexplained infertility. This procedure is more invasive and costly than IVF-ET, with which it shares many features, because of the need to undergo laparoscopy (incision in the abdomen and introduction of a small viewing tube to guide the transfer into the fallopian tube).

The availability of these technologies means that the birth mother may or may not be the biologic mother and has even raised questions as to how to define "biologic" in this context. Surrogate mothers may be egg donors, sympathetic relatives, friends, or paid volunteers who agree to donate eggs and/or nurture the embryo throughout gestation. These technologies, with the aid of hormonal replacement, also make it possible for postmenopausal women to become pregnant and carry the pregnancy to term. The ethical and legal implications are growing as fast as the technology and invoke decision-making skills of biblical proportions.

Despite remarkable advances in the field of ART, more than 75 percent of treatment cycles still do not result in a birth. The success rate varies with the experience of the center performing the procedure, the cause of the infertility, and the age of the female partner; rates are higher in younger women (American Fertility Society, Ethics Committee, 1994). The financial and emotional costs of infertility and its treatment remain enormous (see also Chapter 7).

Contraception

Unfortunately, since the development of the Pill, contraception has, de facto, become the responsibility of women. Some might argue that this has always been the case, but history tells us otherwise. The Bible describes the use of withdrawal (Himes 1963: 71) and periodic abstinence. The forerunner of the condom in the form of a decorative sheath was worn over the penis as early as 1350 B.C. (Hatcher et al. 1990: 159). Some women take the position that women *should* bear total responsibility for contraception because they are the ones to bear the greatest consequences should it fail, in terms both of pregnancy and of STDs, including deadly HIV. "Can you trust someone you hardly know to care as much about you as you do, yourself?" is a common refrain among young women. The judicial and welfare systems are trying to force men to take more responsibility for their offspring, but this does not necessarily translate into greater contraceptive responsibility for men. The following discussion addresses both female-controlled and male-controlled methods of contraception.

Both efficacy and safety are critical issues in evaluating birth control methods. When we consider the possible side effects of each method, as well as potential complications, it is important to remember that pregnancy itself is not without risk (see above). In fact, for the population as a whole, there are more deaths from complications of pregnancy than from any contraceptive method. But for individual women, the risk from a particular method may be greater than that from pregnancy.

Before we review available birth control methods, a few words about the way in which they are typically evaluated. Pregnancy rates are the usual end point of evaluation of any contraceptive method. This seems logical, but it is by no means straightforward. For example, this rate is usually expressed using the "Pearl Index," calculated as the number of pregnancies per 100 woman-years of exposure to pregnancy risk. This could represent the experience of 100 women each using the method for one year, or 50 women using it for two years, or even, theoretically, one woman using it for one hundred years. Actually, however, the risk of pregnancy isn't evenly distributed over time. Failure rates for most methods decline with increasing duration of use (Trussell et al. 1990). This suggests that experience with a method improves its effectiveness.

Moreover, some studies of contraceptive efficacy have been fraught with methodological problems that make their results difficult to interpret. For example, there have been very different criteria for entry into the studies, with some excluding and others including women who have not been sexually active and others setting a minimum frequency of intercourse as an entrance requirement. Obviously, differences in frequency of intercourse can affect the risk of pregnancy and, accordingly, conclusions about a method being tested.

In addition, the FDA, at least for its expedited review process, does not require that study participants be randomly assigned to a group using the device under study and to a control group. This may result in differences in outcome that have nothing to do with the specific method being tested, but rather that reflect behavioral differences among study participants who chose one method over another. Only with random assignment can these individual differences be neutralized and the method itself be tested.

A third methodological problem is that different studies define and determine the end point, pregnancy, differently. For example, some determine pregnancy by pregnancy tests, others by clinical confirmation.

Under the second method, a pregnancy would not be counted if there is a spontaneous miscarriage after a positive test but before an examination.

Finally, a limitation of many studies is the way they deal with subjects who drop out and are lost to follow-up. If these subjects are excluded from data analysis as if they had never entered the study, there may be too few subjects left to draw valid conclusions. If the dropouts are counted as method failures, the method will appear to be less effective, which may or may not be true. Yet it isn't valid to count these subjects as method successes, because the researchers do not know whether they became pregnant while using the method being tested.

With these limitations in mind, we will review what is known about the efficacy and safety of different birth control methods.

BARRIER METHODS

There are currently three barrier methods of contraception that are controlled by the woman: the female condom, the diaphragm, and the cervical cap. A fourth female-controlled method, the contraceptive sponge, is no longer available. There is also one male-controlled barrier method, the condom.

In the age of AIDS, interest has grown among women in having more female-controlled methods of protection against both STDs and pregnancy. In response to this need, the female condom has recently been developed. This device combines features of the diaphragm and those of the male condom. The data are not conclusive, but with a failure rate for pregnancy of 12 percent when tested in the United States and 22 percent in Latin America, its effectiveness appears to be comparable to that of the other barrier methods currently available. One study (Trussell et al. 1994) reports a six-month 2.6 percent probability of failure with "perfect use," defined as "correct use according to instructions at every act of intercourse." Based on this analysis, the authors rate the female condom equal in effectiveness to the diaphragm, equal or superior to the cervical cap, and superior to the sponge. They further speculate that the efficacy of the female condom is close to that of the male condom without added spermicide, and that it has high potential for reducing the risk of HIV. If there are disadvantages to the female condom, they are not yet known. Each female condom costs approximately $2.50.

One of the oldest female-controlled methods is the diaphragm, a rubber circle with a flexible rim that is inserted in the vagina to cover the cervix, providing a barrier to the entry of sperm. The diaphragm's effectiveness is greatly strengthened by the addition of spermicidal jelly, given its tendency to move around during intercourse, rendering the cervical opening exposed as often as covered. This suggests that it is the spermicidal jelly that is doing the yeoman's work of pregnancy protection, rather than the device itself. It is not, therefore, surprising that the failure rate for this method is about 15 percent. On the other hand, some studies have found that women who use a diaphragm seem to have a lower incidence of STDs (Hatcher et al. 1990). It is uncertain whether this reflects some self-selection bias, in which case it would be other behaviors of the women who chose this method, rather than the method itself, that are responsible for their lower STD rate.

The diaphragm has several disadvantages. Its use has been implicated in some cases of toxic shock syndrome. Also, some women experience an increase in bladder infections, presumably because of irritation of the urethra during insertion of the diaphragm. Another disadvantage is that the diaphragm requires initial fitting by a trained health practitioner and periodic checking by a professional thereafter, especially after weight gain and/or pregnancy.

The cervical cap is similar to the diaphragm, except that it looks like a solid rubber thimble and fits snugly on the cervix. It, too, is filled with spermicidal jelly before being inserted. It has the advantage of being suitable for use for more than 24 hours, without having to have the jelly reapplied, but this practice may increase the risk of toxic shock syndrome (TSS). Some who experience increased bladder infections with the diaphragm feel that they fare better with this method.

Like the diaphragm, the cervical cap must be fitted by a skilled professional. Although this method has been used for many years, it is only recently that rigorous studies have been undertaken to evaluate its efficacy. Therefore, few data are currently available for judging its potential advantages and disadvantages.

The contraceptive sponge is a device that was until recently sold over the counter and was potentially readily available to women of all ages. It resembles a diaphragm in shape and is made of a spongelike material impregnated with a spermicidal chemical. It is associated with an increased risk of TSS. Its production was terminated in 1994, and it is now generally unavailable.

The only barrier method available for use by males is the condom. Condoms are available over the counter and are made out of animal skins, latex, or rubber. The first is allegedly most comfortable, but the latter two are more effective in preventing transmission of STDs, including HIV. Used alone, the condom has a failure rate of around 15 percent. When it is used together with spermicidal foam, this rate falls dramatically and approaches that of some oral contraceptives (about 2.5 percent). The combination of condom and foam has the added advantage of providing excellent protection against STDs.

HORMONAL METHODS

Several hormonal methods of contraception are available for women. At present, no such methods are available for men.

Hormonal Contraception for Women

Oral contraceptives, commonly known as the Pill, contain either a combination of estrogen and progesterone or progesterone alone. The estrogen used in birth control pills is synthetic estrogen, whereas that used by postmenopausal women in ERT is conjugated estrogen. The combination pill acts by inhibiting ovulation; progesterone alone acts mainly by altering the mucus of the cervix to make it inhospitable to sperm.

The combination pill is quite effective in preventing pregnancy, with a failure rate of 0.8 percent. The all-progesterone pill has a failure rate of 2.5 percent. Each type has advantages and disadvantages. The combination pill not only is more effective but also can regulate the menstrual pattern of women whose menses are irregular, and is quite helpful in preventing menstrual cramps. By preventing ovulation, the Pill eliminates the production of progesterone, which acts as a primer for the prostaglandins that cause the painful contractions of the uterus with menses. In addition, the Pill decreases the build-up of the lining of the uterus, the same tissue responsible for manufacturing these prostaglandins. The Pill also decreases the incidence of anemia and noncancerous breast disease. Some recent data suggest that it also decreases the rate of ovarian cancer by almost 50 percent and that of cancer of the uterine lining by

40–70 percent in women who have used it for a minimum of three years (Hatcher et al. 1990) (see Chapter 3).

The disadvantages relate to possible side effects and rare, but serious, complications. Common side effects of estrogen include breast tenderness, nausea, weight gain (which can be up to ten pounds in adults and averages two pounds in teenagers), and amenorrhea. The first two of these usually disappear after one or two cycles; the weight gained is often lost again; and the amenorrhea usually disappears within months after a woman stops taking the Pill. (On the potential interactions of the Pill with other drugs, see Chapter 14.)

Medical complications, most of them rare, include cancer of the liver, high blood pressure in susceptible women, increased clotting of the blood, and worsening of glucose control in diabetics. Women particularly susceptible to high blood pressure include those who have had toxemia in pregnancy, those with a family history of hypertension, and those with kidney disease. It is not certain which of the two hormones in these pills, estrogen or progesterone, is responsible. It is generally agreed, however, that blood pressure should be watched in all women taking oral contraceptives and that their administration should be stopped if blood pressure rises above acceptable levels.

The increased clotting can cause heart attacks, strokes, and blood clots in the legs; these last can travel (embolize) to the lungs and cause death, particularly in smokers and women over the age of 35. Estrogen generally increases blood clotting, and nicotine causes blood vessels to constrict. Age, smoking, and Pill use independently increase the risk of heart attacks, blood clots in the legs and lungs, and strokes, and the risk is significantly greater when they are taken in combination. In women over the age of 35, the combined effect is to increase the risk of heart attack and stroke 170-fold. For this reason, women smokers over the age of 35 are advised not to use the Pill. It is worrisome, therefore, that a study of the advice given by physicians to their patients who smoked showed that almost half of women who smoked and were taking the Pill denied ever having been told to stop smoking (Frank et al. 1991).

Concerns about these possibilities were responsible for the earlier recommendation that women not use oral contraceptives containing estrogens after the age of 35. This recommendation was revised in 1990 by the FDA in the belief that the benefits of oral contraceptives may outweigh any possible risks for healthy, non-smoking women over 40. These benefits include the protective effect of these hormones against ovarian and endometrial cancer, as previously discussed.

Taking birth control pills that contain estrogen has been found to elevate HDLs, whereas the progestin in such pills tends to elevate LDLs (Hatcher et al. 1990). The significance of this finding, however, is still unclear.

The jury is also out on the matter of breast cancer, but the weight of current evidence is reassuring. Studies that have included almost 20,000 women have not found the risk of breast cancer to be increased by the age of 60, even with long-term hormonal contraceptive use (Thomas 1991). Most studies now agree that the risk is not increased, but that hormonal contraceptives should be used with caution by women with a family history of breast cancer in a close relative.

With the progesterone-only pill the side effects and complications owing to estrogen in the combination pills can be avoided. But their failure rate is higher, and they are responsible for side effects of their own, including irregular menses, depression, high blood pressure, and acne.

The cost for a year of use of oral contraceptives is about $300.

After many years of deliberation, in 1993 the FDA approved Depo-Provera (medroxyprogesterone) for use as a contraceptive agent. This is a long-acting progesterone that is injected into a muscle every three months. During that three-month period, it prevents ovulation; after that period, its effects are completely reversible. It is extremely effective, with a pregnancy rate of 0.08 percent. Among its rare side effects is weight gain, and it has only rare complications, including chemical hepatitis and possibly a decrease in bone density. It is currently the most widely used hormonal contraceptive in the world and is increasing in popularity in the United States because it doesn't require daily vigilance. Currently, it costs about $120 each year for the four necessary injections.

Also recently approved for contraceptive use by the FDA is Norplant. This is a system of tiny Silastic tubes filled with long-acting progesterone that are inserted through a small incision in the arm. They inhibit ovulation for five years and have a failure rate of 0.03 percent. Their effect is rapidly reversible after removal. Complications have included local pain (and, rarely, infection), nipple discharge, weight gain or loss, and hair loss.

Currently, the price of the Norplant kit is $365 in the United States. The additional cost of insertion and removal doubles the cost of the kit. Although some states will cover Norplant use through Medicaid and the manufacturer has set up a foundation that has donated more than 10,000 kits, cost still represents a barrier to a sizable number of women. Particularly problematic are those state Medicaid programs that cover women only for 60 days after delivery. This would cover insertion of Norplant during this period but would not cover later removal should a woman desire it.

The availability of Norplant has generated considerable controversy because of its potential for coercive misuse. Nonvoluntary insertion has been ordered by some judges intent on preventing pregnancy in some women, a drug-abusing mother in one case and a child-abusing woman in another. Some have advocated its use as a condition of receiving welfare. In some areas of the world, lack of availability of resources for removal has led to concern.

"Morning after" or "emergency" contraception (EC) refers to the use of a device or medication after an episode of unprotected intercourse that will prevent the implantation of a fertilized ovum and thus prevent pregnancy. EC is widely used in Europe; it is estimated that about 343,000 courses of it were sold in 1991 in Great Britain alone (Wentz 1994). Morning-after pills will soon be available to British women without a prescription, yet in the United States most women don't even know about them. In this country, many doctors are reluctant to prescribe them because of concern that they will steer women away from consistent contraceptive use. Doctors will, however, often prescribe EC to prevent pregnancy after a rape. All women deserve to know of the availability of this method of contraception and how to use it. "What if every female of reproductive age in this country had one course of EC in her medicine cabinet: What would be the down side?" (Wentz 1994: 82).

The most popular approach to EC is called the Yuzpe regimen. This involves taking two birth control pills (Ovulen is the brand name that has been best studied) immediately and another two pills twelve hours later, all within 72 hours of unprotected intercourse. This regimen is effective in preventing pregnancy 75 percent of the time. It does, however, often cause nausea and vomiting, which can be controlled by simultaneous use of an antiemetic.

Before the FDA can list this method of birth control as an "approved use" for birth control pills, manufacturers must make a formal request for approval. Although such a request would require little money and time, it is suspected that the manufacturers are reluctant to make it, lest the attention they attract stimulate retaliatory boycotts by "right-to-life" groups of their entire product line (The best kept secret 1993). No drug company has undertaken the marketing of birth control pills for the Yuzpe regimen. Therefore, in June 1996 the FDA took the unprecedented step of publishing this type of use of oral contraceptives in the Federal Register.

Other EC agents include Danazol (600 mg given twice) and RU-486. A single dose of 600 mg of RU-486 given by mouth within 72 hours of unprotected intercourse is more effective in preventing pregnancy than the Yuzpe method. Moreover, it was associated with fewer side effects than the Yuzpe regimen.

RU-486, or mifespristone, is the controversial drug developed by the French pharmaceutical company Roussel-Uclaf in 1980. It acts by blocking the action of progesterone, resulting in the shedding of the lining of the uterus, much as occurs during menses. Should a fertilized egg be implanted in the uterine lining, this, too, will be shed. For this reason, RU-486 has been referred to as the "abortion pill." (It is discussed further below under Abortion.)

Hormonal Contraception for Men

Production of sperm is dependent upon secretion of the same pituitary hormones that control ovulation. The hormonal methods in common use in women might potentially be effective in preventing pregnancies when used by men. This possibility has been under study for more than twenty years, yet no male hormonal contraceptive has been developed in the West. The logical question is, why? There are many answers given.

The biologic issues relate to a major difference between males and females. In women, ovulation can be inhibited without decreasing levels of estrogen. In men, on the other hand, suppressing sperm production by interfering with pituitary production of hormones will also have the effect of lowering testosterone. This will result in loss of libido, as well as of ability to have an erection and to ejaculate. Although some might call this the perfect male contraceptive, it is obviously unacceptable. This is not, however, an insurmountable problem, because tests on other primates have shown that testosterone can be replaced through an implanted source without sacrificing the contraceptive benefits (Bremner, Bagatell, and Steiner 1990). Currently, however, there is no practical system for delivering testosterone over long periods of time, and the cost of mechanisms tested in other primates would be prohibitive. There have also been some serious side effects of the inhibitor, and it isn't entirely clear that the process of inhibiting sperm production is truly reversible. Moreover, it may potentially result in dangerous complications, including cancer of the prostate and alterations of the sperm, which could cause birth defects. Obviously more research is needed to address these limitations and concerns. It is not at all certain that such research will be done, owing to its enormous costs. Potential manufacturers may be reluctant to commit their research dollars to a product with questionable commercial potential, particularly at a time when their income stream is being threatened by the possibility of governmental controls. Nor have marketing surveys shown American men to be clamoring for such devices.

THE INTRAUTERINE DEVICE

IUDs have been in use since the beginning of the twentieth century. The first was a ring-shaped device fashioned from silkworm gut. By the 1970's, IUDs ranked among the most popular of contraceptive methods, used by an estimated 10 percent of women using any form of birth control (Hatcher et al. 1990: 355). Their subsequent fall from popularity followed the widely publicized complications of one IUD, the Dalkon Shield. Because its attached removal string was composed of a filament that drew bacteria into the uterus, this IUD caused an increase in the rate of pelvic infections, some of which were fatal in women who became pregnant. Not only did the publicity surrounding the lawsuits frighten and discourage women and their physicians, but the multibillion-dollar legal settlements caused the manufacturers of most other types of IUDs to remove their products from the market, even though they were not implicated in causing these complications. However, two types of IUDs are available.

The precise way in which IUDs exert their contraceptive effects is not certain. There is evidence that they irritate the endometrium (the lining of the uterus) so that it increases its production of prostaglandins, which stimulate the muscles of the uterus to contract and interfere with the production of certain enzymes and hormones. The combined effect is to make the uterine lining inhospitable to implantation of a fertilized egg. Recent evidence suggests that the effect on muscular contraction extends beyond the uterus to the fallopian tubes, where it affects the passage of the ovum.

The presently available types of IUDs vary in composition and contents. The Copper T 380A is composed of fine copper wire wound around a polyethylene core that is filled with barium (so that it can be spotted in an X ray should it become necessary to locate it) and shaped, as its name suggests, in a "T." Following insertion by a trained professional, this device may safely remain in the uterus for four years. Its failure rate of 0.8 percent is among the lowest for any currently available birth control method. Its small size allows it to be well tolerated, even among women who have never been pregnant, with fewer side effects, such as menstrual cramps or bleeding, than other IUDs. It has also been suggested that the small amount of copper that leaches out of this device may kill some agents that cause STDs.

The other type of IUD in current use is the Progestasert Contraceptive System. This is a T-shaped device made of ethylene vinyl acetate copolymer and filled not only with barium but with progesterone. The latter is responsible for the observation that users of this IUD may experience less severe cramps and less menstrual blood loss than users of other IUDs. Its disadvantage, however, is that it must be replaced each year to maintain its efficacy. The lowest expected pregnancy rate with use of the Progestasert is 2.0 percent (Hatcher et al. 1990: 357). In the unlikely event of pregnancy, users of this type of IUD have a six- to tenfold higher rate of ectopic (tubal) pregnancy than users of the Copper T (Alza Corporation 1986).

Despite their relative safety, even these newer IUDs should not be used by women with current, recent, or recurrent pelvic infections, those with multiple sex partners who do not practice "safe sex," or those who might be pregnant. There is also concern about their use in women with abnormal uterine bleeding, abnormal Pap smears, history of problems of blood clotting, or history of ectopic pregnancy, and those in locations where emergency treatment may be difficult to obtain, should a problem arise. Any woman with an IUD should see her physician immediately if she misses a period or has any other reason to suspect that she is pregnant. Such pregnancies have a 50 percent chance of ending in miscarriage. Early removal of the IUD can reduce this risk by half (Lewit 1970). The risk of infection, sometimes fatal, is higher in pregnant women with IUDs than in other pregnant women.

SURGICAL BIRTH CONTROL METHODS

Voluntary surgical contraception (VSC) is currently the most commonly used family planning method in the developing and developed worlds. It is not only also the most effective method, but also the safest and least expensive. Over the last two decades, more than one million such procedures have been performed in the United States alone, approximately two-thirds of them on women. The procedure for the female is tubal ligation or tubectomy; for the male, vasectomy.

Tubal ligation creates a block in the fallopian tube that prevents the sperm and egg from uniting. This procedure can be performed safely immediately following delivery or miscarriage, as well as at any other time. It is performed by a trained person in an outpatient setting, either by a "mini" laparotomy (a small incision in the abdomen above the pubis) or through laparoscopy (insertion of a light and surgical instruments through a small incision in the upper abdomen). The tubes are blocked by clips, electrocoagulation, or surgical separation. A newly patented method involves nonsurgical insertion of a blockage directly into the fallopian tubes through the uterus.

This is a safe procedure with a risk of death less than 25 percent of that which results from pregnancy alone (3 per 100,000 versus 14 per 100,000). Other complications are rare (less than 1 percent) and mostly preventable with good surgical and anesthetic techniques. The overall risk of subsequent pregnancy is extremely low (between 0.2 and 0.4 percent), but the risk of ectopic pregnancy is significantly higher in sterilized women who become pregnant, particularly those in whom the electrocoagulation technique was used. Studies have shown that women who have undergone tubal ligation have a lower chance of developing ovarian cancer (see Chapter 3).

Vasectomy is the male counterpart of female tubal ligation in that it blocks the tube leading from the testis to the penile opening, thus preventing the exit of sperm. It is a safer procedure than tubal ligation because it is performed without having to enter the abdominal cavity. Accordingly, the death rate is much lower (1 per 300,000 procedures). Other complications are also rare, despite periodic reports in the lay press to the contrary. For example, recent reports that men are at greater risk for developing heart attacks or prostate cancer following this procedure have not been supported by careful research (Hatcher 1990: 412). More than half of men develop antibodies to their sperm following this ligation procedure, and this may have some implications for future childbearing should the man later decide to have the procedure reversed.

Should circumstances change, either the male or the female procedure may sometimes be reversed through microsurgical techniques in the hands of highly skilled surgeons. The chance of reversal is low and unpredictable, leading to the recommendation that these procedures be chosen only by those who have truly decided not to have future children.

THE FUTURE OF BIRTH CONTROL

It costs approximately $250,000,000 for a new drug or product to be developed and tested. In today's climate of economic downsizing and fear of liability suits, it is unlikely that any new methods of birth control will be developed. Moreover, fears of boycotts by "right-to-life" groups have caused some manufacturers of birth control devices and medications to consider ceasing production out of concern that their entire line of products might be jeopardized. The challenge now is not so much to encourage research on development of new contraceptive methods, but rather to preserve those we now have. The public in general, and conservative political leaders in particular, must understand that any restriction of availability of contraceptives will lead to a marked increase in unintended pregnancies. Combined with restrictions on abortion, this will inevitably lead to a tremendous social and economic burden on our society to care for children whose parents often lack the resources to do so themselves.

Abortion

In 1992, 1.6 million of the 6.4 million pregnancies in the United States ended in therapeutic abortion, the lowest rate since 1979. Although this figure represents about one-fourth of all pregnancies, it is estimated to include half of unintended pregnancies. At the present rate, almost half of all women will have had at least one abortion by the time they reach 45 years of age (Forrest and Henshaw 1993).

Since the landmark Supreme Court decision *Roe v. Wade* in 1973, the availability of safe, legal abortions has contributed significantly to improved physical and mental health of this country's women. No longer do they risk the infection and/or death that previously resulted from unskilled and unsanitary illegal abortions, or the emotional and, often, economic burden of bearing unwanted children. In contrast to the statements of opponents of abortion services, their availability has not led to abandonment of contraception. In fact, almost half of the women who have unintended pregnancies each year are currently using contraceptives, according to Janet Freedman (1994), speaking on behalf of the American Medical Women's Association. The problem is that no available method is foolproof.

Nor do women generally regard abortion as a satisfactory method of birth control. For any woman who has undergone an abortion, it has been a difficult decision and an experience she will never forget. That notwithstanding, the weight of the evidence is that, for the majority of women who have undergone the procedure, there has been no serious emotional complication (Adler and Tschann 1993).

A recent study has suggested that the risk of breast cancer is increased among women who have had an abortion (Daling et al. 1994). The authors of this study themselves note its limitations and possible biases. For example, the data collection consisted of interviewing women with breast cancer in detail about their histories and comparing the findings to those from another group of women contacted at random by telephone. Possible explanations of the higher reporting of abortions by the breast cancer patients might be their guilt about having had the procedure and worry that it has caused their cancer, and their greater willingness to disclose information than the comparison group because they trust interviewers they have met in person. Further research is needed, as there is no scientific basis for the connection.

Continued availability of abortion is critical to the health and safety of women, regardless of their socioeconomic and ethnic background. Moreover, there is no aspect of health care for men that is as precarious and subject to scrutiny and intrusiveness as is this one for women. Decisions regarding continuation or termination of pregnancy should be made between a woman patient and her physician, as are all decisions for male patients.

There are increasing threats to the current availability of safe abortion in this country. These include objections of powerful religious and political leaders; terrorist tactics of intimidation, and even murder, of providers of abortion; threats to sources of payment for abortions for poor women; and decreasing ability and willingness of health care providers to perform abortions. Presently, 31 percent of women in the United States live in the 83 percent of counties that are without any provider of abortion services (Freedman 1994). This situation is likely to worsen, if only because few doctors now in training are being taught how to perform abortions (Darney 1993). Darney believes that

> the solution to the dearth of abortion providers is to incorporate education about abortion as a part of women's health care into the under- and postgraduate training of all health care professionals and to make training in the performance of abortion routinely available to all who want to do abortions for their patients. Laws against harassment and violence should be enforced. Compensation for doing abortions should be comparable to other medical procedures. (Darney 1993: 161)

An alternative to surgical abortion, RU-486, is completely effective in emptying the uterus of an established pregnancy about 80 percent of the time. When it is used within nine weeks after a missed menstrual period, in conjunction with a dose of prostaglandin taken 36 to 48 hours later, the success rate rises to 96 percent. It is relatively safe, with few side effects and complications. It is definitely safer than a surgical abortion (especially an illegal one).

The advantages of using RU-486 are many. As highlighted by Boston's Feminist Majority Foundation in 1991, these include the following:

1. Pregnancy termination with RU-486 is a non-invasive procedure, requiring no anesthesia and putting women at far less risk of infection.
2. RU-486 affords women relative privacy—both in making and in carrying out their reproductive decisions.
3. RU-486 can be administered to a woman as soon as she knows that she is pregnant and wants to have an abortion. RU-486 is a more effective method than surgical abortion in terminating pregnancy during the first seven weeks.
4. Many women prefer RU-486 because it allows them greater psychological control over the termination of pregnancy.

In addition to its role as an abortifacient, this drug has many other potential medical uses, including treatment of endometriosis.

Because RU-486 is not available for use in the United States, researchers have been working to find a substitute. In a recent report, the combination of two drugs, methotrexate and misoprostol, has been shown to be effective in inducing abortion in 90 percent of patients. However, it caused more pain than does RU-486 (Creinin and Vittinghoff 1994).

In the current national debate about health care reform and managed care, one of the most contentious issues has been that of coverage for abortion. If private insurance were replaced by a national insurance program that did not cover abortion, millions of women who now have such coverage under their private health insurance policies would lose this protection. Seventy percent of all private insurers provide such coverage. In these discussions, compromises have been offered, including that of a so-called "physician's conscience" opt-out. This would provide coverage but allow providers to refuse to perform abortions, providing they refer the patient elsewhere for the service. With the current scarcity of providers and the decreasing likelihood of ready access in the future, any such provision must be coupled with financial support for transportation and even lodging for a woman and her children, should she have to travel a long distance to obtain necessary care. Another proposed compromise would be for women to pay an extra yearly premium for abortion coverage in the event that they might ever need it in the future. According to the American Medical Women's Association, this is tantamount to "asking women to anticipate an unintended pregnancy, and to consequently pay more for their health care" (Bemmann 1994).

Reproductive Issues of Adolescence

The United States has the dubious distinction of an adolescent pregnancy rate that is the highest in the entire industrialized world and higher than that of some countries in the developing world. It is not that U.S. teenagers are more sexually active than those in other industrialized countries (in fact, they are less so), but rather that they use birth control methods less often (Alan Guttmacher Institute 1976).

In 1990, 835,000 (10 percent) of the nation's fifteen-to-nineteen-year-old women became pregnant. The reported pregnancy rates for women aged fifteen to nineteen ranged between 56 and 111 per 1,000; for those aged fifteen to seventeen, these rates ranged from 25 to 75 per 1,000 (CDC 1995a). The denominator for these rates includes all females in the age groups, not only those who are sexually active. If one were to include only those girls who are sexually active, using a conservative estimate of 50 percent, the pregnancy rates would be double those above. Black adolescents have the highest rate of pregnancy (23 percent), Asians the lowest (6 percent). For those under the age of fifteen, the birthrate is seven times higher for blacks than for whites.

It is estimated that 95 percent of adolescent pregnancies are unintended. About half of them result in live births, with the others being terminated by abortion or spontaneous miscarriage; the rate for the latter is significantly higher in adolescents than in older women.

The U.S. rate of abortions among adolescents is also the highest among industrialized countries; in 1990 it ranged from 6 to 49 per 1,000 fifteen-to-nineteen-year-olds and from 3 to 34 per 1,000 fifteen-to-seventeen-year-olds (CDC 1995a). Here, again, the denominator is all women in this age group, not just those who are pregnant.

In recent years, teenage abortion rates have decreased faster than teenage pregnancy rates; in other words, a smaller percentage of pregnant teens are having abortions. From 1980 to 1990, pregnancy rates decreased in about half the states and increased in thirteen states. Meanwhile, from 1986 to 1990, the ratio of abortions to live births decreased by approximately 21 percent. During the 1980's, the decrease in both pregnancy and abortion rates was greater for whites than for blacks. No comparative data were collected for Hispanic adolescents during this period (Litt 1996).

Pregnancy in an adolescent is fraught with problems for the young woman and her baby and family, as well as society. Compared with an adult woman, the pregnant adolescent is at higher risk for complications such as toxemia (one of the most serious complications, which may kill the mother and/or the fetus, and which is often the reason for emergency premature delivery), miscarriage, infection, blood loss, difficult labor, and even death. Her baby is at greater risk of being stillborn, premature, or underweight. Her own lifelong educational, social, and economic outlook is gloomy. She will probably contribute to the cost to taxpayers, which in 1990 amounted to $25.1 billion, for support of families started by teen births. If every birth to a teenager in 1990 could have been postponed until she reached the age of twenty, it is estimated that the country could have saved $10 billion each year between when the teenagers gave birth and when they turned twenty (Center for Population Options 1992).

The high pregnancy rate among adolescents is hardly surprising, given all the impediments to their using effective birth control. The response of the Reagan and Bush administrations to the rising adolescent birthrate has been, "Just say no." Were it only this easy! As parents, teachers, and doctors, we wish it were possible to influence teenagers to postpone sexual intercourse until they become adults. Reality, however, has shown us that abstinence will not work for many of today's teenagers. By the age of eighteen, 50 percent of girls will have had at least one experience of sexual intercourse. Our national naïveté in promoting abstinence to the exclusion of other effective methods of pregnancy prevention has left these young women without the information and equipment to protect themselves, not only from pregnancy but also from sometimes deadly STDs (see Chapter 5).

Moreover, physicians in general have been poorly informed about contraceptive issues specific to adolescents. Many doctors seem to be more concerned with the possible side effects and medical complications of some birth control methods than with recognition that for an *adolescent* woman, pregnancy poses a higher risk of complications and even death than does any birth control method.

Certain psychosocial and biologic considerations regarding use of contraception are unique to adolescents. In general, the psychosocial factors relate primarily to the initial challenge of persuading adolescents to use birth control at all; the biologic factors relate more to the choice among specific birth control methods.

Motivation, knowledge, and communication skills are all necessary to achieve effective birth control. This combination is a tall order for an adolescent. The first psychosocial impediment relates to cognitive development. To take precautions, one must be capable of thinking abstractly and of putting oneself in hypothetical situations. The concept (obvious to most adults) that intercourse leads to pregnancy requires such thinking, particularly for those teenagers who have had intercourse and *not* become pregnant. This leap of faith requires that an individual be at the cognitive stage of formal operations. This level is rarely achieved before midadolescence, and some people never reach it.

A related problem is that those lucky teenage girls who have had intercourse without becoming pregnant often don't feel relieved, but rather become concerned that they may be unable to have babies. They may then proceed to prove that they can. In the adolescent medicine clinic at Stanford University Medical Center, for example, more young girls fear they cannot become pregnant than fear they will do so before they are ready. For them, discussions of birth control seem totally irrelevant and may fall on deaf ears.

Another group that is difficult to motivate are the many teenagers in denial. They do not self-identify as sexually active but rather believe that each act of intercourse was accidental ("I was swept off my feet by my love") and will never happen again. And then there are all the myths about when, and under what circumstances, one can and cannot become pregnant. Some girls have been told by their boyfriends (and believe) that as long as they have sex every day without a break, they won't get pregnant; that they can only get pregnant if they have sex during menses; and so forth. "It can't (or won't) happen to me" is another common theme among adolescents, who tend, in general, to feel invulnerable. These feelings, although more common in younger adolescents, are not limited to them or to those from impoverished educational or economic back-grounds. Similar attitudes and misinformation are found among university students.

Even among those young women who identify with the need to be protected against pregnancy, using that protection is not always easy. The younger they are, and the poorer their self-image, the less likely they are to be able to discuss the need for birth control with a potential sexual partner. "Good girls" don't carry condoms or in any other way admit to being knowledgeable about such matters. Adolescents at our clinic ask questions such as, "Do you risk losing a great boyfriend by raising the subject?" "How do you do it without sounding like you don't trust him to be free of infection?" Moreover, many teenagers reject methods that involve touching their genitalia, as well as the premeditation involved in their use.

Finally, many adolescents who overcome all these obstacles and begin using contraception do not continue to do so. We have found that only half of the young girls who receive contraceptives in the Stanford clinic continue to use them for more than four months, although those who stop using them continue sexual activity (Litt, Cuskey, and Rudd 1980). They often stop for reasons such as the disapproval of their sexual partners, real or imagined side effects, a change of sexual partners, or discovery by parents. And studies report a failure rate for oral contraceptives in adolescents as high as 18 percent, owing to their noncompliance (Hillard 1992).

The best ways to overcome these barriers to the use of birth control are communication and education, particularly within the family. Parents play a critical role in determining the outcome of their daughters' sexual experiences, often without knowing it. Studies, including that of Inazu and Fox (1980), have shown that young girls who have had open communication with their mothers about sex and birth control are more likely to postpone sexual activity and to use birth control when they begin. Contrary to the opinions of opponents of teaching about birth control, there are more pregnancies among teenagers who know the least about it, rather than the most. Most teenagers want information about sexuality from their parents, as long as it is presented in a factual manner. Unfortunately, not many parents feel comfortable in this role. Interestingly, "more than 75% of parents feel that schools should play a role in family life education" (Carnegie Task Force 1994: 29).

There are, however, no good studies evaluating the effect on young boys of open communication about sexual activity and its consequences. Such research is critical if we are ever to achieve gender equity in sexual responsibility.

In addition to the psychologic barriers discussed above, adolescents may have difficulty accessing contraception, particularly if they do not wish their parents to know about it. Although it is still legal for physicians in most states to prescribe birth control to minors without their parents' consent, many teenagers do not know that. This misconception has resulted, for the most part, from the threat of the "squeal law," a proposed regulation that, if enacted, would have made it mandatory for clinics receiving federal funding to inform parents of adolescents' requests for birth control. Although the regulation was never passed, the associated publicity was so widespread that we still hear teenagers referring to it as though it is the law. Unfortunately, although most states do not require physicians to inform parents, some do not prohibit them from doing so; thus, some teenagers may justifiably fear that their confidentiality might be breached. Inadvertent breaches may also result when bills for health care go to the health insurance policyholders, the parents. Some health care providers make special arrangements with teenagers for payment, so that a bill is never rendered. Other teens, such as those who live in California, may obtain their own coverage under Medicaid for "sensitive" services, which include birth control (as well as treatment of STDs, substance abuse, and mental illness). Some physicians in private practice who have established long-standing rapport with both parents and adolescents have obtained parental permission and promise of payment for confidential treatment with no questions asked.

The biologic uniqueness of adolescence and puberty introduces other considerations into contraceptive choice. Some of these factors relate to the Pill in particular. For example, during the eighteen months after the first menstrual period, ovulation may not occur each month. The delicate system of checks and balances between the production of hormones by the pituitary and the ovaries is still immature and in need of some fine-tuning. Taking hormones, such as those in birth control pills, may prolong the maturation period. In fact, it takes adolescent women many months longer than older women to resume ovulation after they discontinue the Pill. This phenomenon doesn't mean that young adolescents should not take the Pill, but rather that they should be aware of this common, but reversible, problem.

When hormonal contraception was first introduced, there was concern about giving hormones to teenagers because of their possible adverse effect on growth during this critical period. This concern grew out of earlier research demonstrating that large doses of estrogen, given to girls who were afraid of being too tall(!), could close the growth plates in their legs and decrease their ultimate height. This is a critical issue, but one that we are now able to address with information gathered in clinical settings as well as research laboratories over the last 30 years. We now know that the dose of estrogen in the pills currently being used is too small to have any effect on growth. In addition, in practical terms, because the growth spurt in height ends at about the time the first menstrual period occurs, very few young women actually request birth control at a time when there might be any effect on growth.

As discussed in Chapter 8, adolescent women are now the fastest-growing group of new cigarette smokers. This is relevant to decisions about hormonal contraception because, as discussed above, estrogen can cause serious complications when combined with the effects of smoking. There is no evidence as yet that this is a problem for teenagers, but the biological effects of both estrogen and nicotine provide a real basis for concern. With the rate of smoking increasing in adolescent women, it is only a matter of time until we see such complications. This is not to say that teenagers who smoke should never use hormonal contraception, only that they should not use birth control pills that contain estrogens. Pills containing progesterone alone should be safe for smokers. Alternatively, these young women should be informed about these (and other) harmful effects of smoking so that they may reconsider their decision to smoke. Realistically, however, most young girls will not be dissuaded by such information, as, according to the American Cancer Society, they are generally well informed about the health risks of smoking. (For further discussion of smoking by adolescent women, see Chapter 8.)

Another factor in adolescents' selection of a birth control method is that teenagers have many more problems with menstrual cramps than do adult women. As discussed above, estrogen-containing birth control pills are very effective in preventing cramps, while the IUD can worsen them; barrier methods obviously have no effect on cramps.

In addition, teenagers have a higher risk than older women of getting toxic shock syndrome. Although most people think this serious disease disappeared when Rely tampons were removed from the market in 1981, about ten cases are still reported each month in the United States. Interestingly, most of these occur in women using birth control methods designed to be inserted and left in the vagina, rather than as a result of menses, which had been the leading risk factor at the time of the 1981 "epidemic" of TSS. The diaphragm and contraceptive sponge have been implicated in many of these cases.

Finally, the high rate of STDs in adolescents (see Chapter 5) must also be taken into consideration when deciding on a contraceptive method. Because hormonal methods provide no protection against STDs, their use should be coupled with that of a male condom, preferably with spermicidal foam. On the other hand, if both teenage partners are willing to use the combination of condom and foam, they are well protected against both pregnancy and STDs, without any of the possible side effects of hormonal methods. The failure rate (i.e., pregnancy rate) of this combination of methods, if they are used correctly, is in the same range as that for the all-progesterone Pill (2.5 percent).

An estimated 95 percent of adolescent pregnancies are unintended and their social, psychologic, and economic consequences are enormous. As discussed above, the health consequences to both mother and baby are great, as well.

In summary, although the biologic factors unique to adolescence must be considered in evaluating birth control methods for use in this life stage, those factors certainly do not preclude sexually active adolescent women from using some contraceptive method. Rather, it is the psychosocial difficulties that pose the greatest challenge to the goal of reducing unwanted pregnancies among adolescents.

CHAPTER SEVEN

Mental Health

The separation between mental health and physical, social, and economic health is an artificial one. Sadly, however, it is built into the structure of the health care system and its related literature. This chapter seeks to re-forge the linkages between emotional health issues and other aspects of women's experience. These issues will be examined at different stages of the life span, but there is continuity among them. For example, depression is discussed extensively under both Adolescence, the time when it often has its genesis, and Young Adulthood, where it is known to take a great toll. Briefer, age-group-specific discussions of depression appear under The Perimenopausal Years and The Older Years.

This chapter provides a number of illustrations of a recurring theme in medical history: In the absence of data about women's health problems, gendered biases drive conceptualization of their cause and result in negative stereotyping, ineffective treatment, or blaming of the victim.

Childhood

Approximately 13 percent of six-to-eleven-year-olds in the United States suffer from a mental disorder. During childhood, males reportedly experience more emotional and behavioral difficulties than females. The under-fifteen age group is the only one in which males outnumber females (three to one) in utilizing mental health services (1989–90 data; Schappert 1993). This difference is accounted for by a higher incidence in males of three types of disorders: attention deficit disorders (ADD), the conditions of having difficulty with organization of schoolwork and group activities because of inattentiveness, with or without hyperactivity; oppositional disorders, manifested by a pattern of hostile and defiant behavior; and mental retardation and other developmental disorders. According to Nolen-Hoeksema, "boys' greater vulnerability to depression and other psychopathology during childhood can be attributed to their weaker constitution, to a greater intolerance in adults of male deviance than of female deviance, to boys' greater reactivity to psychological stress, to their more maladaptive explanatory styles, and perhaps to a greater pressure by parents for boys to succeed" (Nolen-Hoeksema 1990).

It appears from these data that girls enjoy better mental health than do boys. However, this view is misleading. It diverts attention from the sad reality that for many girls in our society the stage is being set during childhood for a number of emotional problems in later life. This reality includes: (1) a higher incidence of physical and sexual abuse of girls and their witnessing of verbal and physical abuse of their mothers, and often grandmothers, in their homes; (2) a school environment in which boys receive more attention and encouragement from their teachers; (3) a society that values thinness as the ideal female form and creates early pressures on young girls to conform to this ideal; and (4) for the 25 percent of young girls who live in poverty with their single mothers, exposure to limited future options for women. Is it surprising, therefore, that as these girls mature, they develop poorer self-esteem and more depressive illness and eating disorders than their male counterparts? To optimize a positive outcome for girls in their later lives, we must eliminate exploitation and victimization of women, as well as poverty and disease.

Until we achieve these lofty goals, however, we can seek to improve girls' living experiences, and hence women's mental health, in other ways. There has been extensive research on how the early experiences of children relate to mental health outcomes. Although little of it focuses on possible gender differences, some of the findings help elucidate the developmental background of the emotional health of girls.

Studies of parenting styles are particularly relevant. Baumrind has examined four different styles of parenting: authoritative/democratic, authoritarian, permissive, and rejecting-neglecting.

Authoritative parents, according to Baumrind,

> by definition, are not punitive or authoritarian. They may, however, embrace traditional values. Authoritative parents, in comparison to lenient parents, are more demanding and, in comparison to authoritarian-restrictive parents, are more responsive.
>
> Authoritative parents are demanding in that they guide their children's activities firmly and consistently and require them to contribute to family functioning by helping with household tasks. They willingly confront their children in order to obtain conformity, state their values clearly, and expect their children to respect their norms. Authoritative parents are responsive affectively in the sense of being loving, supportive, and committed: they are responsive cognitively in the sense of providing a stimulating and challenging environment. Authoritative parents characteristically maintain an appropriate ratio of children's autonomy to parental control at all ages. However, an appropriate ratio is weighted in the direction of control with young children and in the direction of autonomy in adolescence. Authoritative parents of adolescents focus on issues rather than personalities and roles, [and] they encourage their adolescents to voice their dissent and actively seek to share power as their children mature. (Office of Technology Assessment 1991: II-40)

Democratic/authoritative parenting also was associated with good emotional health during adolescence. Baumrind describes democratic parents as "highly responsive, moderately demanding, and not restrictive. They are less conventional, directive, and assertive in their control than authoritative parents, but like authoritative parents are supportive, caring, personally agentic, and manifest no problem behavior or family disorganization" (Office of Technology Assessment 1991: II-40).

Authoritarian parents are those who exert rigid control over their children. Studies have found these children to be generally less socially competent than children from other families, although this finding has varied with gender, race, and social class. For example, authoritarian upbringing was more harmful to middle-class boys than girls, to preschool white girls than black girls, and to white boys than Hispanic boys (ibid.).

Permissive parents, as the word suggests, are uninvolved with their children or lax in controlling their children's behavior. Baumrind found that preadolescent girls from such families were less self-assertive than those from authoritative families. Both boys and girls from permissive families were also found to be less cognitively competent than those from authoritative families (ibid.). However, it was rejecting-neglecting, or indifferent, parenting that was associated with production of the least socially competent adolescents and those with the most interpersonal problems.

Educating and supporting parents in parenting would address the issue of primary prevention of some psychopathology and behavioral problems. Another approach would come under the heading of secondary prevention, which addresses ways to limit damage to children who have been exposed to stresses in early life. Research in this field focuses on understanding why some children who have these stresses do not develop negative outcomes. A number of psychiatrists, psychologists, and foundations have given such research the highest priority. Emerging from their work is the view that these "resilient" children have developed a sense of connectedness to at least one caring and competent adult, who is not necessarily a parent. Children with certain personality characteristics, such as an internal locus of control, spirituality, and a sense of humor, seem more likely to be resilient than others. This line of research is too new to provide clear guidelines for developing proven interventions to help girls develop resiliency, but it suggests some promising possibilities.

In other research on secondary prevention, Colton and Gore (1991) found sports participation to be a significant buffer for girls. They were less depressed and had higher self-esteem when they were involved in either personal or team sports. Michael Rutter's work (1994) stresses the importance of life turning points, when people on maladaptive paths turn onto more adaptive ones. For young men from disadvantaged backgrounds, this opportunity often came from joining the armed forces. For young women, such a turning point was a harmonious marriage to a nondeviant spouse. As Rutter sought to understand earlier determinants of this finding, he discovered that it was the girls who had had positive experiences at school who developed the ability to plan their futures and subsequently had such marriages. The positive school experiences were not necessarily in academics, but as often in sports, music, arts, or social responsibility. He speculates that such success gives people positive self-esteem or self-efficacy, which in turn gives them "the confidence to take active steps to deal with life challenges in other domains of their lives" (Rutter 1994: 42).

Adolescence

The popular image of adolescence as a time of turmoil and rebellion is not supported by the findings of systematic research. Quite to the contrary, there appears to be continuity of emotional and behavioral characteristics, as well as of temperament, between childhood and adolescence (Offer et al. 1989). In other words, disturbed teenagers are likely to have been disturbed children. Nonetheless, a number of mental health conditions may become apparent during adolescence, and others may develop then, because of either biologic factors or psychosocial stressors at this time in a young person's life.

Perceptions of teenagers' mental health problems vary. For example, parents' views may differ from those of an adolescent; they may have different thresholds of tolerance for different symptoms and even different definitions of mental health problems. One study found that parents and adolescents report different symptoms, and that adolescents often report more symptoms (Kashani et al. 1987). And we found in a recent study of high school students in a middle-class community that the leading reason for their not getting mental health care was not lack of money or insurance coverage but parents' resistance (Cynthia Kapphahn, personal communication, 1995).

Reports of mental health problems also vary with factors such as socioeconomic status, ethnicity, place of residence, and family structure. Studies have found white, non-Hispanic parents more likely to report such problems than black or Hispanic parents. More problems have been reported in teenagers from urban families of lower socioeconomic status and from families headed by a biologic mother and a stepfather.

For these reasons and others, the precise number of teenagers with mental health problems is difficult to determine. We know about those who seek and receive treatment, but we are ignorant about the general population of adolescents whose behavior has failed to attract attention or who lack the resources to get needed help. Estimates of the rate of mental disorders in nonclinical samples have ranged from approximately 18 to 21 percent. Despite this high rate, fewer than 2 percent of adolescents receive mental health services (Office of Technology Assessment 1991; 1986 data).

One common emotional difficulty faced by adolescents is stress. In a study (Pitts and Steiner 1994) of eighth- and tenth-grade students, more than 45 percent reported difficulty coping with stress at home and at school. In this study, the females were more likely to report experiencing distress than the males. A study from the University of Minnesota (Minnesota Women's Fund 1990) found that approximately 25 percent of seventh- to twelfth-graders experienced what they considered to be extreme stresses and strains, dissatisfaction with their personal lives, emotional insecurity, and feelings of being tired or worn out in the month prior to the survey. Feeling tired and worn out was reported by almost one-third of the females, compared with less than one-quarter of the males. This widespread and serious subjective emotional stress does not, however, qualify as a mental health disorder, according to the *Diagnostic and Statistical Manual of Mental Disorders* (*DSM-IV*) (American Psychiatric Association 1994), the "bible" used to diagnose mental illness, determine whether to admit patients for care, and decide whether insurance should reimburse them for that care.

The most common diagnoses in the adolescent age group are, in decreasing order of prevalence: oppositional disorders, conduct disorders (more serious than oppositional disorders, these include hostile and defiant behavior for more than six months and violation of the rights of others and of age-appropriate social norms), separation anxiety (irrational fears or panic about being separated from the parent or others to whom the adolescent is attached), attention deficit disorders, overanxious disorders (generalized anxiety about future performance or events), and major depression (prolonged, sustained, disabling depression, characterized by feelings of hopelessness, helplessness, worthlessness, and thoughts of death and suicide).

Adolescent females experience more mental health symptoms, such as those of depression, anxiety, and eating disorders, than males (Schappert 1993). As mentioned above, however, the majority of patients under fifteen receiving mental health services are males. For example, almost three-quarters of adolescent patients in psychiatric residential treatment programs are males. Even for outpatient care and short-term inpatient psychiatric hospitalizations, male adolescents outnumber females. This undoubtedly reflects the fact that boys have more acting-out behaviors that frighten people and cause parents and schools to refer them for help. Because the types of mental health problems that affect girls don't pose similar threats to society, girls are less likely to receive help with their emotional problems. Several of the disorders to which adolescent girls are most prone are discussed below.

EATING DISORDERS

Eating disorders are not new. From biblical times, there are references to bulimic behaviors, and since the twelfth century there have been descriptions of young nuns and other religious women who starve themselves to achieve their goals. But never before in history have the women doing this been so numerous or so young, and never before have they acted in the name of beauty rather than piety.

Over the last three decades, the incidence of eating disorders has increased dramatically, paralleling an increase in emphasis on thinness as the idealized female form. Although there has been some slight increase in the number of boys with bulimia nervosa, eating disorders continue to preferentially affect women in societies like ours that equate thinness with beauty for women. About ten years ago, it was estimated that 1 percent of sixteen-to-eighteen-year-old women in industrialized countries had anorexia nervosa and that more than 10 percent had bulimia nervosa. These are likely to be underestimates, because most young women with eating disorders never seek treatment and because there is no systematic record keeping for such conditions in this country. Once limited to middle- and upper-class Caucasians, eating disorders now occur across the socioeconomic spectrum and in every racial and ethnic group, although anorexia nervosa continues to be rare in African-American women. The age of onset has also fallen recently. It is no longer rare for ten- and eleven-year-old girls to have this condition, and the eating disorders program I work with has had one patient whose anorexia nervosa began around the age of seven.

Of course, not all young women exposed to societal pressures for thinness succumb. A number of risk factors have been identified or postulated, including family history of eating disorder or substance abuse, control struggles within the family, antecedent physical illness and resulting weight loss, pressure from a ballet teacher or athletic coach to lose weight, teasing from a brother, chemical imbalance in the brain, and early feeding patterns. There are likely many causes and different stresses for different young women. Although a lot has been written about so-called anorexic families, and although some of the risk factors are family-related, it is far from proven that anorexia nervosa is caused by certain family traits.

Although the earlier psychoanalytic literature took the position that young girls with anorexia nervosa starve themselves because they reject their feminine role and their sexuality, this does not appear consistent with the experience at our program. Most of our patients express concern about their lack of menses and, as they improve, are very anxious that their breasts and menses return. What they abhor is the fullness of their buttocks and thighs.

Diagnoses of anorexia nervosa and bulimia nervosa are based on the criteria listed in Appendix D. Although both conditions reflect the desire to lose weight, it is in anorexia nervosa that we find extreme emaciation. Girls with bulimia nervosa tend to be of average weight and typically experience wide fluctuations in weight. Not surprisingly, those with anorexia nervosa restrict their caloric intake greatly, often exercise to burn calories, and may also engage in purging. Those with bulimia nervosa, in contrast, consume huge quantities of food and then purge to get rid of it. Many young women meet one or more of these criteria, but not enough of them to be diagnosed as having either anorexia nervosa or bulimia nervosa. It is critically important for them to receive help, however, to prevent progression to the full-blown disease. The earlier the onset of treatment, the better the outcome.

Eating disorders involve not only serious psychologic considerations, but also the possibility of life-threatening medical complications. Even in this day and age, about 10 percent of patients with anorexia nervosa die from these complications; the risk is higher in the younger patients. Death may result from imbalance of electrolytes, the chemicals necessary for the body's normal functioning. Potassium, for example, which is often lost through vomiting, is critical to the heart's action; when it is low, there is the risk of heart stoppage. Another cause of death is the ingestion of large amounts of the drug ipecac, which is available in most homes to induce vomiting in toddlers who accidentally consume poisons, and which is now popular among people with eating disorders. It is extremely dangerous, however, attacking heart muscle when taken in large amounts or even in small doses over time. Death may also result from sudden overeating or drinking by a severely malnourished person. The unaccustomed increased volume of food and/or liquids causes heart failure. This typically happens in hospital settings when patients rapidly try to gain sufficient weight to be discharged to the privacy of their customary purging and/or starvation routine. Other patients die when severe malnutrition affects the electrical activity of the heart, causing an abnormality in its rhythm that results in complete stoppage. In older patients with chronic anorexia nervosa, suicide may occur.

In addition to these life-endangering complications, anorexia nervosa has many other adverse effects on the body, particularly for the young. Virtually every organ is affected in one way or another. For example, people with this disease often wear layer upon layer of clothing, even when the weather is hot. They do this partly to try to cover up what they consider to be their fat bodies, and partly because they are always cold. There are a number of reasons for their low body temperature. For one, they have lost the insulating fat layer beneath the skin owing to their malnutrition. For another, their bodies produce less thyroid hormone; this is presumably the body's way of lowering its metabolism in an effort to conserve calories. When they are exposed to cold under experimental conditions, those with anorexia nervosa don't respond the way healthy people do. They do not, for example, develop gooseflesh. Low body temperature can further lower heart rate, particularly during sleep, when body temperature drops still more, as it does in all of us. This places the electrical conducting system of the heart in even greater jeopardy of developing an irregular rhythm that can lead to sudden heart stoppage and death. Finally, low body temperature, as well as a lowering of the levels of some components of the blood that are often used by physicians to determine whether there is an infection or inflammation, makes it more difficult for these conditions to be appropriately recognized when patients with anorexia nervosa develop other illnesses.

Other hormonal problems also develop in these markedly malnourished women. The most dramatic of these result in cessation of menses or, if the patient is young enough, in inability to undergo puberty and even achieve her first menstrual period. The same factors also inhibit ovulation, so there has been concern about the future fertility of young girls with early onset of anorexia nervosa. Although there needs to be more research, what we now know suggests that about half of them have return of menses (usually more than three years after they are weight-rehabilitated) and normal fertility. Those at greatest risk for impaired fertility seem to be the girls who get anorexia nervosa before they have entered puberty.

The same hormonal changes are also responsible for extremely low levels of estrogen, much as occur in menopause. Like their post-menopausal counterparts, these young girls undergo weakening of their bones, similar to osteoporosis (Bachrach et al. 1990). The good news is that, unlike that in postmenopausal women, the loss of bone mass and density resulting from malnutrition in these young adolescents seems to be reversible with weight gain. Low levels of estrogen also cause breasts to shrink to some extent. This, too, generally improves with sufficient weight gain.

Other hormones affected by anorexia nervosa include the two that control growth during puberty. Although one (growth hormone) seems to be produced in greater amounts than normal, the level of the other (somatomedin-C) is significantly decreased. The net result is that growth is retarded. Very young girls are at risk for diminished height if they do not get treated and reverse their malnutrition before closure of the growth plates in their legs.

Another, less dire effect of anorexia nervosa is that it causes growth of fine, downy hair all over the body, much like that which covers the bodies of newborn babies. It is called lanugo hair. It is thought to insulate the body in the absence of the fat layer, although this has not been proven. In our experience, young women with the disease find this hair growth worrisome. They are reassured to learn that it will disappear when normal weight is restored. Another frequent effect of anorexia nervosa is dry skin, presumably the effect of deficient dietary intake of zinc, which is found in meat, something rejected by most of these youngsters, who favor vegetables and nonfat yogurt if they eat anything at all.

Bulimia nervosa is life-threatening when self-induced vomiting lowers the blood level of potassium to the point where the heart suffers or when ipecac is used to induce vomiting. The other effects of this condition on the body include swelling of the parotid glands (the same ones enlarged by the mumps) and loss of the gag reflex, as well as some of the consequences of rapid weight loss, even if it does not cause actual malnutrition as in anorexia nervosa.

Treatment for an eating disorder should consist of individual psychotherapy by someone with extensive experience with the condition and the age group; family therapy, preferably by a different therapist, for younger and immature older adolescents; nutritional rehabilitation; and medical surveillance. Some patients also benefit from group therapy.

PANIC DISORDERS

Although panic disorders typically are not diagnosed until adulthood, if at all, they are most likely to begin during adolescence. Nearly one-half million visits to psychiatrists each year are from people who suffer from panic symptoms (Schappert 1993). They are much more common in females. One recent study, conducted in northern California, found that the risk of developing panic disorders is greatest after puberty has begun, especially in girls who enter puberty before their peers. That study also found Latinas to have a higher incidence of panic disorders than girls of other ethnic groups (Hayward et al. 1992).

Some reports (Alpert et al. 1992) suggest that panic attacks occur more commonly in people with a condition called mitral valve prolapse. This condition, which is more common in women than in men, involves redundancy of the leaflets of the mitral valve that causes them to continue upward movement into the left atrium after normal closure. It may cause no problems, but it has been implicated in a wide range of symptoms, from chest pain to palpitations and fatigue.

Although panic disorders are common, fewer than 2 percent of their victims ever get diagnosed, either because the symptoms are not considered severe enough for the patient or family to seek care or because they are misdiagnosed as an organic condition. The latter possibility is understandable when one considers the many symptoms of panic attacks: faintness or dizziness; shortness of breath; a feeling of being about to smother; palpitations or a racing heart; profuse sweating; tremors or feelings of shakiness; choking; numbness or tingling of hands or tip of nose; nausea;

chills or hot flashes; and/or chest pain or pressure. These can be so severe and overwhelming as to make the person experiencing them feel that he or she is going crazy with terror of impending catastrophe or death. The attacks occur without any warning or apparent precipitating cause and typically last only a few minutes, although they may feel as if they have gone on for an eternity.

Obviously, some of these symptoms may occasionally occur in otherwise healthy people. The diagnosis of panic disorder requires at least four of the symptoms mentioned above, as well as four attacks within one month or one attack followed by overwhelming fear of its recurrence. Also, it is important to recognize that these symptoms are the same as those that may occur with conditions such as heart attacks; arrhythmias; asthma; severe allergic reactions; "bad trips" from abused drugs such as amphetamines, cocaine, and certain hallucinogens; thyroid disease; menopause; and hyperventilation. Because of all these possibilities, a skilled physician must be consulted to figure out the cause of the symptoms. Most often, especially in adolescents, it is not difficult to make the right diagnosis with a careful history, physical examination, and possibly some simple laboratory tests to exclude other possible diagnoses.

Once the panic disorder is diagnosed, treatment is very effective. For adolescents, cognitive-behavioral therapy appears most helpful in overcoming their fear that they will have another attack. One approach consists of a trained psychotherapist inducing the symptoms ("implosion") and helping the youngster to handle the physiologic state that results. Medications including fluoxetine (Prozac) are effective in most patients. A recent study showed that with a lower dose (10 mg) of Prozac than that traditionally prescribed for other conditions, most patients improved and didn't experience the common side effects of nervousness and insomnia (Louie, Lewis, and Lannon 1993).

DEPRESSION

From adolescence on, women have twice the incidence of depression that men do. A 1989 national survey of eighth- and tenth-graders found that 34 percent of females and 15 percent of males had felt "sad and hopeless" in the previous month; 21 percent of females and 11 percent of males reported that it was "very hard" for them to cope with stressful situations at school and at home; and 18 percent of females and 9 percent of males often felt that they had nothing to look forward to (American School Health Association et al. 1989). The earlier depression starts, the more severe it is in later life and the higher the risk is of later drug use, according to Christie et al.(1988).

Although there are more deaths among adolescent males as a result of suicide, females are responsible for many more suicide attempts. It has been estimated that 20 percent of adolescent girls attempt suicide (Office of Technology Assessment 1991). In the Minnesota Adolescent Health Survey, it was reported that 7 percent of males and 14 percent of females in grades seven through twelve had made at least one suicide attempt (Auclaire and Schwartz 1986).

Some subgroups are at more risk of depression and suicide than others. For example, the rate of suicide for Native American females 15–24 years old in 1984–86 was approximately twice that for all races in the United States (7.8 per 100,000 versus 4.4 per 100,000) (May 1987). For teenagers of both sexes, this rate is lower in tribes with more traditional values. Family connectedness appears to be particularly protective for teenage girls.

Lesbian adolescents are another potentially vulnerable group. However, there are few good data. One study found adolescent lesbians to have three times the rate of attempted suicide of adult lesbians (McGrath et al. 1990). The latter rate itself is high: A national survey of about 2,000 lesbians in the mid-1980's reported that over half had thought about suicide at some time and that 18 percent had actually attempted suicide (Bradford, Ryan, and Rothblum 1994). Three-fourths of the sample reported having received counseling; of these, half had done so because of sadness and depression. (Other factors in their lives provide background for these statistics: 19 percent had been involved in incestuous relationships while growing up, nearly one-third were regular users of tobacco, and about one-third drank alcohol more than once weekly.) Most experts on this subject agree that adolescent lesbians experience a sense of isolation. Some cope by trying to hide their sexual orientation by getting a boyfriend, thereby often placing themselves at risk for complications of unprotected heterosexual activity. For those who cope by connecting with a multigenerational community of strong, self-defined women (Zemsky 1991), the outlook is more positive than for other lesbian adolescents. Similarly, friendships of all kinds provide a boost to self-esteem and ability to come out (Savin-Williams 1990).

The reasons for the higher incidence of depression in females in general, and in female adolescents in particular, are not entirely clear. A number of factors seem to contribute, and various theories, including those focused on biology, personality, development, social role, coping style, and temperament, have been offered to explain these phenomena.

Biologic Theories

Biologic explanations for the higher incidence of depression in women are of two types. The first focuses on the hormonal differences between the sexes and at different points in a woman's life cycle. The second looks to genetic differences between the sexes. It is also important to realize that depression may result from (although it may also cause) other factors, such as lack of sufficient caloric intake, drug or alcohol use, or sleep deprivation, all of which may be problems for adolescent girls. In addition, some forms of depression tend to be familial.

The biologic process of puberty itself is related to the timing of depression. Not only does depression characteristically make its appearance after puberty has begun, but it occurs earlier in girls whose biologic maturation begins early relative to their peer group (Killen et al. 1992). It may not be puberty per se but rather its timing that is the critical factor in the appearance of depression during the second decade of life for girls. Hayward et al. (1997) found that young girls studied over the course of two years from before to after puberty were more likely to develop depression if they matured earlier than their classmates, regardless of their weight. Other studies have also shown that early puberty can be problematic for girls (see Chapter 1).

It is possible that the depression is the result of hormonal effects or of some psychosocial effect of a change in appearance associated with puberty. The first possibility is problematic, given evidence of an association in both directions between levels of certain female hormones and symptoms of depression. For example, depression is a major feature of PMS and occurs at the time in the menstrual cycle when levels of estrogens are at their lowest. Similarly, the timing of postpartum depression coincides with a fall in estrogen and progesterone levels, and for some women, depression is a feature of menopause. On the other hand, some women develop depression when they are given birth control pills that contain both estrogen and progesterone. So the connection between hormone levels and depression is not clear-cut.

Another possible explanation for the association between puberty and depression is that the physical changes that puberty effects in a girl's body are responsible for the mood change. As we have already seen, puberty for girls means an increase in body fat. Society's emphasis on thinness may, therefore, lead to dissatisfaction with appearance and subsequent depression.

The genetics of depressive disorders has been studied because of the observation that they run in families. Such observations are always suspect, because family members share environmental influences as well as genes, so studies of twins reared separately are useful. These studies examine concordance rates, the percentage of cases in which, when one twin has a condition, so does the other. Reviewing the literature on twin studies of affective illness, the broader term that includes depression, Allen (1976) found that nonidentical (dizygotic) twins had a concordance rate of 11 percent for depression. For identical twins, this rate increased to 40 percent. For manic-depressive disorders, these rates were 14 percent and 72 percent for nonidentical and identical twins, respectively. These high concordance rates for depressive diseases in identical twins argue for a genetic basis. On the other hand, if genes were the only factor, the concordance rate should approach 100 percent. The fact that it does not suggests that there must be other contributing factors.

One genetic theory seeking to explain the higher incidence of depression in women is that depression results from a mutation on the x-chromosome. Because women have two of these chromosomes and men only one, women have twice the chance of having the defective "depression" gene (Winokur and Tanna 1969).

However, theoretical issues, as well as the methods used by these researchers in analyzing their results, have raised objections to their conclusions. Others have therefore approached the question differently, focusing on different patterns in fathers' and mothers' transmission of depression to their offspring. This line of investigation reasons that if depression is the result of a mutant gene on the x-chromosome, a father who is depressed will transmit the gene to all of his daughters and none of his sons, the latter only getting his y-chromosome. A mother with the mutant gene on one of her two x-chromosomes will have a 50 percent chance of transmitting it to both her sons and her daughters, each of whom gets an x-chromosome from her. Thus, if a mutant gene on the x-chromosome were the explanation, depression would be more likely in father-daughter pairs than in father-son pairs and equally common in mother-daughter and mother-son pairs. The actual studies have found father-son pairs of depressed people, evidence against the x-linked theory (Fieve et al. 1984).

In short, the weight of the evidence is that genetic factors are not the most important in determining the higher incidence of depression among females. Environmental factors must play a greater role.

Psychosocial Theories

Social roles theory focuses on the activities, behaviors, and occupations that are deemed appropriate for different groups within a given society. Women's traditional roles in all societies include child care, food preparation, and home maintenance. In addition to these domestic roles, certain additional jobs in the paid labor force have become acceptable for women in most industrial societies in the last half-century or so. These include clerical, service, and teaching positions. It has been argued that the lower status of these roles and those who hold them, as well as the absence of choice and power, render women vulnerable to depression. Seligman (1975) has coined the phrase "learned helplessness" to explain the connection between having no control over outcomes and becoming sad and developing less motivation, which he believes to be a common route to depression. Nolen-Hoeksema (1990) believes that social role theories may help explain the greater vulnerability to depression of young adolescent girls because it is during adolescence that they are choosing their later occupations. To the extent that they are steered toward low-status jobs, they will feel undervalued.

Similarly, the traditional gender differences in the courting rituals of our society place girls in a passive role, waiting to be called by boys, which Nolen-Hoeksema feels may contribute to their learned helplessness and subsequently to depression. Of interest in this regard is the observation that there are no sex differences in the incidence of depression among college students. Nolen-Hoeksema thinks that this reflects the self-selection of the emotionally healthiest of women for college, as well as the fact that their presence reflects their having overcome traditional obstacles to achieve the promise of greater career opportunities and choices. "Thus college may be a setting in which the roles and status of men and women are as close to equal as they ever are. If social-role theories of depression are correct, this equality should help to equalize the rates of depression in the sexes" (1990: 103).

Just as there are stereotypic views of gender differences in social roles, some argue that women and men possess different personality traits. Personality theories have evoked some of these differences to explain the higher incidence of depression in women. Women have been characterized as being more modest, nurturant, dependent, passive, and empathetic than men. The three major theories of personality development—psychoanalytic, behavioral, and cognitive developmental—"hold that nonassertiveness, dependency, and the tendency to be self-effacing put an individual at risk. Because these characteristics are supposedly more common in females than in males, females are more vulnerable to depression than males" (Nolen-Hoeksema 1990: 130). Nolen-Hoeksema goes on to explain the mechanisms by which personality differences may effect a higher rate of depression in women. For example, psychoanalytic theorists believe that those who cannot openly express anger and who need external validation of their self-worth will direct this anger inward and become depressed. According to behavioral theorists, lack of assertiveness results in lack of control over important events, and this helplessness leads to depression. A variation on this theme holds that those who blame themselves when things go wrong and fail to take credit for positive events are more likely to be self-effacing and less assertive, and more likely to become depressed. Finally, cognitive theorists take the position that women, being more sensitive to the opinions of others and less likely to have the confidence of their own convictions, develop a sense of incompetence and lack of self-efficacy, both of which foster depression.

Basic to these theories is the belief that women, as a group, possess different personality traits than men do. There is good reason to question this assumption. Nolen-Hoeksema does this very effectively and finds ample evidence to preclude such simplistic and facile explanations for an extremely complex situation. She concludes:

Although we should not dismiss clinical experience as an important source of information about the different types of problems men and women face, we must be cautious about basing any theories of men's and women's personalities on such information. Like other researchers, clinicians are vulnerable to the biases that may lead them to gather evidence in such a way as to bolster their initial hypothesis about a situation. . . . Clinicians who begin with the assumption that there are differences in men's and women's personalities may use this assumption to guide their search for information about the causes of depression in their male and female clients. They may look for signs that a woman who is depressed tends to be nonassertive or dependent, for example, while ignoring potential sources of depression in women that do not fit common beliefs. Thus, we should insist on clear evidence from objective studies of the causes of depression in men and women that the sex differences in depression are due to sex differences in personality traits. (1990: 158–59)

Developmental theories focus on the extent to which men and women accomplish the tasks that are central to various stages of life. The development of self-image is one of the major tasks of adolescents of both sexes and has been widely studied for that reason. Poor self-image is one of the important predictors of depression.

According to the National Girls Initiative (1990), "between ages 9 and 11, girls have confidence and a clear sense of their own identity. But then, as they reach the brink of adolescence, they receive powerful messages from adults that undermine their self-confidence, suppress their self-identity, and force them to conform to limiting gender roles." The role of the educational system in creating a gender gap in self-esteem during adolescence has been powerfully demonstrated. Girls with good self-esteem during childhood often experience falling self-esteem as early adolescents in coeducational classrooms (American Association of University Women Educational Foundation 1991).

Ethnic considerations play an important role in the development of self-esteem. African American adolescent girls appear to have better self-esteem than those of any other ethnic group. One report found that in elementary school 65 percent of black girls have high self-esteem, and that by high school 58 percent continue to feel happy with "the way I am." In the same study, white and Hispanic adolescent girls showed marked decreases in self-esteem with regard to their appearance, self-confidence, talents, family relationships, and school achievement (American Association of University Women Educational Foundation 1991). According to Nancie Zane (1988), this strong self-esteem of black girls results from family and community reinforcement.

Latinas have been found to have lower self-esteem than white or African-American girls by the time they reach high school; according to one report, 38 percent fewer Latinas had high self-esteem in high school than in elementary school (American Association of University Women Educational Foundation 1991). No research has looked at possible differences among Hispanic subgroups, although there is a study under way by Sumru Erkut of self-esteem in Puerto Rican adolescent girls (Schultz 1990; see also Garcia Coll and de Lourdes Mattel 1989).

In addition to puberty, the second decade of life is the time for major changes in cognition and in school, peer, and family pressures, as well as for solidification of sex role and object preference. Any one of these may precipitate depression. For example, sexual abuse during childhood and/or adolescence is a factor in causing depression during the adolescent years, when young girls may for the first time have the cognitive abilities to recognize and confront the reality and implications of their earlier experience. Because so many sexually abused adolescent girls run away from home, the gender breakdown among the homeless is different for adolescents than for adults. Approximately half of homeless youths are females. Many of these have symptoms of mental illness, and an estimated one-third of them are suicidal, according to one report (CEWAER 1993).

Up to this point, we have been focusing on the gender differences that contribute to mental health problems for adolescent girls. It is equally important to examine the ways in which adolescent females are advantaged in relationship to males at this period of life. Girls have a significant advantage over boys in personality development that is obvious by late childhood and lasts through middle adolescence. In his extensive "meta-analysis" of sex differences over the course of personality development, Cohn found that during adolescence, "although young boys remained bound by egocentric concerns, young girls moved toward a period of social conformity; as boys entered a conformist period, girls approached a period of emerging self-awareness. . . . Ironically, it is adolescent boys who are granted earlier dating privileges, independence, and freedom from adult supervision . . . although it is adolescent girls who display greater maturity of thought" (Cohn 1991: 261).

Early Adulthood

After adolescence, females not only experience and report more mental health symptoms but begin to constitute the majority of mental health patients. For example, in 1989–90, 59.1 percent of all visits to office-based psychiatrists were made by women. However, women were less likely than men to be served in publicly funded mental health facilities, and they were better represented in outpatient than inpatient or day treatment programs.

The distribution of diagnoses in patients seen by psychiatrists also differs with patient gender (Schappert 1993: table 7). The most notable differences include a higher prevalence of mood disorders, including manic-depressive, depressive, and anxiety disorders, among women. Men, on the other hand, have a higher prevalence of substance-related disorders, adjustment disorders, and personality disorders. A study of 18,000 American adults who were not in psychiatric therapy concluded that there are no gender differences in prevalence of mental disorders, but confirmed differences in types of disorders. This study found somatization disorders (those in which emotional distress is manifested in physical symptoms) and panic disorders to be three times as common in women as in men and found a significantly higher prevalence of eating disorders, major depression, and phobias among women. Men, on the other hand, had a higher incidence of antisocial personality conduct disorders. Schizophrenia and obsessive-compulsive disorders were equally represented among men and women (Burke et al. 1990).

Recognizing these differences helps to explain why, if men and women are equally likely to have mental disorders, women are more likely to be under treatment. For example, estimates are that approximately 17 percent of women seek treatment for depression during their lifetime, compared with approximately 11 percent of men. It is possible that men truly have a lower incidence of depression and are instead more likely to experience emotional problems that less frequently result in their seeking help. In addition, there may be differences in the ways women and men are socialized to handle distress. Depressed women may ask for help, whereas men may cope by drinking alcohol, abusing other drugs or their wives or children, or becoming workaholics or compulsive exercisers. It has also been suggested that men may regard low levels of positive feelings as normal, whereas women typically equate this experience with depression. Or part of the answer may be that women see their physicians more often than men, providing greater opportunity for their depression to be diagnosed.

Another possible explanation is physician gender bias in making diagnoses. Male physicians are also more reluctant to question male patients about possible depression (Brody 1991). This may result from gendered perceptions of personality or pathologic differences or from actual bias in the criteria used by psychiatrists for making certain diagnoses. Kaplan (1983) believes that the *Diagnostic and Statistical Manual* (American Psychiatric Association 1994) contains male biases resulting in the labeling of some behaviors as healthy in males but sick in females. The edition of the manual that Kaplan evaluated, the *DSM-III*, has been revised twice since that study was done. It will be interesting to see if these gender biases have changed.

In addition to the criteria being subject to bias, some of the tests that are used to diagnose mental disorders have been developed and tested on male populations. For example, the CAGE test for making the diagnosis of alcoholism includes an item that inquires about the frequency of physical fights. Few women engage in physical violence, even when inebriated. As a result, women would be less likely to be correctly diagnosed using this test. (See Chapter 8 for more on gender differences in problem drinking.)

More likely, however, the CAGE test would not even be administered to a woman, because many health professionals do not consider the possibility of alcoholism in women. This blind spot exemplifies a broader aspect of gender bias: the assumption by male physicians that females are likely to suffer from particular types of disorders and not from other types. Another example is provided by Warner (1978), who presented psychiatrists with identical vignettes of actual patients, differing only in whether they identified the patients as male or female. When the vignette was presented as female, the psychiatrists were more likely to make a diagnosis of "hysterical" personality; when the identical vignette had male personal pronouns, the diagnoses were equally divided between "antisocial" and "hysterical" personality. These differences cannot result from gender-neutral examination of the facts of each case; rather, they reflect the gender difference in prevalence of these two disorders. Even the name of the "hysterical" disorder reflects a long-standing bias against women by the medical profession. Its root is the Greek word for uterus; the centrality of women's reproductive role to the exclusion of everything else led early physicians to believe that the uterus and ovaries controlled every aspect of a woman's health.

TREATMENT OF MENTAL HEALTH PROBLEMS IN WOMEN

There are also gender-based differences in treatment of mental health problems. At all ages, females are more likely than males to be given medication during a visit to an office-based psychiatrist (54.4 percent versus 44.1 percent). This gender difference begins as early as the age of fourteen (Kandel and Logan 1984). This may reflect gender bias in prescribing practices among physicians, as some have suggested, or more frequent diagnosis in women of diseases that are more responsive to medication. There is evidence for both possibilities. Studies of treatment practices for the same condition in men and women show that women are more likely to be given a prescription. However, there have also been major advances in the pharmacologic treatment of depression and anxiety disorders over the last decade, and these conditions are more common in women than in men (or at least, as discussed above, they are more commonly diagnosed).

In 1981, Anderson showed that there was a statistically significant difference in the frequency with which tranquilizers were prescribed by family physicians for 25–44-year-old men and women with the same psychosocial diagnoses. The women received 1.6 times as many drugs. He did not find a significant gender difference for prescription of antibiotics, although the trend was in the same direction with women in the "middle years" receiving more. Not only are more psychotropic medications prescribed for women, but nonpsychiatrists are more likely to renew prescriptions for women than for men. Benzodiazepines (including

such brand names as Librium, Halcion, Xanax, and Valium) are dispro-
portionally prescribed to women. So is electroconvulsive therapy; for example, 70 percent of patients receiving ECT in California in 1991 were
women (CEWAER 1993).

Prescribing patterns reveal not only gender bias, but also age and
racial bias. According to the findings of the NIMH Epidemiologic
Catchment Area Study (Regier 1990), more women with Hispanic surnames over the age of 60 receive prescriptions for such psychotropic
drugs as Valium and Librium than men, Caucasian women, or younger
women do. The reasons for this divergence need to be studied. Is the prescription of a drug for a woman a reflection of stereotypic diagnosing, a
clear way for the doctor to end the visit, a consequence of the physician's
perception that women patients expect to receive medication, or a result
of drug company advertisements for psychotropic medications, which
typically depict women?

Particularly given that women are more likely than men to receive
psychoactive drugs, it is alarming that these medications were not tested
on women in the required Phase I trials, those during which drug dos-
ages were determined (see Chapter 14). There are many reasons to be
concerned about our lack of information regarding the effect of these
drugs on women at the different biologic stages of life. It is clear that the
current practice of prescribing based on information from male drug test
subjects is responsible for potentially dangerously improper (that is, either ineffective or toxic) dosing of psychoactive medications for women.
The biologic reality is that women's bodies will have different effects on
drugs (and vice versa) than those of men (see Chapters 8 and 14).

Yonkers and her colleagues (1992) have pointed out the need for
studies of possible gender differences in drug metabolism in order to better understand ultimate drug levels and proper dosing schedules for
women. Their review of the 49 English-language medical journal arti-
cles they could locate that dealt with possible gender-related differences
in the processing and effects of psychotropic drugs revealed that most
studies that included women as subjects failed to inquire about the phase
of the menstrual cycle or even if the subjects were pre- or postmenopausal. These omissions make it difficult to separate out the effects
of the drugs themselves compared with other factors that might influence drug metabolism, and there were such small sample sizes as to make

it nearly impossible to draw definite answers to the important questions posed in those studies. Despite these limitations, however, they concluded that there was sufficient information to suggest that these drugs affected women differently than men. Their findings included "1) the potential for women to have higher plasma levels of psychotropic drugs (especially when given with oral contraceptives)" and 2) greater efficacy and response at lower doses to antipsychotic agents and benzodiazepines in young women, compared with young men and "a greater likelihood of adverse reactions, such as hypothyroidism and, in older women, tardive dyskinesia" (Yonkers et al. 1992: 593).

Yonkers et al. stressed the need for research: "Too little basic and clinical research has been conducted on sex differences in therapeutic effects and side effects of psychopharmacological treatments. Addressing these differences as well as similarities will lead to safer and more effective treatment for all patients" (1992: 587). On the subject of depression, they stated, "Given the literature citing the higher prevalence of depressive disorders in women . . . the paucity of studies addressing sex-specific medication effects is surprising" (1992: 592). The few studies that have been done come to different conclusions, and their interpretations are confused by the fact that other drugs or substances (such as cigarettes) that can affect drug levels were also used in many cases. In fact, antidepressants have never been appropriately tested in women to determine the safe or effective dose at different phases of the menstrual cycle or during or after menopause.

Indeed, recent studies of specific psychotropic drugs have confirmed some of these theoretical concerns about possible gender differences in their effects. The levels of some of these drugs have been found to be higher in women than men, independent of weight and age (Simpson et al. 1990; Chouinard, Annable, and Steinberg 1986).

As already mentioned, benzodiazepine drugs are overwhelmingly prescribed for women without much information about how gender affects drug levels. One study found that diazepam (Valium) is metabolized by the oxidative system of the liver more rapidly in young women than in young men (Greenblatt et al. 1980). That study did not find this sex difference for women over the age of 62, and another study found metabolism to be slower in women of all ages than in men (MacLeod et al.

1979). It has also been found that Valium is preferentially stored in fat. This may mean that the drug level in the blood is maintained at a higher level over a longer period of time in a woman than in a man, because women have more body fat than do men.

Valium was recently tested in a small number of women and was found to have different effects, depending on the phase of the menstrual cycle. Psychoactive drugs are always prescribed with a constant dosage regimen, because that is the way they were studied in men. When women were prescribed a steady dose of Valium, their performance on certain comprehension and behavioral tasks varied with the phase of the cycle. It was consistent with "intoxication" during the menstrual phase (Ellinwood et al. 1983).

In general, according to Yonkers et al. (1992), this group of drugs is eliminated more slowly from the bodies of women than of men. The simultaneous use of birth control pills that contain estrogens inhibits their clearance from the body and decreases the rate of their absorption from the gastrointestinal tract. For example, it was found that simultaneous use of birth control pills containing estrogen prolonged the effectiveness of one commonly prescribed antidepressant, imipramine. A steady dose of imipramine may result in a blood level that is too high in the first half of the cycle and too low to be effective in the second (Abernathy et al. 1984). This is particularly significant because symptoms of depression are often worse in the latter part of the menstrual cycle, especially for women who have PMS. The implications of these findings for women taking ERT are unknown because they have never been studied—another area in need of research.

Lithium, the major drug used for treatment of manic-depressive disorders, may also affect women differently than men. Women with this condition often complain of worsening of symptoms in the second half of the menstrual cycle. Of the two studies of lithium in relationship to menstrual cycle phase, one found levels to be higher in the first half of the cycle, and the other reported no phase differences. Yonkers et al. (1992: 592) criticize this research on methodologic grounds and suggest that studies should be done that "correlate lithium levels to symptoms throughout the menstrual cycle." It has also been reported that women with manic-depressive illness are more likely than men with the same condition to discontinue their prescribed medication (lithium) because they miss the "highs" of the disease.

Recently, menstrual cycle differences in levels of two other psychoactive drugs (clonidine, an antihypertensive, and Dilantin, used to treat epilepsy) were studied by Dr. Michelle Harrison at the University of Pittsburgh. Dr. Harrison found that with a constant dosage regimen, levels of both clonidine and Dilantin were too high in the first half of the menstrual cycle and too low in the second half. This observation regarding Dilantin is particularly important because the frequency of epileptic seizures is also influenced by hormone levels and many women experience an increase in seizure frequency premenstrually.

DEPRESSION

Some estimates put the number of adult patients with depression in the United States at fifteen million, with women outnumbering men two to one. The annual economic burden of nontreatment of depressed people in this country, in terms of loss of work and poor productivity, has been estimated to be about $44 billion (Bemmann 1994). A 1991 report of the Pharmaceutical Manufacturers Association attributes 15 percent of the cost of depression to the amount lost by society owing to suicides. These figures do not include the cost of medical treatment that depressed people seek for their somatic symptoms, such as pain and loss of appetite. And there is no way to measure the cost to society of failure to treat those depressed people who commit violent crimes through direct anger or drunken driving.

The signs and symptoms of depression are quite varied. They may include loss of interest in things that once brought pleasure, extreme fatigue, difficulty falling asleep at night and/or awakening in the middle of the night, inability to get out of bed in the morning, loss of appetite, or aches in the abdomen, head, or extremities. It is, therefore, not surprising that depressed people who do seek professional help typically start with their general physicians because of concern about organic pathology. It is not uncommon for people who commit suicide to have consulted their general physician within six months of the event without their depression having been diagnosed. A 1989 study by the Rand Corporation found that nonpsychiatrists miss the diagnosis of severe depression in their patients half the time. Male patients' depression more frequently goes undiagnosed, because of physicians' bias toward suspecting depression in women and not in men (Brody 1991). In fact, women with organic disease (including heart disease) are more likely than men to be given an erroneous diagnosis of depression, especially if fatigue and appetite loss are symptoms.

As discussed above, the causes of depression among women are many. Biochemical changes in the brain, hormonal changes, situational stresses, and lack of social support may all be contributing factors. Women with depression are typically married and have children, but being single and/or childless does not protect a woman from depression. Awareness is growing of the role played by domestic violence against women in precipitating depression. It is impossible to know the extent of the problem, as most cases of this type of abuse remain unreported and/or undiagnosed (see Chapter 9), but as several million women are estimated to be abused each year, abuse may be a contributing cause in many cases of depression. Another growing cause of depression among women relates to the increase in female homelessness. Although the most visible and largest percentage of the adult homeless consists of men, 35 percent are women. Of these, the majority are single mothers with young children. For them, depression is both a common cause and a common consequence of being homeless.

Types of Depression

Women are particularly prone to several subtypes of depression. These include PMS, seasonal affective disorder, and postpartum depression.

The diagnosis of PMS is based on the occurrence during the week before menses of five or more symptoms of depression (such as fatigue, sadness, or anhedonia) that are so severe that they interfere with normal functioning and that abate shortly after menses begins (American Psychiatric Association 1986). There is considerable controversy about the existence of PMS as a distinct pathologic entity. Criteria have been variable and subjective; psychologic and biologic research has suffered from major methodologic flaws; and treatment has been largely unsuccessful (Nolen-Hoeksema 1990: 50–61). Until well-controlled prospective studies are performed using standardized assessment instruments with appropriate biochemical markers, and until there is the possibility for effective treatment, it is probably safest not to make or accept this "diagnosis." According to Nolen-Hoeksema (1990: 61),

> It is dangerous to imply through the choice of the label that an aspect of women's reproductive biology is central to a psychiatric illness—particularly in view of the unsubstantiated folklore about the effects of menstruation on women's mental health and competence. When an official label fosters negative stereotypes of women, it clearly seems premature to apply that label to a set of symptoms that are poorly understood and may not constitute a distinct disorder in themselves.

Seasonal affective disorder (SAD) is characterized by recurrent bouts of diminished energy and depressed mood in the winter that improve in the spring and summer. SAD is found predominantly in young women. Its symptoms have been found to decrease with travel toward the equator or with bright light treatments (Morin 1990).

Although women have been aware of the "baby blues" for generations, only in the last 30 years has there been any research on the condition. Three psychiatric diagnoses are now described in the postpartum period: postpartum "blues," postpartum depression, and postpartum psychosis.

The most common of these, postpartum blues, occurs in 50–80 percent of mothers, beginning within two to four days of delivery and lasting a few days. The typical symptoms are fatigue, headache, confusion, tearfulness, anxiety, lack of concentration, mild depression, and irritability. These symptoms may be natural responses to the physical stresses of childbirth (including anesthesia) and its aftermath. It has also been suggested that falling hormonal levels following delivery are responsible for feelings of sadness, as they may be in the case of PMS. The frequency and possible naturalness of these symptoms provide cause to consider whether giving them a psychiatric label is justified or even useful. The danger of assigning the label is that it may have an adverse effect on some women's self-image and may also prompt some physicians to offer treatment when none is needed.

Although it is given a separate name, postpartum depression appears to be a more severe form of the blues, affecting 10 percent of mothers and lasting six to eight weeks (Jermain 1992). The symptoms of depression are worse in the evening and include difficulty falling asleep, decreased appetite, despondency, feelings of inadequacy, decreased sexual interest, and fear about the sufferer's and her baby's health. Suicidal ideation is reportedly rare (Hopkins, Marcus, and Campbell 1984). Some of these symptoms are part of the experience of all new mothers, and here again I question the value of a psychiatric label unless it translates to improved support and care. The question of efficacy and safety of antidepressant medication for this condition is unresolved. Of particular concern is the potential adverse effect of these drugs on infants of breast-feeding mothers. There are no good data to guide the decision about their use under these circumstances (Buist, Norman, and Dennerstein 1990).

The most severe, and happily the rarest, of the three postpartum psychiatric diagnoses is postpartum psychosis. This is said to affect one to two per 1,000 mothers within two weeks of delivery. It is characterized by extreme emotional lability, mania, disorganization, and hallucinations. A major debate in the literature has revolved around whether this type of psychosis is unique to the postpartum period or part of a larger spectrum of the illness. Because it has been found that many of the women who experience this disorder have a family history of psychosis, and that in 30–40 percent of cases there is a later recurrence unrelated to pregnancy, the general feeling is that "childbirth is a significant enough psychological and physical stressor to precipitate a psychotic episode in some women, but probably only in women with a substantial underlying vulnerability to psychosis" (Nolen-Hoeksema 1990: 62).

The cause of these conditions is far from clear. Studies have produced conflicting results; researchers do not even agree on what factors are associated with their occurrence. Most important, studies have failed to establish any link between these symptoms and the hormonal environment following delivery. The risk that symptoms will recur with subsequent pregnancies is also uncertain. Various studies quote this risk as anywhere between 9.5 and 35 percent (Pitt 1975).

Treatment of Depression

Now that so much is known about the biochemistry of the brain in depression, a number of extremely effective medications exist for its treatment. It has been estimated that more than three-quarters of depressed patients can achieve symptomatic improvement from the use of these drugs, with or without brief cognitive psychotherapy (relatively short-term counseling that seeks to change negative self-perceptions and/or conflictual relationships with others). More controversial is the efficacy of electroconvulsive therapy (ECT, or electroshock therapy).

As with other mental health problems (see above), women, beginning in adolescence, are more likely than men to receive medication for their depression. One might ask whether they benefit or suffer from this practice. The few studies that have examined gender differences in treatment response have found that men have a better prognosis than women when treated with most antidepressants (Yonkers et al. 1992). This information should, however, be considered in light of possible menstrual cycle fluctuations in drug levels (see below), which had not been measured in these studies. It may be that adjusting the dosage of antidepressant medications to accommodate these variations, such as giving a lower dose in the first half of the cycle and a higher dose during the second half, would result in an effective drug level and better responses among depressed women.

PSYCHOLOGIC ISSUES OF INFERTILITY

Frequently, when the cause of a woman's health problem is not understood, the woman is blamed. From the mid-1940's to the 1960's, a time when the medical profession was attributing other conditions such as menstrual cramps to neuroticism or rejection of the feminine role (Lennane and Lennane 1973), psychologic explanations for infertility were common. Infertile women were the focus of such psychologic evaluations because of the widely held belief that they and their reproductive systems were more vulnerable to emotional stress than were their male partners. The burden of these judgmental attitudes was thus added to the sadness of their inability to bear children. It is only rather recently that appropriate research has vindicated infertile women with results that show them to be psychologically no different from their fertile peers. Moreover, women with an organic explanation for their infertility have been found to be no different as a group from those for whom no explanation can be found (Mazure et al. 1992).

Although it is now clear that emotional factors do not cause infertility, its emotional consequences are tremendous. Women have been found to react with guilt, anger, depression, lowered self-esteem, anxiety, and sexual difficulties. Marital stress is not uncommon as a consequence of repeated cycles of goal-directed intercourse, followed by hope and then disappointment. (The husband of a friend who was trying unsuccessfully for years to conceive told her, "You only think of me as a stud.") Although both partners are significantly impacted by the situation, research suggests that the impact is more profound for the woman (Collins et al. 1992). Her historic role as childbearer, first and foremost, has left its legacy.

Although failure to produce a child is not grounds for divorce in our society, many of our subcultures and ethnic groups carry judgmental attitudes toward infertile women, but not men. Studies have shown that infertile women in our society are more profoundly impacted by the stress of infertility than by other sources of stress (Andrews, Abbey, and Halman 1992). Furthermore, regardless of which of the partners is found to be infertile, women appear to be more emotionally burdened than their partners (Collins et al. 1992).

Couples electing to use ART (assisted reproductive technologies) have been found to score high on measures of independence, ambition, and creativity (Given, Jones, and McMillen 1985), as well as to exhibit need for orderliness and predictability (Hearn et al. 1987). It is also possible that these traits characterize those with the economic ability to pursue the expensive ART. The gender differences in these personality traits have not been well studied.

The advent of ART has provided infertile couples with renewed hope for conception (see Chapter 6), but it has also brought additional emotional burdens, especially during those periods of suspense while a couple awaits the outcome of technical interventions. Not surprisingly, the disappointment and grief when ART fails are similar to those experienced with any loss of a hoped-for child (Vaughan 1996). Women with a history of anxiety and depression and those without other children have a higher risk of severe emotional reactions to ART failure (Mazure et al. 1992).

The Perimenopausal Years

There remains a good deal of mythology about the mental effects of menopause. Stereotypical thinking about women and menopause led to the creation of a psychiatric diagnosis called involutional melancholia, which gave scientific credibility to the notion that loss of estrogens at the time of menopause caused depression. The symptoms of this "disease" were insomnia, apathy, anxiety, and excessive guilt. In response to studies that found no increase in depression among postmenopausal women and no unique symptoms in depressed postmenopausal women, the diagnosis of involutional melancholia was finally dropped from the 1980 edition of the *DSM*.

In a recent Pittsburgh/Duke study of 541 perimenopausal women studied prospectively for three years, no differences were found in the prevalence of anxiety, anger, depression, stress, or excitability after menopause. There were slightly more depression and somatic concerns among those postmenopausal women taking replacement estrogen, but the differences were not statistically significant. Those not on ERT, not surprisingly, reported more hot flashes (Matthews et al. 1990). This is one of the few studies that looked at women both before and after menopause. Most others focus on women who are in treatment for emotional problems and therefore self-selected for depression, or who are asked to recall events and feelings after the fact. More prospective studies are needed, preferably with random assignment of women to ERT, to avoid the possibility that women with certain mental health features are more likely to choose ERT and that these differences, rather than the hormone itself, might influence findings.

The effect of retirement, a common cause of depression among men, is just beginning to be studied among women in the United States. The findings in other countries have been mixed. It is interesting to speculate about U.S. women's reactions, in the absence of much real data. My hunch is that they would fare much better than men. Working in the paid labor force is just one of women's multiple roles; if their partners are in good health, and particularly if they are financially secure, women's connectedness with their domestic identity would not only continue but possibly even become more enjoyable. They may have the chance to travel, see grandchildren, and get back to gardening and other projects.

Women whose financial situations are not secure may face more depressing scenarios upon leaving the work force. Sadly, many women do not leave their jobs by choice; they either are laid off or must leave in order to care for dependent spouses, elderly parents, grandchildren, or all of the above. Retirement benefits for women are usually considerably less than for men because they have been paid less, because they have not been contributing to a retirement benefit for as long, because their entry into the paid labor force was delayed or interrupted by childrearing, or because they work part-time or in occupations without such benefits. Lack of adequate health insurance goes hand in hand with these problems and adds to the stress of not having a paycheck. (For more on women and health insurance, see Chapter 11.)

The Older Years

Sadly, the mental health problems of older women are often ignored or misunderstood. During their younger years, women's medical conditions are often misdiagnosed as emotional in origin. After they reach the age of 65, however, women with symptoms of mental illness are rarely given mental status evaluations by their physicians. Despite estimates that more than 20 percent of the noninstitutionalized elderly have diagnosable psychiatric illness, fewer than 2 percent of psychiatric outpatients are over 65 (Meyers, Weisman, and Tischler 1984). Of these outpatients, more are women than men; the gender difference in visits to private psychiatrists was most pronounced for those over the age of 65 (Schappert 1993: table 7). The Jacobs Institute of Women's Health (1992) reported that "tranquilizers are prescribed for elderly women at a rate 2.5 times that of elderly men." Development of the new field of geriatric psychiatry is a major step in the direction of gaining understanding and tools for prevention and treatment of some currently understudied critical issues for older women.

DEPRESSION

The true incidence of mental illness in older women is nearly impossible to estimate. For example, figures for depression in women are given as approximately seven million, but depression tends to be reported mostly in women between 25 and 44. A 1990 study in southern California found that about 5 percent of the population over the age of 65 had depression, with the prevalence approximately twice as high in women (Palinkas, Wingard, and Barrett-Connor 1990).

Although those over 60 constituted about 12 percent of the U.S. population, they committed almost one-quarter of all suicides in 1980 (McIntosh, Hubbard, and Santos 1981). It is not surprising that many older women self-medicate with alcohol or drugs and/or commit suicide when faced with depression. Although our society has focused on substance abuse and suicide as problems of adolescence, these problems are often unrecognized and poorly understood in the older age group.

Some possible causes of depression in older women are fairly obvious. Because women often outlive their husbands or become divorced, profound loss is often part of their experience. Loss is a common precipitant for depression, and if it is accompanied by loss of functional capacity, as is often the case with advancing age, women become even more vulnerable to depression. Fear of serious physical illness is another source of severe depression, as is a feeling of diminished self-worth associated with relinquishment of work roles in the home or in the paid labor force.

Some studies suggest, however, that women are less vulnerable to depression than men as they age (Nolen-Hoeksema 1990: 34). An alternative explanation for the lack of gender difference, or even slight preponderance of depression among older men, is that the depression rate of men rises relative to that of women. These findings have been explained by social role theories that suggest that men derive satisfaction, a sense of worth, opportunities for self-expression, and structure for their daily lives through the workplace (Nolen-Hoeksema 1990: 103). For men, work also provides a literal and figurative escape from pressures and problems at home. Retirement disrupts this order and deprives a man of usual sources of praise and satisfaction.

Moreover, men who typically cope with feelings of depression by distraction have fewer distractions after retirement and have more opportunities for rumination. According to Nolen-Hoeksema (1990: 103),

These enormous changes in men's lives, compounded by the physical deterioration they may experience, may be enough to make many men depressed.

For a woman who has not been working in the paid labor force, older life brings few changes in her daily routine except for the now-constant presence of her retired husband at home. But her sources of meaning and worth—namely her family and home—remain the same.

I am reminded of the comment of a friend on the occasion of her husband's retirement party, when asked what she was planning to do now that he would be home all day. She replied, "I plan to extend my part-time job to full time."

Of course, the impact of retirement on the mental health of the growing numbers of women who are now themselves in the paid labor force is yet to be well studied. If distractions are critical, however, to effective coping with feelings of depression, it is likely that older women, with their traditionally greater responsibility for homemaking, will fare better than retired men.

Malnutrition, which may occur in the elderly because of poverty, can also cause symptoms of mental disorders such as depression and personality disorders. Personality disorders are particularly associated with deficiency of riboflavin. Dementia, with symptoms ranging from confusion and disorientation to hallucinations, seizures, and frank psychosis, can result from deficiency of niacin, whether from inadequate intake or from alcoholism. Many of these problems are more common among the elderly than in other age groups.

Many of the women who receive antidepressants are post-menopausal. As is the case with younger women, antidepressants have so far seemed to be less effective for older women than for men. Because no studies have been done on blood levels (or effectiveness, for that matter) of antidepressants following menopause, the poorer outcome reported for women may simply be a reflection of their not receiving the correct dose, rather than any sex difference in response, per se.

There is a higher rate of serious complications from antipsychotic medication in women over the age of 67; although this has not been studied, it may be the result of their having lost the protective effect of estrogens (Smith, Kucharski, and Oswald 1979).

The use of the controversial ECT as treatment for depression has been growing among the elderly. In California in 1991, for example, more than half of patients receiving ECT were over 65 (CEWAER 1993). Although no gender breakdown was provided in this study, it is highly likely that ECT recipients over 65 are mostly women, given the larger number of women in that age group, the fact that more women than men over 65 see psychiatrists, and the generally higher number of depressed women than men in all age groups. This is of great concern because of the questionable effectiveness and side effects of ECT and the possibility, because most of the people prescribed this treatment (at least in California) were women covered by Medicare, that poor women are receiving a different standard of care than men and more affluent women. This problem will surely worsen with managed care owing to the increasing amounts of copayments, caps on psychiatric treatment, and exclusions.

ALZHEIMER DISEASE

Alzheimer disease is a progressive degenerative disorder that causes the brain to atrophy, with degeneration most apparent in the areas responsible for intellectual functioning, including memory. It is associated with loss of chemicals such as acetylcholine that are needed for communication between nerve cells. The cause is unknown. Although it does not directly cause death, over its average duration of about eight years it renders the sufferer more susceptible to other causes of death.

Alzheimer disease strikes men and women equally, yet more than 60 percent of deaths from Alzheimer occur in women, making it the tenth leading cause of death for women over 65 (at least in California in 1988). As the underlying cause of death, its rate among women rose from 0.3 per 100,000 in 1979 to 3.9 per 100,000 a decade later. Until recently, the explanation has been that more women live to the age range at which the disease is likelier to strike. Some recent intriguing research suggests that estrogen is critical to maintaining the integrity of the neurologic connections in the brain and that when these levels fall after menopause, the nerve cells are more likely to degenerate and die (Sohrabji, Miranda, and Toran-Allerand 1994). That may explain why young women are pro-tected and older women more vulnerable to Alzheimer disease. It appears to suggest that the disease should be more frequent among men, because of their lower levels of estrogen, but this research finds that testosterone is converted to estrogen in the brain. Since testosterone levels stay high until perhaps after the age of 80, men have more protection throughout their lives than do women. A recent study (Tang et al. 1996) of 1,124 elderly women found a 5.8 percent incidence of Alzheimer disease among women who had taken ERT and a 16.39 percent incidence among those who had not. Moreover, this study concluded that the longer women take estrogen, the lower the risk.

Another interesting finding is that fatter women may have a lower incidence of Alzheimer disease than those who are thin. It appears that estrogen is processed in fat tissue and slowly released, which possibly maintains a higher effective level of estrogen (Tang et al. 1996).

What is the meaning of this research for consideration of ERT? A study of more than 2,400 women found that those who took replacement estrogen had a 40 percent lower chance of developing Alzheimer disease than those who did not (Henderson and Buckwalter 1994). This finding supports those of a long-term study of women who had undergone surgical menopause, half of whom were placed on estrogens and the other half on placebo pills. This study, conducted by a psychologist who did not know which pill the subjects were taking, found that the women who were taking estrogen had better verbal memory than those who were not (Sherwin 1988). A later randomized, more extensive study of well-adjusted women who were placed on medication or placebo just for the study did not find any difference in memory as a result of estrogen, but it did find less depression and an overall improvement in quality of life for the women taking it (Ditkoff et al. 1991). (See Chapter 3 for further discussion of ERT.)

Scientists are now trying to extend these studies and learn how estrogen might affect the brain. Studies in rodents suggest the possibility that estrogen stimulates nerve growth factors, as well as the enzyme choline acetyltransferase, which is needed to produce acetylcholine, the transmitter of messages between nerve cells in the area of the brain responsible for memory. Both of these factors are thought to be impaired in humans with Alzheimer disease. For example, in the brain of a patient with Alzheimer, the level of choline acetyltransferase is between 60 and 90 percent of normal. This finding is thought to be responsible for the deficits in memory and cognition, as well as the psychosis, that characterize this condition. Tang et al. (1996) postulate that estrogen may promote the growth and survival of the nerve connections that facilitate transfer of information and may decrease the deposition of amyloid in the cerebrum.

In summary, throughout the life span of women, their biologic uniqueness and social circumstances combine to produce a variety of mental health problems. Not enough is yet known about the precise causative factors, prevention, or best treatment at different stages of life.

CHAPTER EIGHT

Substance Abuse

In this chapter we examine the phenomenon of women using potent chemicals that have not been prescribed for medicinal purposes but that meet some self-defined need, either physiologic, psychologic, or social. The chemicals to which we will devote the greatest attention are two of those that are most commonly used: alcohol and nicotine. As is done throughout this book, differences among women at different stages of the life cycle will be explored.

Adolescence

Abuse of illicit substances by teenagers has historically been the almost exclusive domain of boys. Recently, however, the gender gap in substance abuse has narrowed considerably, and for some substances, teenage girls are actually surpassing the boys in prevalence of abuse. Girls' use of these substances reflects different motivations than boys' and has different effects on their performance and emotional state. The special biologic features of some drugs also lead to unique complications for young girls.

The reasons for the observed increase in substance abuse by adolescent women are many. Some have invoked changing social attitudes toward traditional gender roles as the explanation (Engs and Hanson 1990). Another perspective points out that women are socialized from an early age to seek chemical solutions to their problems. Physicians more frequently prescribe antidepressants to adolescent females than to adolescent males, thus sanctioning a chemical response to women's depression, which often begins in adolescence. Along similar lines, use of illicit substances and alcohol may be viewed as "self-medication" giving depressed adolescent women temporary respite from their pain.

In addition, the pressure to conform to society's standard of female thinness also helps to understand abuse of substances such as cigarettes, amphetamines, and cocaine, as well as over-the-counter medications such as diuretics, laxatives, and ipecac to promote weight loss. The still rare, but growing, use of anabolic steroids among adolescent females can also be understood as being aimed at change in appearance (as well as improved athletic performance), in this case development of a body that is more muscular.

As with male adolescents, there are additional factors, such as peer pressure to abuse some of these agents, as well as the perceived assistance derived from agents such as alcohol in decreasing anxiety and inhibitions in some socially stressful situations. Poor self-image, more commonly a problem for adolescent females, further contributes to the need for artificial bolstering under these conditions. Desire to appear more mature also contributes to the use of some substances, such as cigarettes, a fact not lost on the advertisers of these commodities.

ALCOHOL

The gender gap in adolescents' alcohol use is narrowing, and for certain categories of use, adolescent females have surpassed their male counterparts. Among young adolescents with chronic illnesses, my experience has been that more girls than boys admit to alcohol use.

Among college women, the age-old gap between male and female drinking rates has recently disappeared. A survey in 1992, for example, found virtually no difference in alcohol use in the past year between male and female college students (89 and 88 percent, respectively) (Johnston, O'Malley, and Bachman 1993). Although both sexes increase their alcohol use during the first year of college, the frequency of use during that year now appears to be greater for women than men (Berkowitz and Perkins 1987). The rate of drinking "abusively" (i.e., drinking in order to get drunk) in women more than tripled between 1977 (10 percent) and 1993 (35 percent). This rate is now comparable to that of men (*New York Times*, natl. ed., May 22, 1994, reporting a study by J. Merrill of the Center on Addiction and Substance Abuse at Columbia University). The Merrill study underscores the increased risk to young women who drink to the point of drunkenness: 90 percent of all campus rapes occur when victim or assailant or both are under the influence of alcohol, and 60 percent of college women who contract STDs do so under these circumstances.

Sex differences in the body's handling of alcohol are important in this regard. When a teenage couple on a date drink the same amount of alcohol, the female will become more intoxicated than the male (because of hormonal and weight differences), and the effect will likely last longer (because of her greater tendency to store alcohol in fat). This sort of information should be more widely disseminated to adolescent women because of its implications for both driving safety and personal safety.

Race-by-gender differences in alcohol use are of interest. For example, among college students attending a Texas university in a border town, no ethnic differences in patterns of alcohol use were found for the men. On the other hand, among the women, Anglos were more likely to be drinkers than Mexican-Americans (80 percent versus 63 percent) (Trotter 1982). Among young pregnant adolescents, another study also found less substance abuse in Mexicans and Mexican-Americans than in Anglos (Mendoza and Litt, unpublished data, 1984). Another study found more alcohol intoxication among white than black women in two southeastern colleges (Humphrey, Stephens, and Allen 1983).

It may be that more males than females continue patterns of excessive alcohol consumption begun in adolescence. Jessor (1987) found that of a group of adolescents who were considered to be "problem drinkers" in 1972, females (26 percent) were half as likely as males (49 percent) to be so categorized seven to nine years later.

But it is difficult to assess the accuracy of such statistics, because even the definition of "problem drinking" is gendered, having been based on the sequelae of drinking in men. Problem drinking is typically defined as drinking that results in property damage, physical injury to others, or blacking out. The first two of these are more commonly related to the male drinking experience. Other criteria for problem drinking are possible, criteria that are gender-neutral. For example, Perkins (1992) found

no gender differences in the consequences of heavy drinking in the categories of physical injury to self, memory loss, or unintended sexual activity. Prendergast (1994: 105), in his recent review of substance abuse
among college students, writes,

> If more attention were paid to such problems . . . of women as depres-
> sion, damage to interpersonal relationships, physical or sexual assault,
> or unwanted pregnancy, it is likely that higher estimates of the nature
> and extent of drinking problems among women would be obtained. If
> more attention were to be given to problems that are less public and
> that are less likely to involve legal action, then differences between
> men and women may narrow substantially.

The causes of alcoholism in male and female adolescents may be different. A study examining the correlates of drinking problems in male
and female college undergraduates found that, compared with their female peers who did not report drinking problems, women with drinking
problems were more likely to perceive a poor relationship with their
mothers, parental rejection, parental depression, maternal drinking problems, physical abuse by a parent, an unhappy childhood, suicidal thoughts,
and a feeling of worthlessness. In contrast, for college men the differences
between problem and nonproblem drinkers involved the former's perceptions of overprotective parents, frequent conflicts with and between
parents, engagement in delinquent behaviors, and feelings of lack of productivity. The only area of overlap was that, in comparison to nonproblem drinkers, problem drinkers of both genders felt tired more often than
refreshed.

The health consequences of alcohol abuse by adolescent females
have not been adequately studied. Animal studies and the experience of
older women suggest that these young women are at increased risk of
menstrual abnormalities such as prolonged menstrual periods.

CIGARETTES

Overall, it is estimated that 16 percent of teenage girls smoke regularly
and another 28 percent try cigarettes occasionally. Currently, there are
more adolescent girls than boys starting to smoke. A higher percentage

of these girls are white than African-American or Latina. There was a 110 percent increase in adolescent females' smoking between 1967 and 1973, according to a recent study (Pierce, Lee, and Gilpin 1994). Most studies report no gender difference in the overall percentage of male and female adolescent smokers. Such general statements mask the reality that in many places in the United States, there are actually more female than male adolescent smokers. For example, in 1991, in Philadelphia, 22 percent of adolescent females smoked and 17 percent of adolescent males did so. In New York City, it was 26 percent females and 16 percent males; in Hawaii, 27 percent females and 25 percent males; in South Dakota, 32 percent females and 30 percent males) (CDC 1992a: 699).

One of the health goals of the U.S. Public Health Service for the year 2000 is reduction of smokers to 15 percent of the population. To accomplish this goal, it is critical to prevent smoking before it begins. Research at Stanford University (McAlister, Perry, and Maccoby 1979) showed that it was possible to prevent smoking if one began early enough and provided young people with the skills necessary to reduce peer pressure on them to smoke. The study showed that intervening at the seventh-grade level and using peers to model resistance behaviors was effective in this regard. Such strategies are and continue to be effective for males, for whom peer pressure is the overwhelming stimulation for smoking.

For females, however, the reasons for smoking are often different. Young women in our society have learned that smoking is an effective way to curb their appetites and hence to help them be thin. A study of adolescents' attitudes about smoking found that 30 percent of smokers and only 13 percent of nonsmokers (of both sexes) believed that smoking helps people to keep their weight down (Teenage tobacco use 1993). Undoubtedly, female smokers would be represented in an even larger percentage had the data been analyzed separately for them. This attitude is fostered by tobacco company advertisements that feature thin, attractive models. According to Pierce, Lee, and Gilpin (1994), there was a correlation between increased advertisements of "women's" brands of cigarettes and increased demand among girls.

Adolescent smokers of both sexes are more likely to be doing poorly in school and to drop out. It is not clear what the direction of the relationship may be. Nonetheless, smoking appears to be a marker for poor school performance.

The health consequences of smoking during the adolescent years are not well studied. For the growing numbers of female athletes, however, the known adverse effect of smoking on lung capacity is surely important. It remains to be seen whether smoking during puberty will have the same adverse effect on bone density as it surely has in later life.

Not only are more adolescent women now starting to smoke, but once women start to smoke, they are more likely than men to continue to do so (Schoenborn and Boyd 1989). It has been reported that although 77 percent of women have tried to quit smoking, only 1.5 percent are successful (Kaufman 1994). This stands in stark contrast with the reported intention of 92 percent of female adolescent smokers not to be smoking the next year. Moreover, the younger a woman is when she begins smoking, the more likely she is to continue (U.S. Department of Health and Human Services 1987b).

Despite the likelihood that smoking will begin in adolescence, a study of physicians showed that they were less likely to discuss smoking and its consequences with their adolescent patients than with other patients (Frank et al. 1991).

OTHER ILLICIT DRUGS

Just as the gender gap is closing for alcohol use, so is it for abuse of other substances. Among college students surveyed in 1992, for example, approximately one-third of both men and women reported abuse of an illicit drug in the past year (Johnston, O'Malley, and Bachman 1993). Use of marijuana was reported by 25 percent of women and 28 percent of men; abuse of inhalants, by 2 percent of women and 5 percent of men; abuse of hallucinogens (largely LSD), by 4 percent of women and 9 percent of men; and abuse of cocaine, by 3 percent of women and 4 percent of men.

Many abused substances (e.g., heroin and anabolic steroids) cause women, particularly teenage women, to stop ovulating, and hence to stop menstruating completely (Litt and Schonberg 1975). Similar information on possible sex differences in the effects of other abused substances is clearly needed.

DIAGNOSIS AND TREATMENT

One consequence of the failure to view substance abuse as a problem of women is the lack, until recently, of gender-appropriate models for treatment and cure of those who become habituated or addicted. This is particularly true for adolescent females; most of the available resources for drug-abuse problems are based on theoretical assumptions that do not generally work for this age and gender group. For example, the common practice of denigrating addicts in order to remove their defenses may be counterproductive for adolescent females whose reasons for turning to drugs in the first place relate to their still-fragile self-image. Those whose depression is rooted in childhood experiences of physical and/or sexual abuse may, in addition, be further traumatized by this type of approach. The paucity of available programs for female adolescent substance abusers is matched only by the paucity of reliable research upon which to build more appropriate approaches.

Even more worrisome than these problems is the realization that substance abuse by adolescent women is rarely even detected by their physicians. One reason for this failure is the infrequency of contact with the medical profession of otherwise healthy adolescents, a problem that will become worse with the spread of managed care. But even for adolescent females with chronic illness, who are in frequent contact with the health care system, pediatric specialists rarely inquire about the possibility of substance abuse (Litt and Wanat, unpublished data, 1996). Pediatricians, when queried about this, often report that their training did not prepare them to diagnose, let alone refer or manage, substance abuse problems; this underscores the need for physician reeducation.

Early Adulthood

The gender gap in substance abuse among adults, as among adolescents, has narrowed considerably in recent years. Many drugs are susceptible to abuse by women. In California in 1989, women accounted for 25 percent of heroin addicts and 40 percent of cocaine users. Benzodiazepines, too, which are disproportionately prescribed to women (see Chapter 7), are often subsequently abused because of their sedative effect.

ALCOHOL

National estimates suggest that between one-third and one-half of all alcohol-dependent adults are women (CEWAER 1993). In California in 1989, almost half of the alcohol-related deaths from diseases and injuries occurred in women.

If a woman and a man consume the same amount of alcohol, the woman will have a higher blood alcohol level, and it will take longer for that level to fall. There are several reasons for this. Women generally weigh less than men, and their bodies contain more fat. Alcohol is fat-soluble, so alcohol is stored and slowly released into the bloodstream, resulting in a longer-lasting effect. Also, blood levels and effects of alcohol vary during the course of the menstrual cycle and in response to prescribed hormones, such as those found in birth control pills. Chronic use of alcohol may cause these hormones to be excreted more rapidly, thereby decreasing their protective ability. Alternatively, the blood alcohol level may be higher because of the chronic use of contraceptive hormones.

Many of the psychoactive drugs widely prescribed for women have potentially serious and dangerous side effects when taken by people who also consume alcohol. Alcohol can affect drug levels in two ways. First, it stimulates the production of enzymes (chemicals that enhance other chemical reactions) in the liver. Some of these reactions control the rate of drug processing. As a result, certain drugs (e.g., certain anticoagulants) pass through the liver more rapidly, which reduces the time that they are in the bloodstream and therefore effective. Second, alcohol enhances the action of other drugs. These include anticonvulsants, tranquilizers, sleeping medications, antidepressants, and certain painkillers, such as Darvon. In turn, many of these drugs interfere with the metabolism of alcohol and enhance its effects. Other medications, such as Flagyl, Orinase, and Antabuse, cause abdominal pain when taken together with alcohol. (This feature is the basis for the use of Antabuse in some alcohol treatment programs.)

Despite these serious potential complications, women patients are rarely asked by their physicians if they drink alcohol regularly, because of the stereotype that alcoholism is not a problem for women. This is another example of gender bias that impacts adversely on women's health.

CIGARETTES

Fewer women begin to smoke after high school graduation than before, but because it is so difficult for those who have begun smoking in adolescence to stop, there are many adult women smokers. After the age of 25, it is estimated that one in three women is a smoker. Between 1965 and 1985, the percentage of female heavy smokers (those who smoke 25 or more cigarettes each day) increased from 13 to 23 percent, despite a 21 percent decline in the total number of adult women smokers during that same time period (Horton 1992: 82). This decline stopped abruptly in 1991, apparently because more young white women began smoking. Looking beyond America, the trend worldwide is toward more women starting and fewer women quitting than men (Pierce 1989).

Many women smoke to curb their appetites and cite fear of weight gain as the reason they don't stop. Women smokers express more concern about gaining weight should they stop smoking than men (Pirie, Murray, and Leupker 1991). The commonly agreed upon explanation for ethnic differences in women's smoking rates is that white women are more likely to use smoking for weight control. Their fears are well founded in that research shows that smokers actually do weigh less than nonsmokers (Albanes et al. 1987) and that weight gain follows smoking cessation in both men (Gordon et al. 1975) and women (Williamson et al. 1991).

A Swedish study (Lissner et al. 1992) confirmed the earlier finding of less obesity in women smokers but found a difference in fat deposition between smokers and nonsmokers. Women who smoked had more upper-body fat than nonsmokers of similar weight. This finding is important because the risk of coronary heart disease, stroke, and diabetes is increased in people with more upper-body fat (the "apple" distribution). The study also found that the weight women gained after they stopped smoking was not deposited in the apple pattern. In other words, that weight should not be considered as detrimental to their health, and the advantage of smoking cessation may overshadow any minor increase in risk associated with weight gain. This may not be sufficient motivation, however, for women who smoke to stay thin out of concern for fashion, rather than health.

If health concerns were paramount in women's minds, they would never smoke. There has been substantial publicity about the serious health consequences of smoking in general, although less about the devastating effects smoking has had on women in particular. The most obvious of these effects has been the increase in lung cancer in women smokers corresponding to the post–World War II increase in their numbers. From 1975 to 1991, the incidence of lung cancer among women increased 65 percent to a rate of more than 41 per 100,000. The death rate for lung cancer among women has similarly skyrocketed to 31 per 100,000, a 31 percent increase. Lung cancer is now the leading cause of cancer deaths among women, with about 55,000 dying each year from the disease, as compared to 44,000 from breast cancer. It is estimated that it takes about fifteen years after a woman quits smoking for her risk of lung cancer to return to that of a nonsmoker (U.S. Department of Health and Human Services 1980).

Some (most prominently, the tobacco industry) have argued that the increase in lung cancer paralleled an increase in air pollution, and have tried to dismiss or minimize the implications of smoking. If air pollution were the culprit, however, we would expect to see an increase in lung cancer in men as well as women. But the rate of lung cancer has actually leveled off for men over the past fifteen years; it has increased 2.5 percent, versus the 65 percent for women. The increase cannot, therefore, be explained by the air we breathe; rather, it strongly incriminates cigarettes.

Moreover, a recent study done by epidemiologists at Yale University (Risch et al. 1993) concludes that cigarettes pose more of a lung cancer threat to women than to men. This study matched more than 400 women with lung cancer with similar numbers of healthy women, healthy men, and men with lung cancer. They expressed cigarette exposure in terms of pack-years, with one pack-year equal to 7,305 cigarettes. They found that for women who were currently smoking and had fewer than 30 pack-years, the risk of getting lung cancer was seven times higher than that of nonsmoking women. For male smokers in this same exposure category, the risk was only five times that of nonsmoking men. For women with 30 to 60 pack-years, the risk of getting lung cancer was 27 times higher than that of nonsmoking women; the risk of men in this category was only 11 times higher than that of their nonsmoking counterparts. Above 60 pack-years, the risks for women and men smokers, compared to their sex-matched peers, were 82 and 23 times higher, respectively.

The risk of lung cancer is also 30 percent higher for women whose husbands smoke than for those whose husbands do not. In addition, the risk is 39 percent higher for women regularly exposed to smoke in the workplace (Fontham et al. 1994). This study did not examine the effect of wives' smoking on their husbands' risk of lung cancer nor the risk of men exposed to workplace smoke.

Lung cancer is not the only cancer whose risk is increased among women smokers. Current smokers have a significantly higher risk of developing cancer of the cervix, according to a recent study that carefully reviewed all studies published in the medical literature between 1966 and 1988 (Licciardone et al. 1990). The rate of cervical cancer is also increased, but to a lesser degree, among women exposed to "passive" smoke (Licciardone et al. 1990).

The cancer risk most recently linked to smoking is that of breast cancer. A higher rate of death from breast cancer in smokers has now been established (Calle et al. 1994). It is not clear if this relationship is due to other behavioral differences between smokers and nonsmokers, such as in diet and exercise, or if there is actually a biologic effect of smoking per se.

Smoking has also been linked to an increased risk for developing polyps in the colon, a precancerous condition in both men and women, but results for the research on colon cancer among women has produced conflicting results. The risk of cancer of the colon and rectum is higher among women doctors in Britain who smoke than those who don't (Doll et al. 1980). But another study found an inverse relationship between smoking in women and their risk of developing colon cancer; the researchers hypothesized that this might reflect the antiestrogenic effect of smoking (Sandler et al. 1988).

Women smokers are also at increased risk for serious diseases other than cancer. The leading cause of death among both female and male smokers is heart disease. Women who smoke have a higher risk of death from coronary artery disease than nonsmokers, likely related to their lower blood levels of HDLs. They run significantly higher risks of sudden death and death from stroke (subarachnoid hemorrhage), chronic obstructive lung disease, and high blood pressure. Although these risks are highest for women over the age of 65, smoking increases the risk of heart attack and stroke in women as young as 35 who are taking estrogen-containing birth control pills (see Chapter 6). For all of these reasons, smoking is considered the single most important preventable cause of early death and disease among women.

Furthermore, pregnancy and smoking do not mix. Smoking can impair fertility; this risk was found to be greatest for women who smoke one or more packs of cigarettes daily and who began to smoke before the age of eighteen (Laurent et al. 1992). The mechanism for this effect is not entirely clear, but in animal studies, nicotine has been shown to reduce ovulation, blood flow to the ovary, and secretion of some reproductive hormones. Laurent et al. suggest that smokers who are having difficulty conceiving should be advised to stop smoking.

The harmful effects of smoking on the fetus are well recognized. The pregnant woman who smokes places her baby at tremendous risk of health problems and even death. The risk of all complications of pregnancy is increased for smokers. For spontaneous miscarriage, for example, the risk for a smoker is 1.7, compared with the risk for a nonsmoker of 1. The relative risks for premature birth and for death of the fetus or newborn are 1.36 and 1.15, respectively, compared to a nonsmoker's standard risk of 1 for both complications. The more the woman smokes, the greater is her risk of miscarriage, stillbirth, and death of her baby after birth. Passive exposure of pregnant women to smoke in the workplace in the first trimester of pregnancy also increases the risk of miscarriage and stillbirth.

Birth weight is one of the most important determinants of the health of the newborn baby. The risk of having a low-birth-weight baby is almost twice as high for smokers as for nonsmokers (U.S. Department of Health and Human Services 1980). Low-birth-weight babies are at increased risk of death. Even among those who are within the normal weight range, babies of smokers weigh an average of 200 g less than babies of nonsmokers.

Mindful of these problems, more than one-third of female smokers apparently stop smoking during pregnancy. While that is encouraging, the lag time until women know they are pregnant results in exposure of many fetuses. In addition, there is a high rate of relapse after delivery, with one report claiming that 70 percent of women who stop smoking while pregnant resume within one year, most of them within three months after delivery (Fingerhut, Kleinman, and Kendrick 1990). Their babies' passive exposure to smoke increases their risk of upper airway problems (U.S. Department of Health and Human Services 1987a).

The Perimenopausal Years

Alcohol continues to take its toll on perimenopausal women, but smoking is the far greater danger (see above under Early Adulthood for more on both). Smoking continues to cause increased risks of heart disease, chronic obstructive lung disease, lung and cervical cancer, high blood pressure, and stroke from cerebral hemorrhage. Because smoking decreases estrogen levels, it is associated with an increased risk of osteoporosis. It also appears to generally suppress the body's defense against a variety of harmful agents by reducing levels of immunoglobulins and naturally occurring killer cells.

On the positive side, there is some evidence that, because smoking decreases estrogen levels, it may also decrease the risk of developing cancer of the lining of the uterus. It was previously thought to be similarly protective against breast cancer, but a recent study (Calle et al. 1994) shows the opposite to be true.

In addition to its major health hazards, there has been concern about the possible effect of smoking on the skin. After reviewing five studies conducted during the past two decades, Grady and Ernster (1992) concluded that there was sufficient evidence that in whites smoking causes skin wrinkling, particularly around the eyes ("crow's feet"). Smoking may do this by lowering estrogen levels, by decreasing blood flow to the skin, and possibly by damaging the connective tissue that maintains the skin's integrity.

The rate of quitting smoking is highest in the older age groups, probably because of health concerns, but more males than females quit. A California study reported that doctors were more likely to advise men with a history of heart disease or stroke to quit smoking than they were women (Frank et al. 1991).

The Older Years

ALCOHOL

Information about alcohol abuse among older women is very hard to come by. Alcoholism has been traditionally viewed by our society as a problem of men, and it is therefore difficult to learn much about it in women of any age. In addition, because our society is more aware and concerned about substance abuse in the young, little research has focused on older men or women. What we do know is that the incidence of heavy alcohol consumption peaks at about the age of 50 and then declines until about the age of 70, after which there is a slight rise. Gender differences in these figures have not been reported (see Abrams and Alexopoulos 1987).

The elderly are more sensitive to the effects of alcohol, suffering functional impairment with smaller doses (Morse 1988). In addition, some of the common nutritional deficiencies of older age may be the result of, or misdiagnosed because of, alcoholism. Alcoholism is the most common cause of deficiency of thiamin (vitamin B_1), which can cause a number of symptoms simulating depression and organic illnesses (see Chapter 10). It is also responsible for deficiency of riboflavin (vitamin B_2), niacin, Vitamin A, and zinc, as well for caloric deficiency resulting when other foods are shunned or not affordable. Finally, failure to consider the possibility of alcohol use in elderly women may put them at considerable risk when they are given prescription drugs.

CIGARETTES

Despite the fact that many women stop smoking when health consequences force them to do so, almost 14 percent of women over 65 still smoke (National Center for Health Statistics 1991). This is of particular concern given the potential harm caused by nicotine, including worsening osteoporosis; increased risk of heart attack, cancer, and stroke; and peripheral circulatory disorders, to say nothing of wrinkles. Those with diminished sense of smell are also at increased risk for accidentally setting fires.

PRESCRIPTION DRUGS

As a group, the elderly receive a disproportionate number of prescriptions of all kinds. Although they constitute only 12 percent of the country's population, they consume about one-quarter of all prescriptions written. It is not unusual for an older patient to have 30 drugs prescribed in one year (Horton 1992). Older women are more likely than older men to be given prescriptions of psychotropic medications. Tranquilizers, for example, are prescribed for elderly women at 2.5 times the rate of elderly men (Horton 1992: 82). The differential rates of tranquilizer prescription are especially striking for Hispanic women.

The frequent prescription of antidepressant drugs in this age group is of great concern, given the lack of information about the proper dosage of these drugs in postmenopausal women. The elderly, in general, have a higher incidence of untoward reactions to prescription drugs (Whitcup and Miller 1987). Women, particularly older women, have been shown to experience more untoward drug reactions than men (Horton 1992: 82). Older women apparently experience more serious complications than younger women taking antipsychotic drugs. Accordingly, it is generally recommended that the dose be reduced considerably in the elderly (Prien and Cole 1978).

It is often reported that the elderly inadvertently misuse prescribed drugs, owing to confusion about instructions. Patients may have multiple bottles of medications prescribed by different physicians who are unaware of each other's prescriptions, and they may be taking drugs that interfere with each other or that combine to cause toxic results. While the patient is typically blamed for these problems, physicians may also be responsible because they lack information about effects of drugs and drug interactions in this age group, in general, and in postmenopausal women, in particular.

Added to these problems are the fact that older women often self-medicate with over-the-counter medications and substances such as alcohol. One study found that 64 to 76 percent of women over the age of 65 used nonprescription drugs. More of these drugs were used by depressed women (Chrischilles, Foley, et al. 1992). Depression was also found to be a factor in the higher use of both prescription and nonprescription pain medications by women over the age of 65 (Chrischilles et al. 1990).

The effects of drug combinations can be disastrous. Twenty percent of geriatric patients (gender not discussed) in one general hospital had been admitted because of side effects of prescription drugs (World Health Organization 1981). Another study estimated that adverse drug reactions among noninstitutionalized elderly people were responsible for 2.2 million visits to doctors, 1.1 million laboratory tests, and 146,000 hospitalizations each year in the United States alone (Chrischilles, Segar, and Wallace 1992).

Another factor that is unstudied but potentially important and that may affect drug levels and effects is poor nutrition in older women. Conversely, the prescription of certain psychotropic drugs (such as chloropromazine, imipramine, and amitriptyline) can interfere with riboflavin absorption and metabolism, further contributing to the malnutrition of older women.

CHAPTER NINE

Violence

It goes by many names: infanticide, sexual abuse, sexual misuse, child abuse, rape, domestic violence, spousal abuse, elder abuse. Although the definitions, the demographics, the geography, the details, and the laws may differ, these are all in the final analysis variations on the same theme: violence against women.

Childhood and Adolescence

Approximately half a million abused and neglected children are reported each year in the United States. The rate of maltreatment increases with age. A 1986 study, for example, found the rate per 1,000 children to rise from six for children under the age of two to ten for those three to five years old and fifteen for those between six and eleven. In the military, the overall rate for child abuse (ages not specified) rose from 6 per 1,000 in 1988 to 6.6 per 1,000 in 1993, paralleling a rise in spousal abuse during the same period (*New York Times*, natl. ed., May 23, 1994).

A recent report of the Carnegie Corporation showed that "one in three victims of physical abuse is a baby less than a year old. In 1990, more one-year-olds were maltreated than in any previous year" (Carnegie Task Force on Meeting the Needs of Young Children 1994). Fifty-two percent of reported cases of abuse of children less than eleven years of age involve physical abuse.

Sexual abuse more commonly victimizes female children, and males are more subject to other forms of child abuse. In 90 percent of cases of sexual abuse, the violence begins before age twelve; a retrospective study of adults who had been victims of sexual abuse in their youth found the average age of onset to be seven and a half (Kendall-Tackett and Simon 1988). Intrafamilial abuse is the most common type for female children, but little girls may also experience violence at the hands of strangers.

In childhood, there is a 9 percent fatality rate from abuse. This totals approximately 45,000 deaths a year! The leading cause of death among children one to four years old is unintentional injury. Nearly 90 percent of children who died as the result of abuse and neglect in 1990 were under the age of five (Carnegie Task Force 1994).

Although adolescents make up just 38 percent of the population under the age of eighteen, they account for almost half of all reported cases of child abuse. This translates to approximately one-half million cases per year in the United States. A 1986 survey of reported cases of maltreatment put the rate at 23 per 1,000 for twelve-to-fourteen-year-olds and 28 per 1,000 for fifteen-to-seventeen-year-olds (Office of Technology Assessment 1991). As with other cases of domestic violence, true figures about the incidence of adolescent abuse are difficult to obtain, because of gross underreporting and the fact that most large surveys aggregate adolescents with children.

There are two schools of thought about the genesis of maltreatment of adolescents. The first takes the position that patterns of abuse are established during childhood and continue into adolescence. The second holds that much of the abuse that takes place in the second decade of life reflects the inability of a previously functional family to adjust to the challenges of adolescence. Both explanations are probably true and additive. For sexual abuse of girls, however, the first theory seems more applicable. Some types of child abuse are likely to stop in adolescence; in more than half the cases in one study, the sexual abuse that had begun during childhood ceased after the age of twelve (Kendall-Tackett and Simon 1988). In contrast, females are more likely to be physically abused in adolescence than in childhood (Office of Technology Assessment 1991: II-45).

Females are also more likely to be abused during adolescence than are males. A 1975 study by the National Center on Child Abuse and Neglect found two female adolescent maltreatment victims for every one male adolescent victim (Olsen and Holmes 1983). Other studies report between 55 and 77 percent of adolescent physical maltreatment victims to be females. For sexual abuse, females constitute 88 percent of cases, according to a study in New York State (Powers and Eckenrode 1988).

One of the most important predictors of abuse during adolescence is the degree and severity of spousal violence in the home (Straus and Gelles 1986). Poverty is a weaker predictor; a 1979 study found adolescent victims to be half as likely as younger children to come from families with incomes less than $7,000 per year (Office of Technology Assessment 1991).

Adolescent abuse rarely ends in death (0.01 deaths per 1,000 adolescents). However, its other consequences can be severe. Almost half of adolescent maltreatment victims have been found to have symptoms of clinical depression, and between 45 and 70 percent had problems such as "nervous habits, isolation, poor social skills with peers, lethargy, low self-esteem, low frustration tolerance, temper outbursts, and stubbornness" (Berdie et al. 1983).

In contrast to adolescent males, who often retaliate by physical attacks on their abusing parents, girls more often run away from home or try to commit suicide. One study reported that approximately 73 percent of adolescent female runaways said that they had run away to avoid further sexual abuse (McCormack, Janus, and Burgess 1986). The dangers posed to these girls by their runaway status are considerable. In one study, for example, 31 percent of female adolescents who had run away from home reported that they had engaged in prostitution (Office of Technology Assessment 1991). In my own experience working in a juvenile detention center, virtually every female runaway who was remanded by the juvenile courts in New York in the 1970's was found to have at least one sexually transmitted disease. According to Garbarino (1990), "a runaway who leaves home to escape abuse and then falls prey to AIDS, or is murdered, or becomes suicidal on the street is, in a very real sense, an 'adolescent maltreatment fatality'" (quoted in Office of Technology Assessment 1991: II-48).

In addition to the possibility of abuse from fathers, adolescent girls also face abuse from partners. Among high school students interviewed in a 1983 study, 13 percent of the girls admitted to having been physically assaulted by a date. Perhaps more alarming was the finding that 41 percent were still dating the abusing partner (Henton et al. 1983). In a 1994 study of two high schools in an upper-middle-class community in California, 8 percent of females had been touched sexually or forced to have sex against their will (Pitts and Steiner 1994).

The issue of date rape has received a lot of recent attention. Other forms of violence directed at adolescent females have not been well studied, largely because violence has been conceptualized as a problem for adolescent males. Although the incidence of male victimization is higher, it is in no way insignificant for females. In 1988, for example, the rate of victimization by rape, robbery, and assault for adolescent women was 9,000 per 100,000 population, compared to 16,000 per 100,000 for males in the same age group. When these rates are broken down to individual crimes, however, it is apparent that female adolescents are more likely than their male peers to be victims of theft (Office of Technology Assessment 1991).

Another form of victimization can be seen in the way adolescent girls are treated by the juvenile justice system. A number of reports have documented that females who are arrested for status offenses (acts committed by minors that would not be considered offenses if committed by an adult, e.g., running away from home, being truant, violating curfew, and purchasing alcoholic beverages) are treated more harshly than males by the juvenile court system. Female status offenders are more likely to be incarcerated, especially in public juvenile facilities, whereas males incarcerated for status offenses are more likely to be housed in private facilities. This double standard likely reflects society's inclination to be more "protective" of girls than of boys, but there is ample evidence that life in detention centers is anything but growth-promoting for them. It is impossible to know, for example, how many girls remanded by the courts to be "taught a lesson" have been raped, as was documented in the made-for-television film "Crime of Innocence," based on an actual case brought against a judge by the San Francisco–based Youth Law Center.

Early Adulthood and the Perimenopausal Years

Wife abuse has been practiced since antiquity. Martins, Holzapfel, and Baker (1992) reviewed some of its history; their evidence included findings of a 30–50 percent higher incidence of skull fractures in female than male Egyptian mummies 2,000 to 3,000 years old, and the fact that nine-teenth-century English common law allowed husbands to beat their wives to punish misbehavior. The term "domestic violence" was not, however, coined until 1980, when Straus, Gelles, and Steinmetz published their landmark study, *Behind Closed Doors: Violence in the American Family*, and brought it to the attention of the public. The psychologic and sociologic features of domestic violence are extremely complex and beyond the focus of this work (see Fincham and Bradbury 1990 for a review of these issues). What will be discussed here are the implications of this abuse for the health and health care of women.

The leading cause of death for young adults (between 25 and 34) is accidents. For men, these are mostly automotive accidents. For women, however, the leading cause of accidental death is domestic violence (Mc-Goldrick 1986). By 1986 C. Everett Koop, the then surgeon general, cited violence as the number one health problem for women in the United States (Surgeon General 1986).

The extent of the problem is impossible to know. One poll of U.S. adults in 1993 found that 34 percent had witnessed a man beating his wife or girlfriend. In the same survey, 14 percent of women admitted being the recipient of a male partner's violent acts (EDK Associates 1993). In 1990, the National Domestic Violence Hotline (1-800-333-SAFE) received nearly 100,000 calls. In 1991, in California alone there were 203,638 calls for assistance related to domestic violence, and 42,318 men were arrested for spousal abuse (CEWAER 1993). These numbers are just the tip of the iceberg, as most women don't report their abuse, fearing further battering, loss of economic support, and/or social stigma. In 1990, the same year that the National Domestic Violence Hotline received 100,000 calls, between 1.8 and 4 million women were physically assaulted by their partners in the United States (CDC 1994a; Flitcraft 1990). It is estimated that every eighteen seconds in the United States, a women is battered. According to recently retired senator Paul Simon (D-Ill.), the number of women abused by their husbands in 1989 was greater than the number of women who got married that year ("American Woman" 1991).

The problem is not limited to the United States. In Canada, for example, one report claims that one in every ten women living with a man will be battered at some time during the relationship (MacLeod 1980).

Stories of "wife burning" in India and 100 million "missing" women in Asia (*New York Times*, natl. ed., Nov. 5, 1991) provide a glimpse of the universality of the problem. As long as women are viewed as the property of their spouses, are denied education and food and equal protection under the law, they will continue to fall prey to the violence of men who need to prove their superiority through physical domination.

Although there have been some well-publicized reports of domestic violence against men, the overwhelming majority of these crimes are committed by men against their female partners, and almost all of the injuries resulting from marital aggression are sustained by women. Ten-year data from the National Crime Survey (1973–82; Jamison et al. 1989) showed that 94 percent of reported incidents of domestic violence were committed against women, and that 95 percent of those resulted in injuries of women that required medical treatment. When both marital partners were injured, as was the case for 35 percent of military couples involved in conflict, injuries were more severe for the women than the men (Cantos, Neidig, and O'Leary 1991). In a study of couples seeking treatment at a marital therapy clinic (Cascardi 1992), 11 percent of wives who had experienced severe aggression reported sustaining broken teeth or broken bones, with or without injuries to sensory organs.

The greater impact of this violence on women is also seen in the fact that more women than men require medical treatment, confinement to bed, and loss of time from work because of abuse (Stets and Straus 1990). Moreover, one study found that 65 percent of abused women interviewed in the community (i.e., women who were not patients) had experienced between three and seven of the following symptoms, listed in decreasing order of frequency: headaches, back and limb problems, frequent colds, fainting and dizziness, stomach and gastrointestinal problems, gynecologic problems, heart and blood pressure problems, lung and breathing problems, and/or skin problems (Follinstad et al. 1991). With increasing severity of abuse by their husbands, there is also increasing incidence of psychosomatic complaints, such as headaches, limb and back pain, fainting, dizziness, reported stress, and depression (Stets and Straus 1990).

In addition to physical injuries, the more subtle, but undoubtedly longer-lasting, sequelae of domestic violence are emotional. More than half of women who experience battering develop depression (Rounsaville et al. 1979). Estimates of the incidence of suicide attempts following battering range from 25 to 42 percent (Nolen-Hoeksema 1990: 91). Wife abuse is responsible for 50 percent of suicides in black women and 25 percent of all women's suicides (Worcester 1988). Moreover, studies by Carmen, Rieker, and Mills (1984) and by Jacobson and Richardson (1987) found that more than half of women hospitalized for depression had been abused as adults. In contrast, the male psychiatric patients with abuse histories were more likely to have been abused as children by their parents and to manifest aggressive, rather than depressive, symptoms. The link between chronic, repeated abuse by one's husband and depression is likely to be through the sense of helplessness that develops in these women, who cannot leave or report the abuse because of fear of further violence and/or economic retribution.

Behind these statistics of the outcome of domestic violence lies a cycle of horror that is difficult for the outsider to imagine. It has been described by Walker (1984) as consisting of three phases. The first is the tension-building phase, during which there is gradual escalation of tension in the batterer and the relationship from small acts that cause friction, resulting in expressions of hostility and dissatisfaction. The woman attempts to placate and calm him. When she cannot, she withdraws, and this withdrawal often triggers his aggression. The second phase is the actual act of aggression, which can be sparked by the smallest of events, often aided by alcohol. In the third phase the batterer is repentant and apologetic, often showing kindness and giving gifts to the victim. This leads her to hope that the relationship is salvageable, and she gives him another chance. Over time, the first stage increases in duration and intensity, the second becomes more dangerous, and the third becomes shorter and shorter as the batterer finds he can control the victim and situation without trying hard to win another chance. Walker describes the demoralization of the victim after these repeated cycles and her inability to leave the relationship as a result.

The risk of battering is not consistent over the course of an intimate relationship. It appears to increase when male partners experience work stress, job loss, and/or increased alcohol consumption. For example, a rise in confirmed cases of spousal abuse in the military from 12 per 1,000 in 1988 to 18.1 per 1,000 in 1993 was attributed, at least in part, to tensions resulting from cutbacks in the military budget and their impact on careers, according to a *New York Times* report (natl. ed., May 23, 1994). Perhaps apocryphal are reports of increased episodes of battering on Super Bowl Sunday.

In addition, women appear to be more vulnerable at certain stages of a relationship. Shockingly, for example, pregnant women are particularly likely to be battered by their intimate partners (Newberger et al. 1992). Estimates based on reports by women receiving prenatal care suggest that anywhere between 4 and 17 percent of women experience violence during pregnancy (CDC 1994a). A higher risk of abuse during the twelve months prior to delivery is associated with lower levels of education, being poor, being adolescent, having an unplanned pregnancy, and receiving little or no prenatal care. However, women without these risk factors are not immune. Approximately 5 percent of abused women in this reported sample were white, approximately 3 percent were well educated, 10 percent were over 20 years of age, 4 percent had intended to get pregnant, and 5 percent had received good prenatal care.

The violence in such households often is not confined to the women. When a woman is battered, her children often are, as well. Two studies report that between half and three-quarters of children of battered women are themselves abused (Walker and Browne 1985; Bowker, Arbitell, and McFerron 1988). Living in a violent household may also lead the battered mother to abuse her children, as occurred in 28 percent of cases (Walker 1984). Moreover, 11 percent of victims of battering have tried to kill their batterer during an attack (Walker 1984).

Not surprisingly, given their frequent injuries, 80 percent of abused women seek medical assistance, and half of them do so on at least five different occasions, according to one study (Morrison 1988). It has been estimated that about 30 percent and 40 percent of women treated in emergency departments (EDs) have injuries or symptoms, respectively, that are related to physical abuse (McLeer and Anwar 1989; Stark and Flitcraft 1991). In the latter report it was stated that 10 percent of repeat visits by women to the ED resulted from repeated domestic violence. Yet, though EDs routinely treat thousands of abused women, they often do not identify the cause of their injuries. Because they do not recognize the source of the problem, they typically discharge their patients to abusive home situations and to an uncertain fate therein.

EDs and their staffs are ill-prepared and educated to recognize victims of domestic violence. A recent study in one metropolitan area, for example, found that only 54 percent of hospital EDs had written policies for treating adults suspected of being victims of domestic violence. Fewer than 25 percent had any sort of educational program for practicing physicians, and only 6 percent had done anything to train physicians-in-training (CDC 1993e). There are no mandated courses on domestic violence in medical schools, although there is a growing movement, largely fostered by female medical students and some physicians (one leader is Karen Johnson, M.D.) to include courses on women's health that would address such issues.

One of the national health objectives for the year 2000 is for at least 90 percent of hospital EDs to have protocols for the identification, treatment, and referral of victims of sexual assault and spouse abuse. One important step toward having EDs develop appropriate policies and educational programs was taken in January of 1992 when the Joint Commission on Accreditation of Healthcare Organizations (JCAHO) mandated that EDs develop and implement policies and procedures for the care of such patients as a condition for hospitals' receipt of accreditation, without which they cannot operate. In addition, the JCAHO requires that hospitals maintain a list of referral agencies; that the medical record document the examination, treatment, and referrals made; and that staff receive education to help them identify and treat abused patients. As yet, there are no laws mandating reporting of such abuse or suspicion of abuse of adult women, as there are regarding children. Such laws are necessary to protect not only women, but also their potentially abused children.

Besides changing accreditation requirements and laws, we need to change the attitudes of physicians. One study, for example, found that physicians did not consider the diagnosis and management of spousal abuse to be "real medicine" (Borkowski, Murch, and Walker 1983). Although the best way to detect physical violence is to ask about it, fewer than 2 percent of women patients in another study indicated that they had been questioned about this possibility in their most recent office visit to a physician (Hamberger, Saunders, and Hovey 1992). Another study found that wife assault was documented in only 1 percent of the charts of family physicians in a Canadian teaching hospital, although questionnaires revealed that at least 8 percent of the women patients seen by them had been physically abused by their husbands (Martins, Holzapfel, and

Baker 1992). According to the report of the Ontario Medical Association's Committee on Wife Assault (1991), the best tools for detecting wife abuse are a high index of suspicion and a nonjudgmental and nonthreatening approach. I would add to these good rapport, sensitivity in interviewing, and a supportive attitude. Not only are few physicians well-trained about and comfortable with this issue, but most would claim not to have the time to explore the possibility of abuse. As managed care becomes more prevalent, time constraints will become more limiting. This will make it even more important to implement appropriate education and training of physicians, as well as mandatory reporting laws.

The Older Years

The possibility of abuse of the elderly is "alien to the American ideal," in the words of the 1981 report of the U.S. House of Representatives Select Committee on Aging. Nevertheless, approximately 10 percent of Americans over the age of 65 are thought to be possible victims, and this is likely to be a gross underestimate. It is obviously difficult to get true figures for a variety of reasons, including the fact that, until recently, the medical profession was unprepared for detection and reporting. Gender differences among victims of elder abuse are unknown, but it is likely that women are overrepresented, because they are more numerous in the age group at risk; because at all ages, they are more likely than men to have been abused; and because they are more likely to be dependent on their families and to lack resources for extricating themselves from abusive situations.

Now that reporting laws exist in all 50 states and medical societies are turning their attention to improving the awareness of physicians (with publications such as that from the Washington State Medical Association), it is hoped that this outrageous practice will be curtailed. Physicians are now alerted to signs of possible abuse. These signs include bruises at different stages of healing and on both sides of the body, the latter unlikely to have resulted from falls; welts that are unlikely to have been self-inflicted; lacerations, puncture wounds, fractures, or burns; evidence of excessive drugging; evidence of physical restraints around wrists and ankles, suggestive of having been tied to a bed; malnutrition or dehydration;

poor personal hygiene; absence of sensory aids, such as glasses or hearing aids; bruising of external genitalia; refusal of family members to allow social visits or comply with medical advice; and diversion of financial resources.

Research is just beginning on this newly recognized form of abuse of women. Critically important, for example, is information about the intergenerational links that lead to a cycle of parents and children abusing each other.

CHAPTER TEN

Nutrition and Exercise

Nutrition Across the Life Span

The latest advice of nutrition experts is to follow the Eating Right Pyramid of the U.S. Agriculture Department, which divides foods into five basic groups: grains; vegetables; fruits; dairy; and meats, dry beans, eggs, and nuts. Adolescents and young adult women should consume nine servings daily of grains, four of vegetables, three of fruits, three of dairy products, and two of meats (6 oz.). Older women should have six servings daily of bread, three of vegetables, two of fruits, two to three of dairy products, and two of meats (5 oz). Serving sizes are as follows:

Grains
> One slice of bread
> One ounce of prepared cold cereal
> One-half cup of cooked cereal, rice, or pasta

Vegetables
> One cup raw leafy vegetables
> One-half cup cooked leafy vegetables or chopped raw nonleafy vegetables
> Three-quarters of a cup of vegetable juice

Fruits
> One-half cup chopped, cooked, or canned fruit
> One medium-sized apple, banana, or orange
> Three-quarters of a cup of fruit juice

Dairy

> One cup of low-fat milk
> One cup of low-fat yogurt
> One and a half ounces of natural cheese
> Two ounces of processed cheese

Meats, dry beans, eggs, and nuts

> Two to three ounces of cooked lean meat, poultry, or fish
> One-half cup of cooked dry beans
> One egg
> Four tablespoons of peanut butter

MACRONUTRIENTS

Protein should constitute approximately 15 percent of daily caloric intake. The body needs nine essential amino acids (histidine, isoleucine, leucine, lysine, methionine, phenylalanine, threonine, tryptophan, and valine) in order to utilize the protein it takes in each day; this suggests a need for mixed sources of protein in the diet. However, some of the amino acids are complementary. In other words, the body's daily requirement for one amino acid may be met by another. For example, tyrosine may partially meet the body's requirement for phenylalanine.

Protein sources vary in terms of digestibility, and hence availability. The most digestible forms also have the highest content of essential amino acids. The best sources of high-quality proteins are eggs and milk. Seeds, nuts, and grains also contain protein, but these are considered to be lower-quality protein sources because they are less easily digested and absorbed and have a lower content of essential amino acids.

Protein adequacy can be grossly estimated from muscle mass assessment calculated by a formula that includes skin-fold thickness at the triceps and the circumference of the arm at the same site. Standards have been established for each age group and sex for people under the age of 75. Malnutrition is diagnosed in anyone who is more than 35 percent below the appropriate reference standard.

Carbohydrates are necessary for energy. If inadequate amounts are consumed, the body uses protein for energy, which diverts it from its important roles in maintaining healthy bodily functions and building structure. Moreover, fiber is needed for healthy bowel function, and inadequate amounts appear to be associated with serious bowel diseases, such as diverticulitis and colon cancer, in later life. For adults, 58 percent of total calories ingested each day should come from carbohydrates. Only 10 percent of total calories should come from refined and processed sugars; the remaining 48 percent should be in the form of complex carbohydrates such as starches, fiber, and naturally occurring sugars.

Fat is one of the most misunderstood and maligned of the dietary requirements. Our weight-conscious society has characterized fat as dangerous and undesirable, especially for women. The reality is that the body needs fat at all ages for energy, for production of critical substances such as prostaglandins, as a carrier for fat-soluble vitamins, and for the stability of cell membranes.

Concern has been raised about the possible roles of saturated and polyunsaturated (and recently "trans") fatty acids in causing diseases such as cancer, heart disease, and gallstones. Accordingly, it appears prudent to limit intake of fats to no more than 30 percent of ingested calories. The American Heart Association and the National Cancer Institute recommend that saturated fats constitute less than 10 percent of this amount, with the remainder composed of mono- and polyunsaturated fats. A recent commentary (Willett and Ascherio 1994) recommends that these be consumed as unhydrogenated vegetable fats in order to avoid "trans" fatty acids.

Two percent of the fat calories consumed each day should come from linoleic acid and 0.5 percent from linolenic acid. These are considered to be "essential" fatty acids and are found only in food; the body cannot manufacture them. Linoleic acid is provided by most vegetable oils, with corn, soybean, cottonseed, and safflower being the best. Linolenic acid is provided by soybean and canola oil. Cholesterol consumption should be restricted to 300 mg each day.

A general guideline for the amount of water needed each day is 1 ml for each calorie consumed. Additional water is needed when extra calories are expended—for example, when there is a fever (add 200 ml for each degree C over normal body temperature of 36.5 degrees C [97.7 degrees F]), strenuous exercise, or elevated environmental temperature (add 500 ml for every two degrees C over ambient temperature of 32 degrees C).

MICRONUTRIENTS

The body needs certain amounts of a number of essential minerals and vitamins. This section will summarize important points about some of these micronutrients; others, particularly calcium, will be addressed below in the context of particular life stages.

For appropriate levels of micronutrients, we can look to the recommended dietary allowances (RDAs) "designed for the maintenance of good nutrition of practically all healthy people in the United States." The RDAs were most recently revised by the National Research Council in 1989. These recommendations are based on all available studies (laboratory-based studies of human populations, and in some cases studies of animals). They represent broad guidelines and the expectation that diets will vary from day to day.

Iron is needed to build red blood cells and muscle tissue. Red blood cells are required to carry oxygen to all parts of the body. In the absence of adequate iron supplies, anemia results, and from it fatigue and reduced stamina. Iron is lost in healthy young women in menstrual flow and, perhaps surprisingly, in perspiration. Athletes are in danger of excessive loss and increased need of iron because of loss in perspiration and utilization in the building of muscles, as well as some loss through the gastrointestinal tract. The last may result from irritation in runners, or, more commonly, from regular consumption of nonsteroidal anti-inflammatory drugs, such as ibuprofen and naprosen. The usual sources of iron in the diet are red meat and green leafy vegetables. Iron supplements often cause irritation of the gastrointestinal tract and should be avoided unless absolutely necessary.

Magnesium is found within most cells in the body and is critical to well-being because of its involvement with the action of more than 300 enzymes (Wyngaarden and Smith 1988). A recent study suggested that low levels of magnesium may play a role in high blood pressure. The recommended daily intake is about 280 mg. Magnesium is found in green vegetables, meat, and fish. Deficiency of magnesium is usually found together with calcium deficiency, and the symptoms of the two are often difficult to separate. Most cases of magnesium deficiency come from poor absorption or excess loss from the body, rather than from poor diet. Alcoholism or use of some diuretics may cause these problems.

Vitamin A deficiency is common worldwide; in the United States it is seen mainly in the elderly, the poor, and alcoholics. In alcoholics, because of the common associated problem of zinc deficiency, less vitamin A is produced. Night blindness is the earliest sign of vitamin A deficiency. Dryness and other changes in the eye and other vital organs may follow, and loss of taste is a common finding.

Alcohol and coffee consumption can interfere with absorption of vitamin B_I (thiamin). Deficiency of thiamin causes nonspecific symptoms such as loss of appetite, weight loss, and irritability, followed by weakness, headache, rapid pulse, and sensations of pins and needles, pain, or loss of feeling in the feet and elsewhere.

Alcoholism can also lead to deficiency of riboflavin (vitamin B_2) or niacin. The early symptoms of riboflavin deficiency include burning and itching of the eyes, mouth soreness, and personality deterioration. Cracking of the corners of the mouth, swelling of the tongue, anemia, and a variety of skin problems follow. One symptom of niacin deficiency is lesions on those parts of the skin that are exposed to sunlight. The full-blown form of niacin deficiency is called pellagra and is characterized by the four D's: dermatitis, diarrhea, dementia, and death.

Women who follow macrobiotic diets or who take oral contraceptives, penicillamine for the treatment of rheumatoid arthritis, or INH (Isoniazide) for tuberculosis exposure are at risk of developing vitamin B_6 deficiency. The symptoms of this deficiency are variable but may include cracking of the corners of the lips, dryness or rashes of the skin, or sores in the mouth.

Prolonged vegan diets may cause deficiency of vitamin B_{12}. The symptoms include megaloblastic anemia and glossitis.

A macrobiotic diet may lead to inadequate intake of vitamin C. Weakness and lethargy are common early symptoms, followed by difficulty breathing and pain in bones and joints. Tiny blue spots below the level of the blood pressure cuff may be seen by a keen observer. As time goes on, larger black and blue marks appear spontaneously or following minor trauma, as does bleeding from the gums. These are the classical findings of scurvy, the "sailor's disease," which for them came from the unavailability of citrus fruits.

At every age, there is also danger from consuming excessive amounts of certain vitamins (hypervitaminosis). Excess vitamin A can cause hair loss, swelling of the brain (a condition called pseudotumor cerebri; symptoms are headaches and visual disturbances), enlarged liver and spleen, painful and fragile bones, dry and cracking skin, and even death. Excessive intake of vitamin C may cause problems, as well. Doses of two grams or more may produce abdominal pain and diarrhea. High intake of this vitamin places some people at increased risk of developing kidney stones and worsening of other kidney conditions. Continued intake of large amounts of vitamin D can also be harmful. The effects can include weakness, lethargy, headaches, nausea, weight loss, diarrhea, frequent urination, and deposits of calcium in soft tissues; extremely large doses can result in formation of kidney stones.

OBESITY

Being obese is not the same as being overweight, though all obese people are overweight. Overweight is the term used to describe people who weigh more than 50 percent of their peers of the same sex and age. Having heavy bones and large muscle mass can make some people overweight, yet not necessarily obese. Obesity refers to having excess fat, typically as a result of excessive intake of food. Skin-fold measurements taken at seven standard sites provide a gross estimate of body fat. The most accurate way to measure body fat involves underwater weighing, a cumbersome method that is unavailable to most.

Obese people have fat cells that are excessive in number, size, or both. A typical fat cell will enlarge to a weight of one microgram and then stop. As the person continues to consume more calories than the body needs, more fat cells will be made. Once a fat cell is formed, it will, to the best of our current knowledge, continue to exist for the rest of the person's life. If weight is lost, fat cells will decrease in size but will not disappear.

Weight is gained more rapidly after accelerated weight loss. The reason is thought to be that with rapid weight loss, there is an increase in the enzyme lipoprotein lipase (LPL), which causes breakdown of circulating fat particles into free fatty acids that get stored in fat cells. This observation argues for slow, steady, weight loss, not to exceed two pounds each week. Serum levels of cholesterol also increase after fasting, another reason to avoid crash diets.

There is a lifelong relationship for women between television watching and obesity. According to Tucker and Bagwell (1991), adult women who watched three or more hours of television daily were twice as likely to be obese as those who watched one hour or less. The direction of the relationship between these variables is not clear, however. It is possible either that obese people are more likely to be more sedentary and therefore to watch television, or that watching television rather than engaging in more vigorous activity makes people obese.

Nutrition in Childhood

For the first six months of life, all of a baby's nutritional needs (except for vitamins A, D, E, and K) may be met from maternal milk, assuming that the mother is well nourished. Administration of vitamin supplements provides the four missing vitamins. (For more information on the nutritional requirements of nursing mothers, see below under Lactation.)

After the first year of life, the growth rate decelerates and children reduce their caloric intake. Self-selection of food usually suffices over time, and it is felt that future eating problems can be avoided by allowing toddlers latitude in choosing foods. Because the body composition of male and female infants and children is comparable, their nutritional requirements are similar until puberty.

There is little formal evidence of gender differences in feeding practices in the western world (unlike in some developing countries, where female children are considered an economic disadvantage, and where their resultant poorer nutritional status leads to a higher death rate from lowered immunity to infections and inability to tolerate diarrheal diseases). Anecdotal evidence suggests, however, that girls are more likely to be given lower-calorie foods and to have their food consumption placed under greater scrutiny, because of society's emphasis on thinness and the desire of some mothers to spare their female children from the weight struggles they themselves have experienced.

For prepubertal girls, the best measure of adequate nutrition is continuous gain in height and weight along the same percentile lines on the growth curves used by most doctors. If necessary, some of the specific nutrients can be measured in the blood. Protein-calorie malnutrition, rare in industrialized societies, can be assessed by measuring the skin folds at predetermined sites on the body. If the skin fold is less than that of children of comparable age and sex, this type of malnutrition is a possibility. There is a formula for assessing muscle mass using skin fold measurements that works best in older children and adults. Lean body mass can be estimated from analysis of creatinine in a 24-hour urine sample.

For children over two, the recommended intake of dietary fat parallels that for adults; no more than 30 percent of the total calories consumed should come from fat, of which no more than 10 percent should be saturated fat, and the daily diet should include less than 300 mg of cholesterol. A recent study of more than 500 children between the ages of two and five found that 80 percent of them consumed more than the recommended amount of every category of fat. The highest consumption of these fats was found in the poorest families and in black children. There were also ethnic differences in the sources of the fats consumed. For example, for Hispanics, the major source of total fat was whole milk, whereas for blacks, it was franks and related meats (Thompson and Dennison 1994).

Little attention was paid to calcium intake in children until recently. Now that it has been recognized that about 30 percent of total adult bone mass is laid down in childhood and 60 percent during the pubertal growth spurt, it is apparent that calcium consumption during those years is critical. Between the ages of one and ten, the average child needs about 1,500 mg of calcium each day. Milk is an excellent source, and five eight-ounce glasses of whole or skim milk will provide this amount.

Sufficient fluoride is essential for building strong teeth. Poor teeth are problems at the extremes of the life span; whereas there are no reported gender differences during childhood, elderly women appear to have more problems with their teeth and gums than do men. Fluoride is best provided as a supplement, either in the form of drops or in the water supply, as well as by applications to the teeth by the dentist. The daily added amount ingested should be 0.25 mg for babies and 1.0 mg for children three years and older.

For most U.S. children, with the exception of those who live in poverty, the diet is adequate to supply the necessary nutrients and vitamins. Children in vegetarian families, too, can generally meet all their nutrient and vitamin needs. Vegans, who ingest neither eggs nor milk, may over time be at risk for vitamin B_{12} deficiency and deficiencies of some trace minerals. Americans' preoccupation with their health has, however, placed some children at risk from ingestion of too many, rather than too few, vitamins. At every age, as previously described, there is danger from consuming excessive amounts of certain vitamins. For very young children, excess vitamins A and D are particular problems.

In children, as in adults, excessive skin-fold thickness is associated with obesity. Particularly in the first year of life, excess caloric intake increases the number of fat cells; as mentioned above, once formed, these fat cells are permanent. Obesity is most likely to appear either in the first year of life, between the ages of five and six, or during adolescence, and it is equally common in boys and girls. There is no sex difference during childhood in patterns of fat deposition.

It isn't always the case that an obese child will become an obese adult, but eating habits tend to be learned during childhood and are likely to continue into later life. There is also a strong familial tendency in obesity, with children of obese parents being more likely to themselves become obese. It is obviously difficult to separate environmental factors from genetic ones, but recent studies of identical twins reared separately support the notion that genetic influences are most important in producing obesity (Wyngaarden and Smith 1988: 1221).

Nutrition in Adolescence

In planning a healthy diet for a teenage girl, there are many important considerations. First of all, she needs sufficient calories to support the pubertal growth spurt. This translates to about 3,000 calories each day at the peak of the growth spurt. (For discussion of when this peak occurs, see Chapter 1.) A strict weight-reduction diet before the peak of the growth spurt deprives the adolescent girl of necessary energy for a healthy body. In general terms, nutrition is felt to be adequate if a young girl reaches the peak of her growth spurt around the age of twelve and begins her menses within a year of that time.

In addition to adequate calories, the adolescent girl needs sufficient protein, carbohydrates, and fats. Many girls avoid "sweets," "starches," and fats, but this approach is based on misinformation. As discussed above, both carbohydrates and fats are necessary for good health. No studies are available on how adolescents' requirements for these nutrients may differ from those for adults.

Good studies upon which to base guidelines for adolescent females' consumption of cholesterol and essential fatty acids (see above) are also lacking. There is no evidence, for example, that consumption of high-cholesterol food affects cholesterol levels in adolescent females, and even less is known about the relationship of elevated cholesterol levels at this age and later risk for developing coronary artery disease. Even what "high" or "normal" levels are for women in this age group is currently unknown. Most physicians do not now recommend screening adolescent females to determine their cholesterol or LDL levels, because they do not know how to interpret the results, or whether anything need be done about elevated levels.

We do know that many things can affect cholesterol levels at this age. Most important among them is the stage of pubertal development. For example, before puberty begins, girls have cholesterol levels between 3.5 and 6.7 mmol/L. By the time puberty is complete, the range has dropped to 3.1 to 6.4 mmol/L. At every stage of pubertal development, these levels are slightly higher in girls than in boys.

The general recommendation of consuming one ml of water per calorie consumed translates to almost 3,000 ml of water for adolescent females at the peak of their growth spurts and about 2,000 ml after pubertal growth is completed. Additional amounts should be consumed under the circumstances described in the first section of this chapter.

Although it is recommended, based on studies in adults, that adolescents limit their salt intake to less than three grams each day, it is still unclear whether this is optimal, or even possible. There are, for example, no long-term follow-up studies indicating whether or not adherence to such a limit will decrease the incidence of high blood pressure in later life. Adolescents' diets tend to be high in salt, and restrictions are not generally well received by this age group. There is some evidence, however, that restriction of salt intake may be helpful to some young women who experience bloating in the week prior to their menstrual period.

The recommended daily allowances of the macronutrients (protein, carbohydrates, and fat) and the vitamin and mineral micronutrients for an adolescent female who is past her growth spurt are shown in Appendix E.

The calcium requirement for adolescent females has been given as one gram of elemental calcium each day, and the current RDA is 1,200 mg. Recent studies show these levels to be insufficient to produce sufficient bone density to protect against osteoporosis in later life. It is probably wiser to aim for two grams of elemental calcium during the adolescent years. This will put a young woman in a better position to endure the inevitable loss of bone density that begins in the twenties and results in osteoporosis in the older years (see Chapter 4). However, only 10 percent of adolescent girls have been found to be meeting even the 1,200 mg RDA for calcium (Albertson, Tobolmann, and Marquart 1997).

The best source of calcium is dairy products. Adolescent women typically shy away from these foods, fearing the accompanying fat. Interestingly, the nonfat version of yogurt has more protein and calcium than the regular, fat-containing variety. For example, a serving of plain nonfat yogurt has 10 g of protein and 350 mg of calcium. Skim milk provides 302 mg of calcium in each eight-ounce glass. At the peak of the growth spurt in height, it is advisable that a young girl eat six such servings of dairy products each day. After menses begin, it is probably acceptable for her to reduce her intake to about four servings daily until she turns twenty.

A condition called lactose intolerance (caused by gradual loss of the enzyme lactase from the intestine) is common, particularly among American Indians, African-Americans, and Asians. For adolescents who are intolerant to milk products, there are alternative sources of calcium. Broccoli (particularly the stems) can provide some calcium, but not enough (175 mg in one cup of cooked broccoli). Supplements of calcium carbonate (the best-absorbed form) are well tolerated and can be useful. The best of these is Tums-Ex, which provides 750 mg of calcium carbonate or 300 mg of elemental calcium in each tablet. This supplement is best taken with meals.

The daily requirement for fluoride in the diet of adolescents is between 1.5 and 2.5 mg. Because adolescence is the time of the second peak for development of dental caries, it is particularly important that teenagers continue to take the equivalent of a 1.0 mg supplement each day. This may be provided in the water supply. Fluoride has been shown to make tooth structure more resistant to acids. Its possible role in strengthening bones during pubertal development has not been adequately studied.

Adolescence is a time of increased requirement for iron. Regularly menstruating adolescent females who are not athletes need approximately 18 mg of elemental iron each day; athletes need more. Fear of fat may keep adolescent females from eating red meat, but one needs large amounts of green vegetables to get adequate levels of iron, and supplements may cause gastrointestinal irritation. Ingestion of lean red meat is preferable. Measurement of serum iron and hematocrit level is often useful because many adolescent girls become deficient in iron without having symptoms. The hematocrit determination is easily and cheaply performed in most health centers, using a few drops of blood. It is recommended that this be done yearly throughout adolescence for girls, especially athletes.

Idealism, love of animals, and health-consciousness often come together for adolescent girls and lead to espousal of vegetarianism. This diet is compatible with normal healthy growth and pubertal development, so long as care is taken to ensure meeting all the nutritional requirements of this demanding period of the life cycle. Macrobiotic or vegan diets can cause vitamin deficiencies, as discussed in the first section of this chapter. Most vitamin deficiencies seen in female adolescents, however, result not from dietary deficiencies but from medications (including oral contraceptive pills and certain anticonvulsants, i.e., phenobarbital and phenytoin). Moreover, excessive consumption of vitamins places more U.S. adolescents at risk than consumption of inadequate amounts. This is particularly true for adolescent females. Because vitamin A is often recommended to treat acne, some girls overdo it. Excess consumption of vitamins C and D is also possible.

Obesity is the physical state most feared by adolescent women, yet the numbers suggest that more of them worry about it than actually have it. For example, one study of adolescent females found that 63 percent thought they were overweight, though only 40 percent actually were (Moore 1988). Another study found that 62 percent of adolescent girls who wanted to lose weight were within their normal weight range (Storz and Green 1983).

The most recent comprehensive study of overweight adolescents (NHANES III; Ezzati et al. 1992) took place from 1988 to 1991. Among the 1,849 twelve-to-nineteen-year-olds selected for the study, 21 percent were found to be overweight using the criterion of having a body mass index (BMI, calculated as weight in kilograms over the square of height in meters) higher than the 85th percentile for a reference group of the same age and sex. For females aged twelve to fourteen, this meant having a BMI at or over 23.4; for those aged fifteen to seventeen, at or over 24.8; and for those aged eighteen to nineteen, at or over 25.7. Interestingly, there was not much difference in prevalence of overweight between males (20 percent) and females (22 percent). These figures represent significant increases over the findings of the previous survey (1976–80) that only 5 percent of adolescent males and 7 percent of adolescent females were overweight (CDC 1994d). Although this increase in overweight adolescents over the past decade has not been definitively explained, it parallels a decrease in participation in physical education (Heath et al. 1994) and a 14–17 percent increase in average caloric intake by females sixteen and older (McDowell et al. 1994) during the same time period. Television viewing patterns, too, have been shown to influence the weight of children and adolescents. One study showed a 2 percent increase in obesity for each additional hour of television over two hours each day watched among a sample of twelve-to-seventeen-year-olds (Dietz, Gortmaker, and Cheung 1985). In a follow-up study, this team found that more than 60 percent of overweight in those adolescents resulted from excessive television viewing (Gortmaker et al. 1996).

The health risks for women who are overweight as adolescents have been poorly studied. The first study to follow overweight adolescents into adulthood was reported in 1992 (Must et al.). In this 55-year follow-up study it appears that women fared better than men. Whereas the men who had been overweight as adolescents had a higher death rate beginning at the age of 45 and twice the expected death rate by the time they reached their seventies, overweight adolescent women did not have an increased rate of premature death as adults.

Both men and women who were overweight as adolescents had double the risk of heart disease and an increased risk for developing non–insulin dependent diabetes mellitus in later life. However, their rates of other diseases differed. The men had an increased risk of colon cancer and gout, whereas the women had more difficulty with activities of daily living and with arthritis.

In addition, a study by Gortmaker et al. (1993) showed that adolescents' obesity had adverse effects on their later self-esteem and social and economic life. Especially for obese female adolescents, their later socio-economic attainment was lower, and their rate of poverty higher, than for their nonobese counterparts.

On the other side of the coin, the effort to be thin can lead adolescent girls to diet excessively, which can also have negative health consequences, such as absent menses. Anorexia nervosa is a well-recognized cause of primary or secondary amenorrhea (see Chapter 7). In a study of more than 2,500 women entering college, Krahn et al. (1992) found that intense dieting (defined as having symptoms in one or more domains of *DSM-IIIR* criteria for bulimia nervosa, but not meeting the threshold criteria for any) was associated with an increased frequency of irregular or absent menses. This was true even when the researchers controlled for the presence of depression, a known independent cause of absent menses, and common in women with eating disorders.

Nutrition in Early Adulthood

Appendix E gives RDAs for the "average" nonpregnant and nonlactating woman in the 25–50-year age group (who weighs 138 pounds and is 64 inches tall). Although women are not following all of these recommendations, some progress is being made. A 1991 study documented a decrease in fat intake over the past two decades, though the percentage of calories derived from total fat was above the target of 30 percent in the national health objectives for the year 2000, and the percentage of fat that was saturated was also greater than recommended. The intake of dietary cholesterol was lower for females than for males, with females aged 20–49 having the highest daily intake for their gender group, 235–49 mg (McDowell et al. 1994).

PREGNANCY AND LACTATION

During pregnancy, nutritional requirements obviously increase. (The RDAs for pregnant women are shown in Appendix E.) The most important determinants of a well-nourished newborn infant are the nutritional status of its mother and the adequacy of the placenta. Despite this obvious fact, we are far from achieving the national health objective for the year 2000 that we increase to at least 85 percent the proportion of mothers who gain the minimum recommended amount of weight during their pregnancies. Currently, it is estimated that only 67 percent of all married women do so. This rate is considerably lower for unmarried women, particularly those who are adolescents and poor. Moreover, in 1991, it was estimated that 8 percent of low-income women of childbearing age have iron-deficiency anemia (Children's Defense Fund 1991). This may result in anemia or cerebral anoxia in the fetus.

The effect of exercise during pregnancy and lactation is another area deserving of further investigation. Most of the evidence thus far supports the continuation of moderate exercise throughout early and midpregnancy.

A little-known fact is that nursing mothers can produce more milk than their infants need. Their diets must, however, contain sufficient calories to compensate for those in the milk, as well as those needed to secrete it. It is estimated that lactation increases energy requirements by 500 calories each day. A nursing mother must maintain her weight for the sake of her health and that of her baby. This is no time for a weight-reduction diet. She should also consume approximately three quarts of water each day and at least one gram of calcium, preferably in the form of milk. Nursing women who are vegans should take additional vitamin B_{12} to prevent a condition called methylmalonic acidemia from developing in their infants. The RDAs for adult women during lactation are shown in Appendix E.

Some infants are distressed by their mothers' consumption of some foods, including certain berries, onions, tomatoes, cabbages, chocolate, and spices. This would be manifested by loose stools and crying. Most babies, however, will not be affected by the particular foods a mother eats. Moreover, there are no particular foods that are capable of stimulating more milk production, despite folklore claiming the contrary for foods such as beer, oatmeal, milk, and tea.

Obviously, lactating women should not eat fish caught in waters contaminated with PCBs or mercury, and should not smoke or consume any drugs not specifically proven to be safe. The latter is problematic because no drugs released for use between 1974 and 1994 have been tested on pregnant women. Sufficient raw and cooked vegetables and fruit, whole wheat bread, and water should be consumed to prevent constipation and thereby avoid the use of laxatives, which can be harmful to the baby.

Lactating women may exercise as long as they consume sufficient water and calories. However, a recent report suggests that babies prefer the milk produced by their mothers before exercise and may reject it afterward, possibly because of the increased concentration of lactate after exercise (Wallace, Inbar, and Ernsthausen 1994). Thus, it is advisable to nurse before exercising rather than after.

DISEASE PREVENTION THROUGH DIET

There is a growing body of data supporting the notion that some cancers in women may be related to their diets. Among these is the finding of a higher incidence of cancer of the colon (responsible for approximately 13,000 deaths each year among women) in those who consume little fiber. One of the national health objectives for the year 2000 is for adults to increase servings of fruits and vegetables from the current average of 2.8 per day to five or more per day. The precise connection between consumption of fruits and vegetables and cancer-risk reduction is unknown. It may be the vitamins, minerals, or other micro- and macronutrients contained in these foods, or even the life-styles of people who eat more of them.

As discussed in Chapter 3, research is ongoing to determine the possible role of diet in breast cancer prevention efforts. Studies of laboratory animals and in tissue culture experiments suggest that large doses of vitamin C may play a role in slowing the growth of breast cancer cells. This research has not yet been extended to human trials, so it is premature to speculate on its potential value. The finding of a higher rate of breast cancer in populations that eat higher-fat diets has prompted investigation of the possible role of fat in causing the disease. Here, too, it is too soon to translate this finding into specific dietary recommendations. An intriguing recent report suggests that olive oil may have some protective effect against breast cancer (LaVecchia et al. 1995).

Because of the observation that high blood pressure is more common among those who are overweight, weight reduction is often recommended to help in the treatment of this condition. The results are generally positive. In addition, there is a large body of evidence that blood pressure levels are related to salt intake. For that reason, a limitation of daily salt intake to less than two grams is recommended.

It will come as no surprise that current recommendations on heart disease and diet include a number of "thou shalt nots": no excessive fat, saturated fat, or salt. But there is some good news for those who are concerned about preventing this common cause of death. Following reports from France that consumption of red wine is the reason that the French have a relatively low incidence of heart disease, despite their high consumption of cholesterol, researchers at Harvard studied this phenomenon. Much to the surprise of skeptics (and the delight of California wine growers), the study found that consumption of a moderate amount of alcohol increases blood levels of HDLs, the "good" cholesterol. A moderate amount is defined as two or three drinks each day, with a drink being twelve ounces of beer, five ounces of wine (which doesn't have to be French!), or one and a half ounces of distilled spirits (Linn et al. 1993). Consumption of more than these amounts, however, can be harmful.

Another mechanism for the beneficial relationship of alcohol consumption to heart health was suggested by a study that showed that levels of the enzyme tissue-type plasminogen activator (TPA), which contributes to the body's ability to break down blood clots, were higher in those who drank one or two drinks daily, compared to alcohol abstainers. As with most other studies of heart disease, the subjects for this study were male doctors (Ridker et al. 1994).

Thus far, we have been discussing the kind of heart disease that includes heart attacks and hardening of the arteries. Another common kind of heart disease involves rapid or irregular heartbeats, called arrhythmias. There are many causes of arrhythmias, and for many young people they are easily prevented by decreasing the intake of caffeine.

Caffeine reduction can also be useful for people with other forms of heart disease, as well as those with ulcer disease, diabetes, or even anxiety. Caffeine intake should be limited to no more than 300 mg each day. That adds up quickly when you realize that each cup of brewed coffee has 200 mg (don't even ask about espresso!); instant coffee, 100 mg; decaffeinated coffee, 2 mg; brewed tea, 40 mg if steeped for one minute, 60 mg if steeped for five; iced tea, 30 mg; regular cola, 35–50 mg.

Gallbladder disease, which is more common in women than in men, is responsible for one of the most common surgical procedures (cholecystectomy) and is a leading cause of hospitalization. A number of dietary constituents have been examined for their possible role in causing gallstones, including cholesterol, linoleic acid, oleic acid, fat, carbohydrates, fiber, and calcium, with inconsistent results. One fascinating study found that an important risk factor for gallstones was not what was eaten, but what was not eaten. Specifically, it documented a high risk of gallstones among women who fasted, dieted, and had low intake of fiber. The researchers postulated that these factors may have decreased the motility of the gallbladder or changed the composition of the bile in it (Sichieri, Everhart, and Roth 1991).

OBESITY, DIETING, AND FITNESS

The definition of obesity in adult women is usually based on height and weight in relationship to those of other females of the same age group. The most reliable of these reference standards is based on the BMI, which equals the weight (in kilograms) divided by the square of the height (in meters). Unfortunately, this seems to be a more reliable index of fatness for males than for females, but it is widely used for both. Graphs are available for comparison of an individual's BMI with that of the reference group to determine if she is obese. For example, a woman between the ages of 25 and 59 with a medium frame and a BMI of 22.5 is at the midpoint for her sex and age and would be considered "just right." In fact, any BMI under 25 would be considered nonobese. For women in the 20–29-year age group, a BMI of 27.3 represents the 85th percentile, and a woman at or above this level is considered obese.

There are many problems with using this system, not the least of which is that it is based on possibly obsolete data, namely, the 1983 tables of heights and weights of the Metropolitan Life Insurance Company. A recent report showed that in just the seven years between 1985–86 and 1992–93, the average adult weight rose ten pounds, unrelated to aging. For example, the weight of white women aged 25–30 rose from 140.6 to 150.8 pounds, and that of black women in the same age range rose from 158.5 to 166.2 pounds (*New York Times*, natl. ed., Mar. 19, 1994). Moreover, the reference standard of the life insurance company is not representative of people of all socioeconomic and racial groups, and the data were obtained from self-report rather than from actual measurements. Past studies show that under such circumstances, in general, men tend to exaggerate their height, and women to underreport their weight. These facts suggest that the Metropolitan Life reference standard is inappropriate.

It has been estimated that 23.4 percent of adults (those over eighteen) are overweight. All Americans tend to gain weight as they age. A study by Smith et al. (1994) followed almost 3,000 women, ages 18 to 30, for five years. They found an average weight gain of 19.4 pounds for black women, and 9.92 pounds gain for white women, who had been pregnant in the interim. Among women who had no pregnancies the average weight gain was 12.79 pounds for black women and 5.95 pounds for white women. Interestingly, the parallel study of young men over a seven-year period showed that they, too, gained weight, to the tune of 17.6 pounds for black men and 13 pounds for white men.

Various factors may contribute to this weight gain. Many women believe that each pregnancy adds to a woman's weight, but the Smith et al. (1994) study suggests that the truth is not as bad as many imagine. Only the first pregnancy added weight over and above that which accompanies aging, and the amount of that extra weight was only six and a half pounds for black women and four pounds for white women. Some differences were noted in the distribution of the weight, with larger waists in proportion to hips in the women who had had babies; this difference may have been the result of abdominal muscle laxity rather than necessarily of increased fat.

Many young women also fear that obesity is accelerated by birth control pills. In fact, these pills may cause weight loss as often as weight gain. Among women who do gain weight with birth control pills, the average amount is two pounds, most of which is water and is often lost over time despite continued use of the pills.

Other possible causes of weight gain are change in exercise and cessation of smoking. These factors did not, however, account for the weight gain in the Smith et al. study (1994). This gain may simply be attributable to diet: A related survey of the diets of Americans showed that between 1980 and 1991, there was a general increase in caloric intake of 100–300 calories per day. The increase was more pronounced for females than for males (14–17 percent versus 1–13 percent, respectively) (McDowell et al. 1994).

An important sex difference relates to the location of fat tissue in the body. In men, fat tends to be deposited above the waist. In women, it is more likely to end up in the lower abdomen, hips, buttocks, and thighs. Besides giving rise to the fruit analogy of men being more "apple-like" and women being "pears," this difference has implications for cardiovascular health. Upper-body fat is worse than lower-body fat with regard to the risk of heart disease, high blood pressure, and diabetes, at least in men. The reasons for this are interesting and suggest that all fat cells may not be equal. When excess calories are consumed, the fat cells in the upper body tend to enlarge rather than to multiply. They are also more affected by the hormone insulin and chemicals called catecholamines. In contrast, the fat cells in the lower body increase more in number than in size.

Regardless of the location of the fat, there is a clear correlation for both men and women between being overweight and having high blood pressure. Among overweight adult women, 40.5 percent had high blood pressure (CDC 1993a).

Because weight gained in the lower body is in the form of a greater number of (permanent) fat cells rather than enlargement of existing fat cells, it is more resistant to attempts at weight loss. There are many other theories about why it is so difficult for women to lose weight. One popular theory that has not been proven in humans is the "set point" theory, according to which each woman has a control system that works to keep weight within a narrow range, regardless of weight-loss attempts.

Recent research has identified a protein called leptin, produced by fat cells, that is elevated in obese people (Hassink et al. 1996). It is thought to regulate satiety, and obese people are thought to be "leptin-resistant." It is interesting that levels are higher in females than in males, regardless of their adiposity.

There are three main approaches to weight loss: diet, behavior modification, and exercise. Drugs and surgery are other options that are distinctly less desirable.

Diets can be effective if they are palatable, nutritionally sound, and geared to limit weight loss to no more than two pounds each week. Crash diets will initially work but are associated with rapid regaining of weight, a number of health hazards (e.g., rebound elevation of cholesterol), and even death. For an adult woman, the minimum caloric intake is about 1,100. The diet should include at least 500 mg of high-quality protein for each pound of desired weight to reduce the risk of loss of nitrogen.

Behavior modification is useful for women who have habits supportive of excess eating. It reteaches patterns and cues to eating that help to control food intake. Some examples include replacing the fork on the plate after each mouthful, chewing each bite 100 times, not serving "family style," serving on small plates, and not going to the market when hungry.

Increasing activity, in combination with judicious dieting, is the most effective and safest way to lose weight and keep it off. To lose one pound, it is necessary either to reduce intake by or to burn up 3,500 calories. Depending on the starting weight, the person, and the activity, more or less exercise will be required to achieve the same amount of weight loss (Wyngaarden and Smith 1988; see Table 10.1).

Until recently, exercise and athletic competition were the nearly exclusively domains of the male in our society. Women recently have become more involved in sports for reasons of recreation, appearance, and health improvement, but we know very little about their health effects. For the most part, results of studies done on men have simply been applied to women, without sufficient consideration of possible gender differences. There are a number of reasons to question the wholesale transfer of knowledge from men to women, relating to differences in body composition and structure as well as hormonal variations during the menstrual cycle and before and after menopause. Examples of the first type of difference include the fact that women have lower lean body mass and less muscle than men, a lower volume of blood (and hence lower oxygen-carrying capacity), lower lung volume, and smaller heart size; these are of potential concern when it comes to sports, as they suggest that women may have less endurance than men. On the other hand, women's higher percentage of body fat is known to be advantageous in giving them buoyancy in swimming and in protecting them against cold exposure.

In response to the paucity of information on these critical factors, a panel of experts was convened to make recommendations for future research into the response of women to acute and chronic exercise (Mitchell et al. 1992). Their recommendations included the following:

TABLE 10.1
Approximate Energy Expenditure in Selected Activities for People of Different Weights (calories per 30 minutes)

ACTIVITY	Weight (pounds)					
	110	130	150	170	190	210
Aerobic dancing						
"walking pace"	99	114	132	150	168	186
"jogging pace"	159	186	213	243	270	300
"running pace"	204	240	276	315	351	387
Basketball	207	243	282	318	357	396
Canoeing—leisure	66	78	90	102	114	126
Canoeing—racing	156	183	210	237	267	294
Carpentry	78	93	105	120	135	147
Cycling—5.5 mph	96	114	132	147	165	183
Cycling—9.4 mph	150	177	204	231	258	285
Dancing—ballroom	78	90	105	117	132	144
Dancing—disco	156	183	210	237	267	294
Gardening	150	177	204	231	258	285
Golf	129	150	174	195	219	243
Judo	294	345	399	450	504	558
Lying or sitting down	33	39	45	51	57	63
Mopping floor	96	105	120	138	153	171
Running						
11.5 minutes per mile	204	240	276	315	351	387
9 minutes per mile	291	342	393	447	498	552
7 minutes per mile	366	417	468	522	573	624
5.5 minutes per mile	435	513	591	669	747	828
Skiing, cross-country	216	252	291	330	369	408
Standing quietly	39	45	51	57	66	72
Swimming						
backstroke	255	300	345	390	435	486
crawl	192	228	261	297	330	366
Table tennis	102	120	138	156	174	195
Tennis	165	192	222	252	282	312
Walking						
3 mph	102	114	126	138	153	165
4 mph	120	141	162	186	207	228

SOURCE: Wyngaarden and Smith 1988.

1.   To investigate the adaptation of heart and skeletal muscle to exercise in women and the molecular underpinnings thereof. This recommendation is based on the fact that these muscles have been found to have receptors for estrogen, the role of which is unknown. Moreover, the panel points out that "knowledge about the role the sex hormones play in the overall functioning of striated muscle is critical to the health-related aspects of physical activity programs" (p. S263).

2.   To study the molecular mechanisms underlying gender differences in uptake of oxygen, the best measure of cardiovascular fitness.

3.   To investigate any gender differences in the body's use of energy sources. This follows from observations that women may use fat as an energy source more than men, thus possibly sparing protein and carbohydrate.

4.   To investigate regulation of blood pressure and reactivity of blood vessels during exercise in women. This is based on the known fact that women's blood vessels are more sensitive and react more and at a lower level of stress in certain circumstances than those of men. "Studies should be designed to identify and examine the gender-related difference in blood pressure regulation during exercise, elucidate the mechanisms underlying these differences, and determine the consequence of these differences in response to a variety of other stimuli" (p. S264).

5.   To determine the body's response to circulating sex hormones, particularly in the context of prolonged physical activity in stressful environments, at different stages of the life cycle, when taking birth control substances, and after menopause.

6.   To investigate the gender-specific responses to exercise in differing environments, particularly with regard to loss of fluids and electrolytes when exercising in hot environments and in women taking birth control pills or hormone replacement therapy.

What has been well studied recently is the effect of strenuous exercise on menstrual function. As previously discussed, strenuous exercise may lead to cessation of menses ("athletic amenorrhea").

A number of medications are abused for the purpose of weight loss. They include appetite suppressants (nicotine), drugs that increase metabolism (e.g., amphetamines), and "water" pills (diuretics). These either become ineffective after a short period of time, become addictive, or cause serious side effects. They have no place in a safe or effective weight loss program.

There are two different approaches to surgery for obesity. One involves "stapling" the stomach, a procedure designed to decrease its capacity. This is still experimental, and a number of serious complications as well as failures have been reported. For that reason, this approach should be reserved for those adults with "morbid" obesity, that is, obesity that exceeds 100 percent of desirable weight and causes severe medical complications.

The other procedure that has become popular is liposuction. This operation involves insertion of a tube, attached to a vacuum, beneath the skin to suck out fat cells. Some deaths have occurred when particles of fat have become dislodged and closed off the coronary arteries. More minor problems include scarring. Liposuction is definitely not recommended.

The Perimenopausal Years

Concern about weight gain often causes women to begin dieting when they reach this age range (approximately 44 to 65). However, some bodily changes that we consider inevitable consequences of aging may actually represent nutritional deficiencies. It is, therefore, critical that women consume adequate amounts of food. Appendix E gives RDAs for perimenopausal women.

Although the RDA for calcium is 800 mg, most experts recommend that women in the perimenopausal years take at least 1,000 mg daily and increase this to 1,500 mg after menopause. This is the equivalent of six servings of dairy products or ingestion of five Tums-Ex tablets. Moderate exercise can also help avert osteoporosis. For example, a recent study of women over the age of 62 showed that women who walked about one mile each day delayed the onset of osteoporosis by four to seven years in later life (Marcus et al. 1992). The risk of osteoporosis is also lower for heavier than for lean women (see Chapter 4). However, the most important protection against further loss of bone mass comes from estrogen replacement (see Chapter 3).

Perimenopausal women should consume no more than 3 g of salt and no more than 300 mg of cholesterol per day.

It has always been believed that menopause caused weight gain. Interestingly, this is not the case, but the news is not all good. Between the ages of 42 and 53, whether or not menopause occurs, women gain an average of 2.25 kg (4.95 pounds), with a wide range that includes women who do not gain at all and some who gain as much as 6.5 kg (14.3 pounds) (Wing et al. 1991). The factors associated with weight gain were found to be less physical activity, black race, and living alone. However, regardless of life-style, it appears that some increase in weight is inevitable with aging, particularly for women. Along with the weight gain comes an increase in the relative amount of fat in women's bodies. At eighteen years of age, about 24 percent of total body weight is fat; at 25 years, 27.8 percent; at 45 years, 30.8 percent; at 65 years, 34.1 percent (Wyngaarden and Smith 1988: 1220).

The Wing et al. (1991) study, which followed women for three years, found that along with the weight gain came worsening of risk factors of coronary heart disease. Specifically, there were increases in blood pressure, cholesterol, LDLs, and triglycerides.

The Older Years

As previously discussed, aging is associated with a normal increase in both body weight and fat content for women. By the age of 65, 34.1 percent of total body weight is fat; by 85, this percentage rises to 36.7 (Wyngaarden and Smith 1988: 1220).

The RDAs for older women (see Appendix E) are based on a number of assumptions, as well as actual studies. For example, the energy requirement is based on the observation that lean body mass declines during the adult years at a rate of approximately 2 to 3 percent each decade (National Research Council 1989: 30). In addition, for those over the age of 65, it has been determined that the previously observed gender differences in expenditure of calories gradually disappear, so that the recommendations for caloric consumption become identical for men and women in this age group. This recommendation also "assumes continued light-to-moderate activity, which should be encouraged in the interest of maintaining muscle mass and well-being. It should not be assumed that the marked decline in activity often observed in the elderly is either inevitable or desirable" (National Research Council 1989: 33).

Despite the realistic concern about osteoporosis and the attention paid to its prevention and treatment, it appears that diet makes very little contribution to this disease by this age. The most important tool for preventing further loss in bone mass is taking estrogens. Nonetheless, it is recommended that women past menopause consume 1.5 g of calcium daily.

Poverty and depression are the most common causes of malnutrition of elderly women in the United States, but alcoholism is also often a hidden cause. The common "tea and toast" diet puts these women at risk for many dietary deficiencies, as do consumption of alcohol and medications. These deficiencies may, for various reasons, go undiagnosed.

In the elderly, dietary intake of vitamin A is often inadequate; the common practice of using laxatives (particularly mineral oil) compounds the problem because vitamin A is fat-soluble and gets excreted in the stool, rather than getting absorbed.

Older women are also subject to deficiencies of several of the B vitamins. Alcoholism is the most common cause of thiamin (vitamin B_1) deficiency in older people, though lifelong patterns of consumption of large amounts of coffee may also be to blame. Because alcoholism is often missed by physicians of older women, the diagnosis of associated thiamin deficiency is rarely considered. Some of its symptoms (see the first section of this chapter) may also be misdiagnosed as being caused by heart disease, neurologic disease, or just "old age." Alcoholism can also result in niacin deficiency, worsened in the presence of deficiency of pyridoxine, with which it shares some symptoms.

Deficiency of riboflavin (vitamin B_2) commonly occurs in this age group as the result of intake of less than the required 1.3 mg each day, owing to inadequate consumption of milk, liver, meat, and eggs. In addition, certain chronic illnesses that occur more commonly in women than men can interfere with its absorption from the intestine or its processing in the body; certain medications can have the same effects. Some of the psychotropic drugs that are more often prescribed for women (e.g., chloropromazine, imipramine, and amitriptyline) interfere with the metabolism of riboflavin.

The weakness and lethargy that are common early symptoms of ascorbic acid (vitamin C) deficiency are obviously nonspecific and easily confused with "aging." The difficulty breathing and pain in bones and joints that follow also mimic other problems in this age group.

Diagnosing malnutrition in the elderly is difficult for physicians for two reasons. First, there are no clear criteria; it is disconcerting that despite their high risk for nutritional deficiencies, there are no standards for diagnosing malnutrition in people over 75 (Wyngaarden and Smith 1988). Second, some of the changes typically associated with malnutrition may also accompany aging. For example, sparse hair, dry skin, atrophy of the tongue, diminished taste and smell, and bleeding gums in someone with poorly fitting dentures are considered effects of aging, but they are also signs and symptoms of possible malnutrition. As physicians begin to study and better understand the aging process, they may learn that some changes that have been considered part of the normal aging process are, in fact, the result of undiagnosed malnutrition.

PART THREE

Health Policy Issues for Women

CHAPTER ELEVEN

Medical Care of Women in the United States

Access to Health Care

Much has been written about the problems of access to health care in America. It is clear that in this country socioeconomic status often determines whether or not health care can be obtained, as well as the quality of that care. For women, even being of high socioeconomic status does not guarantee access to care, but surely the problem is worse for those who are poor.

The concept of access is more complex than it might appear at first. Access has been described by Pechansky and Thomas (1981) as consisting of five relationships: availability, accessibility, affordability, accommodation, and acceptability. Each of these is problematic for women patients.

Availability is the relationship between supply and need. This is a problem because, in contrast with that for men, the extent of the need has not yet been determined for women. The more we investigate the true status of women's health, the more we realize that they need far more services, particularly in the areas of prevention and screening. The adequacy of the current supply of physicians who are appropriately trained to meet these yet-to-be-fully-determined needs awaits further study. Regarding the well-defined health needs of women (that is, those that relate to their reproductive health), we already have evidence of disparities between supply and need. For example, the high cost of malpractice insurance for obstetricians has caused many to retreat from the delivery rooms, creating a shortage of sorts. A resurgence of midwifery in this country might fill this void were it not for restrictive legislation in many states that bars many otherwise qualified midwives from practice. The decline in training to perform abortions is another area in which supply is unable to meet demand (see Chapter 6).

Accessibility is the relationship between the locations of services and the populations being served. This aspect of access is problematic for women for many reasons, primarily related to their multiple roles as caregivers for children, spouses, and parents and as participants in the paid labor force. These responsibilities greatly limit the time women have for obtaining the health care they need for themselves and their families. Moreover, some health services are not provided anywhere near certain populations of women. The inability to find convenient sources of health care often precludes women from ever getting it. For women to get the care that they and their families need, more thought must be given to providing care in more convenient locations, as is now done with school-based health clinics for adolescents. The work place, the day-care center, the senior center, and even the shopping mall are alternatives to be explored. The growing numbers of neighborhood "urgent care centers" and of doctors returning to the practice of making house calls suggest that some providers have gotten the message. The federal government has also recognized that a house call may be more cost-effective than having a patient come to a hospital or doctor's office. For example, Medicare is now paying doctors almost twice their office fee for the average house call (*International Herald Tribune*, Aug. 9, 1992). Such action provides an incentive for more doctors to follow suit.

Affordability is the relationship between the price of health care and the financial resources of the patient. This critical issue is discussed below under Health Insurance. Suffice it to say here that women are less likely than men to have adequate health insurance, which in this country remains linked to job and marital status.

Accommodation describes the relationship between the organization of health care resources and the use patterns of patients; it is closely related to accessibility. Not only are health care facilities not typically located in sites accessible to busy women, but their hours are rarely convenient for women in the paid labor force or those dependent on others for transportation.

Acceptability is the important relationship between the characteristics of the health care provider and the attitudes, preferences, and expectations of patients. Although there has been a lot of research into the satisfaction of patients with their health care, it has only recently considered the genders of the patients and the providers. (These factors will be explored in greater detail in Chapter 12.) The weight of the evidence suggests that women are less satisfied with the care they receive than are men. For example, a 1993 survey by Louis Harris and Associates for the Commission on Women's Health of the Commonwealth Fund found that 41 percent of women and only 27 percent of men surveyed had changed doctors because they were dissatisfied with their care (Commonwealth Fund 1993).

Cost of Women's Health Problems

According to data from the Department of Commerce and the Department of Health and Human Services, spending on health care in the United States in 1991 reached a record level of $738 billion. It rose to $817 billion in 1992, equivalent to 14 percent of the gross national product (GNP). By comparison, in Canada, which has a plan of national health insurance, the cost of health care represents only 8.6 percent of GNP.

Between one-half and three-quarters of the total health care expenditures in the United States are attributable to women, according to estimates made in 1988 (Litt 1993). While it is difficult to verify the components of these expenditures under the present system of care, the total represents an amalgam of costs for medications and other services, time lost from the paid labor force, terminal and residential care for the elderly, and other costs. Table 11.1 provides an estimate of costs related to women's illnesses.

It has been estimated that more than 50 percent of lifetime health care costs are expended in the last six months of life. These costs could be significantly reduced by effective screening for prevention of illness, early detection of curable illness, and referral for early prenatal care. These measures would reduce the number of chronic conditions that require hospitalization. Long-term cost reductions would also eventuate from an increase in current research expenditures.

TABLE 11.1
Estimated Cost of Women's Health Problems

Arthritis (Osteoarthritis, rheumatoid arthritis)	$36 billion/yr
Osteoporosis	over $10 billion for care of fractures (1987)
Cancers (all)	$104 billion (1990)[a]
Atherosclerosis	$34.2 billion (1987, direct costs)
Congestive heart failure	$4.7 billion (1987, direct costs)
Coronary artery disease (e.g., heart attacks)	$14 billion (1987, direct costs)
High blood pressure	$13.7 billion (1991, estimate)
Stroke	$25 billion/yr
Urinary tract infections	$4.4 billion/yr[b]
Alzheimer disease	$88 billion (1985)
Migraine	over $50 billion/yr (workdays lost and medical expenses)
Eye disorders	over $16 billion/yr
Depression	over $27 billion/yr[c]
Asthma	$6.8 billion/yr (1986)[d]
Chronic obstructive pulmonary disease (e.g., emphysema)	$10.2 billion (1988)
Diabetes mellitus	$20.4 billion/yr

[a] Approximately one-third for direct medical costs, less than two-thirds for mortality costs, one-tenth for lost productivity/morbidity
[b] Includes physician, hospitalization, and lost productivity
[c] 15 percent of this amount lost owing to suicides
[d] One-third for direct medical costs

SOURCE: Adapted from Litt 1993.

Health Insurance

Thirty-seven million Americans had no health insurance in 1990, and an additional seven to ten million had insurance considered to be inadequate. By 1994, it was estimated that an additional ten million people had lost their health insurance.

One-quarter of American women aged 18–24, and 13 percent of those aged 18–44, are uninsured. Even these figures are deceptively low; many women in the childbearing years are defined as "insured" because they get Medicaid coverage that is limited to pregnancy-related care. Among those aged 45–64, twice as many women (13 percent) as men (7 percent) have no health insurance. Older women are also less likely than older men to have private group health insurance. They must therefore rely more heavily on individual private health insurance policies, which cost more (Older Women's League 1991). In fact, this type of insurance is purchased by 24 percent of women and only 17 percent of men in the over-45 age group (U.S. Bureau of the Census 1990).

Women figure prominently among the uninsured and underinsured for a variety of reasons. Health insurance coverage in the United States is typically linked to employment status. Census Bureau data from 1991 show us that, regardless of the criteria used, women in the paid labor force are at a clear disadvantage when it comes to health insurance coverage. This has been acknowledged in the past and rationalized on the grounds that women enter the labor force later than men because they often have their children first, or that they work fewer hours each week because of competing domestic obligations, or that they work for employers who have businesses that are too small to provide health insurance. The 1991 study controlled for all of these factors and compared men and women who have worked the same length of time, work the same number of hours, and work for companies of the same size. It found that "at any point in the employment spectrum, men are more likely to be covered than women" (*New York Times*, natl. ed., May 22, 1994).

Here are the details: Of those who have been working less than one year, 52 percent of men but only 41 percent of women have health insurance; of those with one to ten years on the job, the figures are 68 percent of men and 57 percent of women; and of those working eleven or more years, 78 percent of men and 70 percent of women.

Moreover, men who work less than 25 hours per week are 7 percent more likely than women working the same number of hours to have health insurance through their jobs. Even for the workers with the longest hours, 35 or more each week, 66 percent of the men are covered, compared with 62 percent of the women.

The greatest gaps are found, however, when one examines company size. In the smallest firms, those with fewer than 25 employees, 35 percent of men but only 23 percent of women have health insurance; in firms with 25 to 99 employees, 63 percent of men and only 48 percent of women; and in the largest firms, those with 100 or more employees, 78 percent of men and only 64 percent of women.

In addition to these discrepancies, women who are in the paid labor force are more likely than men to work part time, to work in temporary and/or service positions, and to work for small businesses, and therefore to be ineligible for health insurance. Only 40 percent of employed women have health insurance, compared with 59 percent of employed men (Commonwealth Fund 1993). According to an Older Women's League study (1991, quoted in Commonwealth Fund 1993), only 55 percent of female administrative support staff, 30 percent of female sales staff, and 24 percent of females in service industries have group health insurance provided by their employers. Moreover, employed women in and after their mid-forties are much more likely than men of the same age to lack health insurance. A recent study showed that only 55 percent of working women, compared with 72 percent of men, aged 45–64 have health insurance from their employers. The situation is particularly bad for black and Hispanic older women. Although women constitute only 52 percent of this age cohort, they pay an average of 62 percent of all out-of-pocket medical costs paid by the cohort (Older Women's League 1991). In sum, three-quarters of the twelve million uninsured women in the United States are employed, and 15 percent of all employed women have no health insurance. The Health Security Act proposed by President Clinton in 1993 would have provided direct access to health insurance to half of all working women, aged 18 to 64.

To the uninsured or underinsured employed women are added the unemployed female heads of households; these women often have no insurance or have meager federal insurance under Medicaid. Twice as many women as men are served by Medicaid, and three-fifths of the Medicare elderly population in 1984 were women (Jecker 1991). According to Jecker, in 1986, women made up 71 percent of what has been referred to as the "crossover population," those who are both poor and elderly and thus entitled to both Medicaid and Medicare (Muller 1991). Such government health insurance is often inadequate because of limited provider participation; restrictions on services, especially for screening and prevention; and, for Medicare, considerable copayment requirements (Commonwealth Fund 1993). An example of these limitations is that Medicaid coverage for pregnancy-related care doesn't apply to other health needs and usually ends within two months after the pregnancy. This often translates to the inability of women to receive contraception for more than two months after delivery. Under the block grant proposal likely to be implemented by Congress, this situation will worsen.

Even women who have health coverage are likely to have it as dependents on their husbands' policies, so they are at risk for losing it as the result of divorce or widowhood (Berk and Taylor 1984). Moreover, women have fewer possessions and financial resources to use in the event of medical need than men (Lewis 1985). These facts reflect the disproportionately high poverty rate for women of all ages (Pearce 1993). They also relate to the continuing wage gap between the genders. Although, in general, women are paid 72 cents for every dollar earned by men, this gap widens with age. According to 1990 figures from the U.S. Department of Labor, women 50 and older earn 63.7 cents for every dollar earned by men of the same age. For the most part, this inequity reflects barriers to entry into better-paying careers and late entry into the work force for women who first bore children in the 1950's. But that is only part of the story. Even within the same careers, men earn more than women of the same age. For example, female doctors 50 years and older earn 84.3 cents of every dollar earned by male doctors in the same age group. Female lawyers fare slightly better at 90.3 cents for every male lawyer's dollar.

When it comes to receiving necessary medical treatment for illnesses, more women than men lack the insurance coverage they need. Even among those who do have health insurance, twice as many women as men have policies with inadequate catastrophic coverage (U.S. Bureau of the Census 1990). A survey conducted by the Commonwealth Fund in 1993 showed that "13 percent of women needed medical care but did not get it, compared with 9 percent of men." Thirty-six percent of uninsured women did not receive needed care, compared with 10 percent of women with employer-paid insurance and 6 percent of those covered under Medicare. Many studies have shown that uninsured women are less likely to have a checkup or even to be hospitalized than women with insurance. A 1991 study showed one shocking result of this disparity in care: Uninsured black women between the ages of 50 and 64 have a 37 percent greater chance of dying than women with insurance. White women in this age group without insurance had a 15 percent higher rate of dying in the hospital (Hadley, Steinberg, and Feder 1991).

Even women who are insured often are not covered for all the services they should receive, particularly preventive services. The importance of prevention to saving lives and reducing the toll of illness, as well as lowering the cost of providing health care to the victims of preventable diseases, is now well recognized. Nonetheless, the majority of insured women have coverage that excludes preventive and early detection screening procedures, which is surely penny wise and pound foolish. In the 1993 Commonwealth Fund survey, one-fifth of insured women reported lack of coverage for preventive services. A 1988 study found that the single most reliable predictor of the failure of women in the 45–64-year age group to receive recommended preventive services (such as blood pressure checks, Pap smears, breast examinations, and screening for glaucoma) was lack of health insurance coverage (Woolhandler and Himmelstein 1988).

Most of the research on the impact of inadequate health insurance on women has focused on pregnancy outcome, with compelling findings. As discussed in Chapter 6, early and continuous prenatal care is the most important determinant of good pregnancy outcome, having been convincingly shown to reduce the incidence of stillbirths, miscarriages, and prematurity, the last being one of the most costly of these complications. This has been shown to be true for all ethnic, socioeconomic, and age groups. Adolescents are the group that is least likely to seek and receive adequate prenatal care; accordingly, adolescents continue to have a higher rate of premature births than any other age group. Although there are psychologic as well as sociologic reasons for this, one contributing factor is clearly their lack of health insurance coverage for maternity-related care. They may have no insurance at all, or they may be covered by their parents' policies. Some of these policies exclude maternity care; others require that the parental policyholders be notified when such care is provided, and this requirement makes teenagers reluctant to use the care.

Many women other than adolescents also fail to receive adequate prenatal care because they lack health insurance. The cost to society of providing health care to the premature babies born to these mothers far exceeds that of simply providing coverage for the prenatal care. Moreover, the human toll of the failure to provide that coverage is tremendous: The fact that the United States has the highest infant mortality rate in all the industrialized world is largely attributable to inaccessibility of prenatal care.

Lack of health insurance for mothers often translates to lack of coverage for their children. Hartmann (1991) found that during the 1980's there was a 3 percent drop in the proportion of married couples with children who had health insurance through their employers. For single mothers, however, this drop was 10 percent. By 1987, half of all single mothers had no health insurance for their children. Even when the inadequate coverage provided by Medicaid is included, children of single mothers are twice as likely not to have health insurance as those of married couples. They are therefore more likely to get sick, due to lack of preventive care (e.g., immunization). In addition to the possible health consequences for the children and the unmeasurable psychologic impact on the mothers, the economic toll of this situation is substantial. Children's illness is a leading cause of their parents' absence from work, a factor that often leads to job loss for single parents, most of whom are women (Hartmann 1991).

Reform of the American health insurance system is clearly needed but must be carefully structured. Health insurance for all people must be provided, not only for humanitarian reasons, but also to reduce the costs of health care. Enhancing the employability of women remains an important step toward improvement in their health status as long as this country is burdened by employment-linked health insurance coverage. Universal health coverage would be the more effective route, provided that it were unencumbered by politicized restrictions of choice and that it permitted access to the needed range of detection, prevention, and treatment options required to protect and improve women's health.

The other issue to be considered in the debate over national health insurance relates to proposals for covering its costs. Among the options being discussed is reduction in Social Security payments. While this may, at first view, appear appropriate, it is another potential land mine for women. Because many more women than men are dependent upon Social Security benefits, any reduction in these benefits will disproportionately impact women. The same is true for the recommendation to contain the skyrocketing costs of Social Security benefits by delaying the payout until the age of 67. Again, because more women are in this age group, they will be disproportionately hurt.

Health Care Rationing

When health care resources are scarce and/or expensive, as they currently are in the United States, decisions about their allocation are made. There is growing evidence that when health care is rationed, women suffer disproportionately. Society's view of the "relative worth" of men versus women appears to influence rationing decisions. As men are still viewed as the primary financial supports of families in this country, our society continues to place a higher value on their lives and appears to be more willing to pay for their health costs and to favor them in rationing of limited resources.

One example is that gender differences have now been found in the length of hospital stay and level of utilization of intensive care. Bernard et al. (1993) found that for the same diagnoses, women were hospitalized for longer periods and were less likely to be placed in an intensive care unit.

Another common example involves coronary artery bypass, an expensive surgical procedure that extends the lives of those who have obstruction of the blood vessels that supply heart muscle. Alternative treatment includes passage of a balloon through the obstruction. Failure to institute any treatment eventuates in complete blockage of the artery, resulting in a myocardial infarction and possible death. In order to know who is in need of these treatments, that is, who has blockage of the coronary arteries, cardiac catheterization must be performed (see Chapter 4). As discussed in Chapter 4, recent research has shown that women over the age of 65 are just as likely to die of a heart attack as are men in the same age group. Among younger people, men have three times the risk of coronary artery disease. It has recently been revealed, however, that women are not three, but 6.5, times less likely than men with the same symptoms to be referred by their physicians for coronary artery catheterization. Moreover, when coronary artery disease is discovered, women are less likely to be referred for bypass surgery.

Surgeons have rationalized these findings on the basis of the observation that women do more poorly and have a higher chance of dying
after bypass surgery than men. While at first glance this explanation seems
reasonable, more careful scrutiny of the situation suggests otherwise. It is
now clear that the reason women do more poorly after bypass surgery is
that they are referred for this procedure later in the course of their disease, when they are sicker than men are (Khan et al. 1990). When men
and women are matched by the severity of disease at the time of surgery,
there is no difference in outcome. There is, therefore, no scientific reason
for withholding this expensive, but life-extending, surgical procedure
from women.

Organ transplantation, too, is affected by considerations of gender.
Because there are so few organs available for transplantation and because
the costs of the procedure are so high, patients who need a transplanted
organ in order to live are at the present time in competition with each
other. The process of deciding who will be accepted for transplantation is
obviously a difficult one, typically shared by physicians, ethicists, clergy,
and social workers on hospital ethics teams. Despite the care that goes
into the process, these individuals are often accused of "playing God" because of the grave implications of their decisions. The factors that enter
into such a decision include the age of the patient (with younger patients
generally being favored), the likelihood that the individual will "contribute to society," whether or not the person is the family breadwinner,
the presence or absence of other illnesses, the likelihood that the patient
will be psychologically able to handle the demands and pressures of the
procedure and necessary long years of follow-up treatment, and so on.
Although gender is never an explicit factor in the decision-making
process, there is evidence that it enters into it indirectly. This is clearly illustrated by a study of patients with untreatable kidney disease for which
kidney transplantation represents the only hope to avoid death. A female
patient with this disease had a 25 percent lower chance than a male with
the same disease to receive a kidney transplant. Among those 46 to 60
years old, a woman's chance was actually half that of a man (Kjellstrand
1988).

More broadly, the age criterion for transplants biases the decision
against women as a group because they are overrepresented among the
elderly, those most often in need of transplantation. A similar argument is

made by Jecker and Pearlman (1989), who point out the potential disparity in effect on men and women of proposed denial of publicly funded life-extending care for the elderly. Not only are there more women than men in the ranks of the elderly, but, as previously mentioned, they rely more heavily than men on publicly funded health insurance. What is rarely taken into account is that denying life-extending care to women would deny them more years of life than men because they tend to live longer.

CHAPTER TWELVE

Women as Doctors

Who says that women doctors are new on the scene? As early as 3,000 years ago, evidence indicates that women practiced medicine, even surgery. It is written that Philista was a professor of medicine in the fourth century before Christ who was so beautiful that she had to lecture from behind a screen to avoid distracting her students (Kiprowska 1978).

In colonial America and during the early republican era, health care was primarily administered by women in and to their families and their communities. Midwifery was the exclusive domain of women in many cultures throughout recorded history. By the mid-nineteenth century, however, this role was usurped by men, who were "professionals" in terms of their scientific training, but unschooled in this, the most female of experiences. It is perhaps ironic that the exclusion of women from this traditional role was caused by the action of a woman. It is said that Queen Victoria's insistence that her childbirth be painless led to the practice of administering ether for deliveries, a task considered too demanding for women midwives.

From their European scientific educational backgrounds, male physicians dramatically transformed the practice of medicine in America in the second half of the eighteenth century. Soon joined by graduates of the few American medical schools, such as those associated with Harvard University, Columbia University, and the University of Pennsylvania, these physicians secured their futures by establishing licensing procedures that effectively foreclosed the possibility that women would ever compete for their patients and practice medicine.

Although her admission to the Geneva Medical College in New York resulted from a class joke, Elizabeth Blackwell nevertheless, on January 23, 1849, became the first woman in the United States to receive an M.D. degree. The thinking of her male medical colleagues was reflected in the remarks of the famous gynecologic surgeon, Dr. Charles Meigs, in a lecture to the students at Jefferson Medical College entitled "Distinctive Characteristics of the Female." He began, "The great administrative faculties are not hers," and concluded, "She has a head almost too small for intellect and just big enough for love" (Women in Pediatrics 1983: 679). Harvard Medical School admitted a woman student (and three "Negroes") in 1850, but all were forced to withdraw after student riots. Women were not again admitted there until 1945 (Clever 1991).

By the last half of the nineteenth century, the medical profession could scarcely be called that, having degenerated into a panoply of sects, with no licensure requirements; medical schools of poor quality proliferated. In such an environment, it became easier for women to train to be physicians, particularly in the many women's medical schools that opened. Accordingly, in 1894, in Boston, 23.7 percent of medical school graduates were women (Rincke 1981). Around the turn of the century, the number of women doctors grew to a level not even equaled in 1992, the so-called Year of the Woman.

Enrollment in medical school did not, however, guarantee access to clinical lectures or the right to observe demonstrations of surgical procedures, as these typically took place in hospitals, where women students were not welcome. It is said that the arrival of the students from the Philadelphia Women's Medical College to observe clinics at the Pennsylvania Hospital in 1868 precipitated a riot by the male medical students.

The Medical School of the Pacific (which later became Stanford University School of Medicine) graduated its first woman student, Alice Higgins, in 1877 and its second, Anabel McG. Stuart, the next year. Clelia Duel Mosher, a Stanford University A.B. in zoology, found after receiving her M.D. from Johns Hopkins School of Medicine in 1909 that she could not get a medical school faculty position. She returned to the Stanford campus with the title of assistant professor of personal hygiene and medical advisor for women. Alice Hamilton became the first woman physician faculty member at the Harvard Medical School in 1919, but she was not allowed to join the faculty club or academic processions, nor could she "exercise the faculty option for season football tickets!" (Clever 1991).

Even with diploma in hand, a young woman doctor continued to face closed doors at hospitals and dispensaries in which she sought to work in order to gain experience and, later, admitting privileges. Some women, including Elizabeth Blackwell, who, in spite of having graduated first in her medical school class, could not get a clinical appointment in this country, went to Europe for training. To earn a living, many women physicians engaged in public health lecturing. Blackwell offered one of the first courses on the physical education of girls in 1852 in support of her belief that women physicians "should be the 'connecting link' between science and the everyday life of women" (Morantz-Sanchez 1985: 150).

While some women found practice opportunities in rural communities, others were relegated to filling the low-pay, low-status positions in institutions rejected by their male peers. Work in "lunatic asylums," almshouses, "water-cure" establishments, penal institutions, and women's schools provided both job security and the experience they could not get elsewhere. Some returning, European-trained women doctors founded their own hospitals and dispensaries, which catered to the poor and immigrant populations of women and children. Seeing the effect of miserable living and working conditions on their patients led many women physicians to activism for social reform and thus laid the foundation for the profession of social work.

The next hurdle for women physicians was membership in medical societies, an opportunity denied them in all but some midwestern states until the 1870's. National professional societies continued this discriminatory practice until the twentieth century. In fact, women were not permitted membership in the American Medical Association until 1915 (at the time of the presidency of Victor C. Vaughan, M.D.). In response, women formed their own medical societies, the first of which was founded in 1898 in Iowa. According to Morantz-Sanchez (1985: 181), these organizations provided support and friendship, and "coached younger and timid or reserved women in self-confidence before they went on to grapple with the forbidding world of male colleagues."

With the closing of most of the women's medical schools early in the twentieth century and with the increasing "professionalism" promulgated by the elite cadre of male physicians, women again faced frustration and quotas. In fact, until passage of the federal equal opportunity legislation of 1974, medical schools in this country (many of them openly) limited to 10 percent the number of women admitted. As a result, only 17 percent of currently practicing physicians are women. From 1975 through 1992, there was an annual increase of 1 percent in women medical school applicants (Bickel 1995). Between the 1992 and 1993 academic years, the number of women applicants increased by 15 percent to 17,957 (compared to 14 percent and 24,851 for men; Association of American Medical Colleges 1994). Of greater interest is the percentage of woman applicants who are accepted for matriculation. In thirteen of the elite medical schools, this figure rose from 38 percent in 1983 to a peak of 51 percent in 1984 and 1985. Since that time the percentages have been falling, and in 1994, the figure was 38 percent, the same as that recorded more than a decade ago. The actual percentage of women in medical schools currently ranges from 40 to 50 percent. In 1993, 32 percent of all resident physicians (i.e., those in specialty training) were women.

Women physicians continue to face intense scrutiny. One question has been whether (as I was admonished when I was accepted to medical school) women take the place of men who would contribute more time and effort to medical practice. A number of studies have concluded that women spend less time in practice in their early adult years but that these apparent deficits are more than compensated for over the course of a woman physician's longer lifetime. For example, a review of five surveys from 1957 to 1971 concluded that 84.3 to 91.1 percent of female, compared with 94 to 99.4 percent of male, physicians were working (Heins et al. 1977). These researchers, in their own survey in the Detroit area, found that women physicians spent 90 percent as much time in medical practice as did the men, "despite the fact that most of the women had full responsibility for homes and families." Recent studies suggest, moreover, that the differences in number of hours worked by female and male physicians are decreasing (Freiman and Marder 1984).

A 1989 study by the American Medical Association found that although women physicians work 8 percent fewer hours weekly than their male counterparts, they earn about 40 percent less (American Medical

Association Center on Health Policy Research 1989). That income disparity has not diminished in this decade.

Women's Practice of Medicine

It is too soon to know what effect the increase in women physicians will
have on the practice of medicine. Some of the preliminary findings are
interesting, however. For example, in a report of a survey conducted at
the Johns Hopkins School of Hygiene and Public Health, female doctors were found to spend more time with their patients than did male
doctors (Ganske 1992). Among internists, the average visit with a male
doctor lasted 18.7 minutes, compared with 23.5 minutes for a female
doctor. One study (Mendoza and Litt, unpublished data) of prenatal care
visits for pregnant adolescents found a similar difference between female
health care providers and male doctors. Of course, these differences are
open to many interpretations. Rather than representing women's greater
interest and work, they may reflect men's greater efficiency or skill. This
latter possibility is, however, challenged by Debra Roter of Johns Hopkins, whose study of gender differences in physician-patient communication was reported by Ganske (1992). Her analysis of 500 visits in eleven
different health care delivery sites showed that the longer sessions with
women doctors were the result of their spending more time discussing
the patients' conditions and of the patients' talking more. Of course, this
study could be criticized for not taking into account the possibility that
patients chose to go to either male or female doctors partly because they
perceived women as being more willing to talk with them, and that the
resulting differences reflected their own preference and comfort rather
than those of the providers. In the smaller study of prenatal visits, however, patients did not choose their health care providers, yet the same
physician gender differences were seen.

Further evidence of gender differences in the medical visit was found
in a videotape study of interactions between physicians and their patients
by Candace West, a University of California, Santa Cruz, sociologist.
West's study showed that female physicians were half as likely as male
physicians to interrupt their patients (Pfeiffer 1985).

In her study of gender differences in communication styles, Deborah

Tannen (1990) finds much to help us understand what goes on in the doctor's office, though she has not yet turned her expert ear to that setting. Since most doctors are male and since most patients are female and many are dissatisfied with their doctors, a lot of what Tannen describes is likely to apply in doctor-patient communication. Tannen characterizes male talk as "report talk," as compared with women's "rapport talk." By this, she means that women talk to express empathy, show support, and build consensus. In contrast, males talk to get facts and solve problems; men are also keenly aware of status differences between parties that demand that the conversation place them in a "one-up" position.

What does this have to do with the doctor's office? Think about what usually transpires in the few minutes of conversation between the typical male doctor and the typical patient. In my experience, the doctor takes a "history," which means that he asks questions about the symptom that has brought the patient to see him. Time constraints and the kind of training he has received demand concise, specific answers to his questions. Male patients typically comply; women are less likely to. After gathering the information he needs to reach a diagnosis, the male physician makes his pronouncement about what is wrong and what has to be done to fix it.

This conversation may take different forms, depending on the sex of the patient. Consider the following exchange:

DOCTOR: When did you first get the pain in your chest, Mr. Jones?
PATIENT: One week ago.
DOCTOR: What were you doing when you first felt the pain?
PATIENT: Shoveling snow.

After a few more similar questions and answers, the doctor concludes that Mr. Jones may be suffering from angina. He gives him a prescription for nitroglycerine and orders a stress test EKG.

How is this conversation different when the patient is a woman?

DOCTOR: When did you first get the pain in your chest, Mary?
PATIENT: I think it was sometime last week. Yes, it must have been on Sunday because that's the day I always speak to my daughter

in New York. You remember her, the one who got married last year when I had that rash that you told me was from my nerves.

After a few minutes of what appears irrelevant and time-consuming talk, the doctor is annoyed and might note in the chart that the patient is "a poor historian." More often than not, the chest pain is interpreted as "psychosomatic," the female patient is given a prescription for a tranquilizer, and no further tests are ordered. The patient leaves the office feeling dissatisfied because the doctor didn't appear to be listening and she didn't have the time (or the courage) to ask other questions about her health.

Poor communication between doctors and patients is responsible for most dissatisfaction with health care. Patients often feel that their doctors haven't listened to their concerns or don't understand them. Doctors, on the other hand, may feel that patients aren't following their advice and blame lack of improvement on presumed noncompliance with their prescription or instructions.

There are other, related reasons why patients are dissatisfied with their physicians. Whenever this topic is studied, there are fairly predictable findings. Dissatisfaction results when patients have to wait a long time before seeing their doctor, when they are forced to see a doctor other than their regular doctor, when they feel that the doctor hasn't spent enough time with them, when the doctor either forgets something about their history or asks for information they assume is available in the chart, when they are not given enough information to understand what is wrong with them or how they are supposed to take their medication, when they believe the doctor to be incompetent, and/or when they feel they have been charged too much money for what they have gotten. Naturally, patients are more satisfied when they see improvement in the condition under treatment.

These complaints are common to both men and women patients. When I talk to women about their experiences with their doctors, I hear more. Women object to the terse, businesslike approach of most doctors. If the doctor asks how they are doing, they feel that he is not really interested in knowing about the things that are important to them (e.g., family events, juggling work and home, and feelings). Missing are the trappings, if not the reality, of connectedness: the nods of agreement, the words of affirmation. The doctor, on the other hand, often characterizes his women patients as being unable to give coherent, logical, and chronologically sequenced descriptions of the reasons for their visits. Women typically tend to enrich their telling of their health story (the "herstory" instead of the more traditional "medical *history*") with associations that are important to them but may seem irrelevant to the doctor. I think these gender differences help explain why women patients are so turned off by doctors. First, by urging that they "get to the point," the doctor cuts off their history telling. The patients then feel that the doctor doesn't have all the information. Tannen believes that men speak in this way in order to be "one-up" on their conversational partners. The doctor then tells the patients what is wrong and what to do about it. This is "report talk," devoid of apparent caring. It may be to the liking of some patients, but often, particularly for women, it is annoying.

What about the growing numbers of women doctors? It is probably too early to see if there will be major differences between their communication styles and those of their male colleagues. Remember, also, that these women have been trained by male teachers and role models. They may, therefore, have been influenced to practice medicine as these men do, in a way that may override their "natural" tendencies to do otherwise. It is also important to recognize that there are individual differences in personalities and communication styles among women doctors, just as there are among all women and men.

Surveys suggest greater idealism among women physicians about their role as doctors; they are more willing to provide care to poor patients than are their male peers. In addition, a study of Boston-area physicians by Isaac Schiff of the Massachusetts General Hospital found women to be twenty times more likely than men to prescribe ERT for menopausal patients (Angier 1992). This same gender difference is seen for the prescription of pain medications, suggesting that women doctors may be more empathetic in responding to their patients' complaints of pain, or perhaps that patients are more willing to "complain" about pain with a woman doctor. These possibilities have not yet been looked at independently. Another interesting study (Borum 1996) found that physicians of both sexes order more screening tests for patients of their own sex. This implies greater identification with patients of one's own sex, just as has been found for race. As a result, women doctors are more likely to order Pap smears and mammograms for their patients than are male doctors. On the other hand, it appears that male doctors more frequently order screening tests for prostate cancer. For a condition that is not linked to sex, such as colon cancer, there also appears to be bias in screening based on physician gender. In one study, female physicians were more likely than male physicians to screen their female patients, and male physicians more likely than female physicians to screen their male patients (Borum 1996).

Female Doctors' Career Choices and Development

Pediatrics, psychiatry, and pathology are the fields of medicine most often chosen by women in the past, with 38 percent, 23.3 percent, and 23 percent in each, respectively, as of 1992. This picture is rapidly changing, however. For example, among the 31,000 women in residency training in 1993, more than 25 percent have chosen internal medicine; 16 percent, family practice; 9 percent, obstetrics/gynecology; and 8 percent, psychiatry (Bickel 1995). In recent years there has also been a tremendous increase in the numbers of women doctors choosing emergency medicine and intensive care. The reasons for these shifts from the primary care areas to the higher-technology fields in which there is considerably less opportunity for continuing patient contact are complicated and not yet well studied. Do they represent women doctors' recent rejection of the traditional nurturant role, the attraction of the controllable schedules and absence of initial financial investment in these hospital-based fields, or reduction of male discrimination against women in their well-guarded ranks? This last possibility seems unlikely; what has changed are not male surgeons' attitudes toward admitting female doctors into their ranks, but their exclusionary tactics, which by all reports are now more subtle.

Although women now comprise about 40 percent of medical students in the United States, their representation on faculties and in academic leadership positions remains problematic. It has long been argued that this is a pipeline issue; that is, that it is too early to expect to see women in higher places. The reality is that women began entering medical school in greater numbers twenty years ago. In other words, there has been sufficient time for women to rise through the academic ranks, were time the only issue. More likely, the pipeline leaks.

Recent figures reflect this interpretation: women compose only 20 percent of medical school faculties, and the great majority remain clustered at the lower ranks (American College of Physicians 1991). In 1989, for example, 71 percent of faculty women were at the level of assistant professor or lower, in contrast to only 43 percent of the men. In a 1994 report, the number of women professors (1,883) was just 10 percent of that of men (18,745). Even within the professor group, there are gender differences in status. For example, 23 percent of the male faculty in clinical departments are tenured, compared with only 7 percent of the women (Bickel 1995). Across all ranks, in 1989 only 6.7 percent of all tenured faculty were women (Eisenberg 1989).

Janet Bickel examined the cohort appointed to faculties in the same year (1976) and found that 12 percent of men and only 3 percent of women had been promoted to full professor by 1987 (Bickel 1988). Over a ten-year period in the 1980s, the percentage of men promoted to professor rose from 26 to 31, while the percentage of women rose from only 7 to 9. This pattern is consistent with that seen in the previous decade. Similarly, a study of academic promotion in four U.S. medical colleges found that the average number of years for promotion to each professional rank was consistently greater for women than for men (Wallis, Gilder, and Thaler 1981). As of 1990, only one woman was serving as a medical school dean in the United States. Lest you think that represents progress, there were two in 1988. In 1990, in the approximately 130 medical schools in the country, 81 chairs were filled by women (47 in basic science departments and 34 in clinical departments). By 1992, women held approximately 104 chairs in medical school academic departments— fewer than 5 percent of the total number. Even in pediatrics, a field in which there have been more women in academia recently, there were only five women chairs at the beginning of this decade. In the pediatrics departments of medical schools nationwide, half of the resident staff, more than a third of the junior faculty, and only 4 percent of the department chairs are women (Shaller 1990).

These data give rise to the obvious question of why women physicians have advanced so slowly in academia. Advancement within the medical school faculty is based on achievement in three major areas: research, teaching, and patient care. Is there systematic (or unintentional) discrimination against women in these areas, or have they simply not made the grade?

For tenure-line promotion to senior rank, excellence in research and an international reputation are minimal requirements. The first is generally evidenced by having many sole- or first-authored research papers published in prestigious, peer-reviewed medical journals. Some have asserted that women scientists in general, including medical researchers, produce fewer publications (Cole and Zuckerman 1984). They base their conclusions on reviews done before 1983. More recent studies focused specifically on medical school faculty do not find a significant difference (Carr et al. 1993), but it may be too early to appreciate trends.

If the earlier studies are replicated, it will be important to examine reasons for lower research productivity among women. One obvious explanation lies in their conflicting roles as mothers and the need to interrupt their research careers for childbirth and subsequent obligations. In examining this possibility, one study of American scientists actually found that unmarried women publish *less* than married women with children, and that the productivity of women scientists becomes slightly less than that of their unmarried women colleagues only after they have three children (Cole 1979). A 1990 study by Kyvik concludes that comparisons between women with and without children can be misleading. This study, which considered the age of the children, found that child care becomes a critical factor in women scientists' productivity. Although women with children less than ten years old "are considerably less productive than their male counterparts, women with all their children older than this are as productive as men in the same family situation and academic position" (Kyvik 1990: 149).

Another interpretation of the allegedly lower publication rates of women scientists is that they are more careful about their published work and therefore less likely to "crank it out" for the purpose of inflating their curricula vitae.

Inequality in allocation of the necessary resources for research productivity may be another explanation for this allegedly lower number of publications by women scientists. This possibility is supported by a recent study of scientists working at the National Cancer Institute (Seachrist 1994). Female scientists were found to have less than two-thirds of both the personnel and the budgets allocated to male scientists at the same level of seniority. The women also had lower publication rates, but when the calculations were adjusted for the staff and budgetary differences, the women performed at least as well as the men.

In most situations, the resources necessary for research are obtained through the awarding of grant money by federal agencies or private foundations. Although this has not yet been documented, I am aware of anecdotal evidence that women are often left out of the information loop and may be less likely to hear about the availability of these grants.

There is a broader problem of less effective mentoring of women scientists than their male peers. Particularly for women with husbands and children, the opportunities to socialize with their colleagues after work are limited, and, conversely, men often are more comfortable "going out with the boys for a beer." And in the absence of sufficient role models of senior faculty women, fewer female medical students consider academic careers. Moreover, the few women on the faculty are frequently asked to mentor the younger women students and faculty. This adds disproportionately to their already heavy burden of committee and teaching assignments.

It has also been alleged that the present system of decision making with regard to what work actually gets published and to whom it gets credited is itself subject to gender bias. For example, women may lack assertiveness in establishing themselves as first author (even when they have done the bulk of the work or are the creative force in designing the study—two usual criteria for assigning first authorship).

Bias may also result from a medical journal's peer review process, which includes an initial decision about whether or not to send a manuscript out for review, and if so, a decision about who should review it. Very few editors of major medical journals are women. Although it has not yet been well studied, there is the possibility that decisions about the quality of the research may be influenced by the gender of the editor.

Moreover, although the reviewers are anonymous to the author, the reverse is not the case; most journals include the names of the authors when a paper is sent out for review. It has been alleged that this system perpetuates the old-boy network and favors senior (usually male) investigators who have name recognition. It is not that women are directly discriminated against under such a practice, but that they are often less well known than their male colleagues for reasons that seem to be gender-related.

For example, women researchers are less likely than men to be invited to talk at prestigious scientific meetings. According to Natalie Angier (1991), at a recent meeting of skin cancer researchers in New York, only one out of 47 invited speakers was a woman. She believes that those who are invited are the "giants" in the field (read "men") and the great raconteurs—again, generally men. She quotes Dr. Florence Hazeltine of the National Institutes of Child Health and Disease, who is often in a position to organize such meetings. Hazeltine states that women often decline invitations unless they are the top experts, whereas men "will talk about anything." This article also reflects on the ambience of many of these meetings, described as being brutal, "scathing intellectual brawls"; women are often poorly socialized "to enter the fray."

In response to this potential bias against women investigators, a few journals (including the *Journal of Adolescent Health*, of which I am the editor) have begun the practice of sending manuscripts out for "blind" review. By not revealing the names of the authors to the reviewers, blind review levels the playing field.

Establishing a national and international reputation is often another criterion for promotion to senior academic levels. To garner such recognition, a faculty member must achieve wide dissemination of his or her work and travel widely to be seen and to join the network. We have already seen how the publication process may disserve women scientists. The same is true for this networking process. As discussed earlier, women are less likely to be invited to present their work at prestigious meetings. Furthermore, women are rarely considered for membership on national and international boards and committees because of the presumption or the reality that they will be less inclined to commit to frequent travel. When I was asked to become an examiner for the American Board of Pediatrics in 1980, for example, only 3 percent of the group were female, although more than one-third of those being evaluated for board certification at the time were women. The explanation given by the leadership was that women were not willing to travel. The reality was that the group had the reputation at the time of being an old-boy club in which women felt distinctly uncomfortable. Happily, this is beginning to change.

The ultimate form of recognition for academic scientists is election to the National Academy of Sciences. This prestigious institution has a long history of underrepresentation of women. Only 4.1 percent of its total membership is female. In 1991, 60 American scientists were elected to the academy. Only six of them were women (Angier 1991).

Even when their work is equivalent in amount and quality, women faculty in medical schools are given fewer rewards than their male colleagues. In a 1993 controlled study of 1,693 faculty in the internal medicine departments of 107 major teaching hospitals in the United States, Carr found that "women in academic medicine have lower rank and pay than their male colleagues even though they do similar work and achieve similar levels of academic productivity" (Carr et al. 1993). Despite comparable success in receiving research grants and publishing papers, the average woman received $7,600 less in annual compensation than the average man (Carr et al. 1993). One of the study's authors, Mark Moskowitz, commented, "This study has dispelled the myth that women make less because they work less. . . . The fact is that, although women are as productive as men, they are being treated differently" (Boston University School of Medicine News, Oct. 31, 1993).

Perhaps the best way to summarize the present situation is this statement by Estelle Ramey, Ph.D., who is professor of physiology and biophysics at Georgetown University: "I have worked all my life with men, and I have discovered that some of them are very smart, some of them are very stupid and most of them are mediocre hacks. Women fall into the same categories. We will have equality when a female schlemiel moves ahead as fast as a male schlemiel. That's equality, not when a female Einstein gets promoted to associate professor" (Women in Pediatrics 1983: 697).

CHAPTER THIRTEEN

Choosing the Right Physician

In the old days, it was easy. You grew up with the family physician and used him until one or both of you dropped. If it was the doctor first, you inherited his successor, who typically bought his practice. All family members used the same doctor, regardless of age or ailment.

All that has changed—except, perhaps, in rural and remote areas. In this age of specialization, there are different doctors for the youngest, the younger, the young, the old, the older, and the oldest, or so it seems. At a minimum, it is expected that there will be a pediatrician (until the age of 21) and an internist thereafter. To them may be added an ephebiatrician for the adolescent years and a geriatrician for the "golden years."

The territory is further divided on the basis of the body part afflicted. Accordingly, there are neurologists, psychiatrists, gastroenterologists, dermatologists, allergists, pulmonologists, ophthalmologists, otolaryngologists, gynecologists, et cetera—23 recognized specialties in all, which in turn are divided into many more subspecialties. As the world continues to grow in complexity, the list expands to keep pace. There are now proposals, for example, for new specialties of underwater medicine and space medicine.

Pediatricians, family physicians, internists, and geriatricians function as primary care physicians, whose role it is to anticipate health problems, to prevent them before they occur when possible, and when not, to treat them. Because it would be daunting for any layperson to have to choose among specialists, another role of the primary physician is to decide which problems require further consultation and to make appropriate referrals to specialists. As we will see shortly, however, cost considerations have impacted this aspect of physician decision making, particularly in prepaid health care delivery systems.

There are cost differences between primary care and specialty physicians. Some cynics might say that this is because of the laws of supply and demand: There are more of the former and fewer of the latter. Although there is some logic in that position, the basic difference relates to the length of training. Medical school requires a minimum of four years of study (at Stanford, however, most students take five years to graduate, and many even six years, because they elect to do research while in medical school). After medical school, one year of clinical experience (and passage of the National Board of Medical Examiners' test or its equivalent) is required of all doctors in order to qualify for state licensure. This year used to be called an internship. Currently it is referred to as PGY 1 (for postgraduate year one). Completion of this year of training does not, however, confer specialty status; that typically requires at least three years of postgraduate training, including the internship and two years in a residency. This is the case for pediatrics, internal medicine, and general psychiatry. For general surgery, four years are required, and some surgical specialties require as many as seven years. At the completion of residency training, a physician must pass a board certifying examination to be considered a specialist. A certificate is awarded that attests that such a procedure has been followed.

In the last decade, in most specialties these certificates have been made time-limited, so that a specialist must renew certification by passing an examination every seventh year. This procedure is a form of further quality control that forces physicians to continue to update their skills and knowledge. Certificates issued prior to 1990 were, for the most part, not time-limited, so physicians who were certified prior to that time are not required to be recertified. Any board-certified specialist of a board that recertifies may, however, voluntarily become recertified.

After completion of residency training, some physicians take further fellowship training and examinations so that they may become board-certified in a subspecialty. Like the board certification itself, certification in most subspecialties is time-limited, so that the physician must pass examinations every seven years in both the specialty and the subspecialty.

It should be noted that there is no comparable certification requirement for nonspecialists. Most state licensure bodies do, however, require any physician who renews a medical license (which must be done every two to three years) to provide evidence of attendance at a minimal number of educational courses or lectures. This is clearly not as stringent a requirement as that imposed by passage of an examination, but it is better than nothing.

The field of family practice was an attempt to resurrect the G.P. (general practitioner), albeit with a longer training period to address the added complexities of current care. The field became very popular in the 1970's, and there is renewed interest in it at the present time, primarily in the move to contain health care costs.

What should you be looking for in choosing a primary care physician? The answer to this question can be found in the four "C's": competence, caring, communication, and cost. The first three of these will be discussed here. Cost issues are personal decisions that each patient should make; for a discussion of some limitations on patient choice, see Chapter 11 on health insurance.

The issue of evaluating physician competence is critically important, yet frustratingly elusive. In deciding whom to admit to medical schools, educators have attempted to define the characteristics predictive of physician excellence. The best we have achieved, however, is the ability to predict that the student who performs well on medical school entrance examinations (the "MCATs") will perform well on the examinations given by the National Board of Medical Examiners. The latter are administered after the second and fourth years of medical school and after the first postgraduate year. The first two exams are basically achievement tests that cover the material taught in the preclinical (basic science) and clinical years, respectively. The third attempts to assess decision-making skills, an imperfect science at best.

As discussed above, the process of state medical licensure, to a minimal extent, and that of board certification, to a somewhat greater degree, are attempts to assess physician competence. You can determine if the physician you are considering is a board-certified specialist and/or subspecialist by consulting the directory of the American Board of Medical Specialists or calling the board. State boards of quality assurance, the bodies that issue licenses to practice medicine, keep files on complaints brought against physicians. If such complaints have resulted in suspension or revocation of licensure, the information may be released to you. Recently, a federal data bank has been created which will maintain this information for the entire country. In 1996, the state of Massachusetts became the first to make this information available to private individuals.

If you have a primary care physician you trust, he or she is surely your best source of information about the competence of a specialty physician. Choosing the primary care physician can be more difficult. It usually falls to word of mouth, that is, getting a recommendation from a friend or colleague. This method is, however, far from reliable and subject to many influences. I first realized this some years ago when I served on a hospital's quality assurance panel and found frequent discrepancies between the professionals' evaluation of the quality of the care received and the subjective experience of the patients. After physician reviewers identified problems in appropriateness of care in selected medical records from the emergency room, the patients were contacted by lay members of the committee and asked what they thought of the care they had received. As often as not, those who received care judged by physician reviewers to be less than optimal said that they had been happy with the care received.

In addition to checking to be sure that the physician's license has not been suspended or revoked and/or asking a friend, what more can one do to assure the competence of a physician? Being on the medical staff of a hospital is another kind of "minimal" standard of competence. For a physician to join a hospital's medical staff, his or her credentials must be checked and letters of recommendation from other physicians must be received. Physicians who admit patients to a hospital are subject to peer review of their medical records and are called to task if deficiencies are found. Though not every record is checked, this adds another layer of evaluation to the process. Staff privileges may be revoked if there are legitimate complaints about the physician.

Having a teaching appointment at a medical school further implies competence, if not excellence, in the eyes of the physician's peers. The process of teaching in medical school places the physician in the position of having to justify and support medical advice and to keep up with the literature in order to answer the frequent challenges of medical students and residents. On the other hand, there are many good doctors who are not on the teaching staffs of medical schools.

After you have entertained or engaged in any or all of these methods of evaluation and narrowed your choice to a few physicians, it's time to schedule an interview. A physician who won't allow (or who will charge) for this is probably not someone you want as your doctor (unless there are extenuating circumstances). If you are told that the practice is closed to new patients, it generally means that the physician is a good one, but one who feels too busy to provide good care to a larger number of patients. Often, under such circumstances, you will be referred to the most junior colleague in the practice. You may accept that recommendation, or you might choose to ask for the name of the physician's personal doctor. If you get that information, you are likely to have a winner.

Once you have an interview scheduled, gather your medical records and a list of any medications you are taking. Ask the physician how comfortable he or she is with any medical condition you may have. Ask about the practice of referral for consultation to specialists and for second opinions. Especially under managed care, many physicians are discouraged from seeking consultations and may, as a result, place a patient at risk if they are not experienced or knowledgeable about his or her condition. Ask if the doctor is eligible for board recertification and, if so, whether or not he or she has been recertified. If the physician is critical of the concept, that should be a warning signal. Determine whether the doctor is on the staff of at least one reputable hospital and/or medical school. Find out if there is a "call-in" hour (a regularly scheduled time when patients can phone in and talk to the doctor) and how emergencies are handled. Find out about night/weekend and vacation coverage practices. You will also want to know how much time is allotted for a visit, how long the waiting time is to get an appointment, and whether all patients get the same battery of routine laboratory tests or if choices vary with the age and sex of the patient.

Interviewing the physician will not only provide factual answers to these questions but will also give you a sense of your comfort with the doctor, a critical factor. If it is your style to read the medical literature (increasingly available to the lay public through health libraries and computerized databases, such as Medline), find out how comfortable the physician will be with your doing that. The doctor who responds along the lines of "Let me be the doctor and you the patient" is clearly not for you. If, on the other hand, you prefer to leave the worrying to your doctor and be presented with a rational recommendation, say so and judge the response you get.

It has been my experience that primary care physicians are arranging to coordinate their care of their female adult patients with that of a gynecologist. This often takes the form of alternating routine checkups, so that a healthy woman might see each every other year to avoid duplication of testing and save time and money. Some form of communication between the doctors and their records is obviously necessary for such a system to work.

Although many gynecologists consider themselves primary physicians as well as specialists, it has been my observation that in general they are not yet as well trained to fulfill this role as an internist or family practitioner. Also, when a gynecologist thinks he or she is the only doctor a woman needs, the message conveyed is that the woman is defined by her reproductive function and that her health needs are primarily those related to her gynecologic system. As we have seen, this attitude has done a great disservice to women and has been a barrier to their receiving the health care they need and deserve.

Once you choose the physician, your search may not yet be over. The first appointment should give you important additional information in deciding if you made the right choice. Your comfort with the physician, your sense that he or she cares about you, and the quality of the communication you shared are critical. The following checklist may be helpful:

1.   How long did it take to get an appointment? Did that seem appropriate, or were you uncomfortable with the wait? Did the office staff reassure you that you would not suffer from the wait?

2.   How long did you remain in the waiting room before you were taken in? Were you given an explanation for the wait? Did the staff try to keep you informed of progress?

3.   Once you were ushered in to the doctor, were you asked to change into a gown immediately or given a chance to meet with the doctor in his or her office before the examination? Most offices are set

up for the former. If this was the case and you requested a meeting while you were still dressed, how was your request handled?

4. Did you feel you had enough time and were made comfortable enough to ask all your questions? It's a good idea to write down your questions before coming to the doctor's office to ensure that you won't forget any. It is often helpful to write the answers next to the questions so that you will have a record should your memory fade and/or you need to ask follow-up questions later (if, for example, the directions on the prescribed medication differ from what you were told by the doctor).

5. Was the doctor supportive and helpful to you in answering questions and giving you time to clarify them, or did he or she seem annoyed or pressed for time?

6. Were you told why tests were being ordered and given an opportunity to question their necessity and cost?

7. Did you receive test results and their interpretation promptly without having to call for them?

8. If you received a prescription, were the instructions explained to you and were you informed about possible side effects and told what to do should any occur?

Women, as health care consumers not only for themselves but often for their parents, children, spouses, and/or partners, deserve respect, support, and information from their physicians. They need to know that they will have this care when they need it, from the physician or her or his well-informed colleague. In order to achieve and maintain optimal health, patients and their doctors need to form a therapeutic alliance in which goals are articulated and shared.

CHAPTER FOURTEEN

Research in Women's Health

Issues in Research on Women and Drugs

A biologic double standard has deprived us of critical information about the effects and proper dose of medications commonly used to treat women. Women have been systematically excluded from Phase I trials in which drugs, after passing tests on animal models, are tested on human subjects to determine the effective dose, in accordance with FDA regulations. The justifications for this exclusion seem reasonable at first glance. First, women may be pregnant, and it might be dangerous to expose fetuses to possible toxicity from the drug; second, levels of hormones, such as estrogen, fluctuate during the course of the menstrual cycle, which might confuse the test results by changing the levels of the drug. This second possibility is deduced from theories about the effects of hormones on drug metabolism, as well as on naturalistic experiments, such as observing different effects of alcohol consumption on men and women. These concerns are certainly legitimate.

However, when a drug tested only on men is prescribed for a woman, the gender differences in the way drugs are processed by the body are not taken into account. In particular, the possible effects of changing hormone levels during the menstrual cycle or after menopause are never discussed. In other words, doctors commonly prescribe drugs to women that have never been appropriately evaluated to determine whether they are effective and/or toxic in the doses used, whether the doses need to be adjusted depending on the phase of the menstrual cycle, and whether there may be dangerous interactions when women are prescribed more than one drug at a time. This is of great concern, because we know that sex differences are possible at every stage of a drug's passage through the body: absorption, distribution, metabolism, and excretion.

There are several sex differences in the way drugs are absorbed. For one, women secrete less acid in the stomach than do men (Grossman, Kirsner, and Gillespie 1963). This gastric acid can affect the absorption of certain substances, including alcohol and possibly prescribed medications. Although their lower level of gastric acid may be the reason that women are less likely than men to suffer from ulcers, it may also mean that they absorb drugs more slowly from their stomachs than do men. This would cause the level of certain medications to be lower and the drugs less effective.

Absorption is also known to be affected by the simultaneous ingestion of other substances, including food or other medications. Calcium supplements in the form of calcium carbonate (such as in Tums) may interfere with the absorption of many medications. Similarly, iron, often prescribed for women who have a tendency toward anemia, will interfere with the absorption of some medications.

The amount of time a drug remains in the stomach, and especially in the intestine, will also affect its absorption. In women, it takes longer than in men for food to leave the stomach and pass through the intestine (Datz, Christian, and Moore 1987). The reason for this difference has been studied, with inconclusive results.

As an added complication, buried in the literature of 40 years ago is the finding that gastric emptying time speeds up in the middle of the menstrual cycle (MacDonald 1956). Delay in stomach emptying may cause drug levels to be either higher (if the drug remains in contact with the absorbing surface of the stomach for a longer time) or lower (if food that interferes with absorption of the drug remains in the stomach longer). Hormones may play a role; it appears, for example, that when progesterone levels are highest (during the second half of the cycle), it takes longer for material to move from the stomach into the intestine, as well as through the intestine (Wald et al. 1981).

Another possible sex difference relates to the distribution of the drug once it is absorbed into the bloodstream from the stomach or intestine. The amounts of water and fat tissue in the body can affect drug distribution. The amount of water in the tissues of women varies according to the phase of the menstrual cycle; in the premenstrual phase, the body retains more water than in the postmenstrual phase. Although this has not been studied as yet, it is possible that in the premenstrual phase the level of drug in the blood may be diluted by the increased water, resulting in lower efficacy. Conversely, the drug will be more concentrated at other phases of the cycle. The fact that women have more fat in their bodies than do men is also relevant here. Many drugs are lipophilic—that is, they are drawn into fat, where they are stored. As a result, they remain in the body for a longer time in an individual with more fat.

Metabolism of drugs involves their breakdown or combination with other chemicals in various organs, most commonly the liver. These processes largely depend on the blood flow through the liver and/or the amount of enzymes, the chemicals that facilitate the chemical transformations, in that organ. At this phase of drug processing, hormones may play an important role. There is reason to think that the activity of two enzymes, the hepatic microsomal oxidase system and monoamine oxidase, may be affected by the levels of estrogen and progesterone. Fluctuating levels of these female hormones throughout the menstrual cycle may be responsible for different drug levels throughout the course of the month.

For example, the activity of monoamine oxidase is increased by progesterone and decreased by estrogen (Yonkers et al. 1992). When production of liver enzymes is increased, the drug will be eliminated from the body more rapidly, and the resulting drug level in the blood may not be high enough to achieve the desired effect. If the patient doesn't get better, she is often accused of being noncompliant, that is, not taking her medication as prescribed. Conversely, if enzyme production is decreased, the drugs processed by that enzyme may be eliminated from the bloodstream more slowly, leaving the blood level of the drugs higher. All this suggests that the same dose of a drug processed by a given enzyme may result in a higher blood level (and a greater effect, even to toxic levels) during the postmenstrual phase of the cycle and a lower blood level (possibly less than therapeutic) during the premenstrual phase.

The pubertal growth spurt in girls also has hormonal implications for processing of medications. This was pointed out by the creative research of Dr. Karen Hein before the AIDS epidemic drew her away from studying this important issue. What she discovered was that as puberty progressed and the levels of estrogens in the body rose, the amount of medication needed by a young girl with asthma to achieve proper effects increased (Hein 1987). More research of this kind is needed in order better to understand the differences in drug metabolism in women at different physiologic stages of life (see Rogers 1994). Moreover, the lower levels of all female hormones after menopause suggest that women at this stage of their lives may need a dosing schedule different from that for premenopausal women to protect them from the resultant changes in drug levels.

Fiset and LeBel's study (1990) of differences in the kidney's elimination of drugs in relationship to menstrual cycle phase was one of the first pharmacologic studies to include this factor. It concluded that the elimination of the substance studied (D-xylose) was faster during the second phase of the menstrual cycle than during the first phase or during ovulation.

Studies that include women but fail to ascertain menstrual cycle phase may come to erroneous conclusions. For example, a recent study showed that blood pressure levels in women who were not taking any medication were highest at the beginning of menstruation and lowest during days 17–26 of the cycle (Dunne et al. 1991). This suggests that studies evaluating the effect of blood pressure–lowering drugs may reach incorrect conclusions if they fail to note the menstrual cycle phase—that is, they may attribute effects to the drug that may simply reflect normal variations over the course of the menstrual cycle. This may also be true for other body systems not yet studied.

Other medications may affect or be affected by estrogens taken for birth control or replacement purposes; these interactions may influence the efficacy of either the estrogens or the other drugs. For example, in a few reported cases, women became pregnant while taking tetracycline along with their regular birth control pills. It is theorized that the tetracycline, being a broad-spectrum antibiotic, reduced the level of beneficial bacteria in the gastrointestinal tract; this loss of essential bacteria interfered with the processing of the ingested estrogen and caused the blood level to be too low to prevent ovulation. Birth control pills have also been shown to raise blood levels of Valium to intoxication level during the menstrual phase of the cycle (Ellinwood et al. 1983). The implications of this finding for women taking ERT are unknown because they have never been studied.

Thus far, we have been concerned mainly with drugs that are pre-scribed by doctors. It is obvious, however, that many of the issues raised here are also important in terms of the way the body handles abused drugs or substances. For example, owing to differences in estrogen levels during the menstrual cycle, the blood alcohol level resulting from the same-sized alcoholic drink is higher in the first half of the cycle than in the second. Similarly, because of estrogen's effects, women taking estro-gen-containing birth control pills have a higher blood alcohol level from the same amount of alcohol than those who are not on the Pill. Alcohol may also affect the efficacy of these pills, lowering the blood level of es-trogen. Studies of the possible effects upon alcohol metabolism of post-menopausal ERT have not as yet, to my knowledge, been undertaken. These are of great importance, given the number of older women who abuse alcohol.

The Past and the Future of Research

Throughout this book, it has been made apparent that there are more questions than answers about the health status and needs of women. In many cases, the absence of gender-specific information has already re-sulted in serious consequences for women's health. In others, the poten-tial for harm exists. Why do we find ourselves, at the end of the twentieth century in the richest and most scientifically advanced country in the world, in this dismal situation? Is it, as some have suggested, that the male-dominated medical establishment, jealous of women's longer life span, has actively thwarted research efforts that might further strengthen the female advantage? Or is it that thoughtless gender stereotyping has limited the view of women's health needs to those related solely to their traditional childbearing role? Alternatively, it has been said that the pa-ternalism of male researchers has kept women out of research studies as a way of protecting their hypothetical unborn children. We have also seen evidence that women were excluded from scientific drug studies because of the likely variation that hormone fluctuation could introduce into blood levels of the drug. This variability could complicate data analysis or require a significant and costly increase in the sample size necessary to control for it. Finally, in the first half of this century, many studies were performed on the most available subjects: medical students. It just so happened that more than 90 percent of these students were males.

At some level, intentional or unintentional, each of these explanations has probably played a role. What is clear, however, is that the absence of women from health research studies until recently has left us with insufficient information upon which to base prevention or rational treatment of many health problems in women, and inadequate knowledge about how to vary therapy to account for hormonal fluctuations during the menstrual cycle, during pregnancy, and after menopause.

To better understand the present situation, it is useful to examine the history of medical research and the concept of protection of human subjects. Prior to the 1940's there were no protections for humans who participated in medical research. The many male medical students who did so were not volunteers in the true sense, as they often felt that they had no choice in the matter. Prisoners, too, were traditionally used as human guinea pigs, or so they felt. Whether or not it was ever stated, incarcerated research subjects expected that their living conditions might be improved if they participated in such studies, and often this was the case. However, often research subjects received medications or were exposed to other potential dangers without their knowledge, much less consent.

Many past abuses of research subjects have been uncovered. Many more likely never will be. Among the more egregiously abusive studies is that of the natural history of syphilis in black men at Tuskegee, which started in 1932. Despite the discovery of a cure for the disease and despite many deaths, this study was continued for almost forty years without treatment being offered to these men. Studies of the effect of starvation on young male conscientious objectors during World War II furnish another example of dangerous research that disregarded potential risk to subjects. The most heinous of all, however, were those experiments carried out in the Nazi concentration camps during World War II. It was in response to revelations of those atrocities that the first attempt at protection of human subjects was forged in 1949 through the Nuremberg Code. This document states, "Research subjects must have the legal and real-life circumstantial power to freely provide consent as well as the information and comprehension necessary to make informed decisions."

It wasn't until four years later that the first U.S. guidelines for the protection of human subjects appeared. The creation of institutional review boards (IRBs) in research institutions was mandated in the United States in 1974. For the first time, a researcher had to submit the research plan, as well as the consent form, for approval before recruiting human subjects. In 1975, the U.S. Department of Health and Human Services directed IRBs to set limits on the conditions for conducting research on pregnant women, who were thus designated a "vulnerable population." Ironically, this limitation followed the revelations about the damage done to fetuses when pregnant women took thalidomide or DES, not in research experiments, but in real life. These medications had never previously been tested on women, pregnant or not.

This protective stance of the U.S. government was further extended the next year to exclude all women of "childbearing potential" from the early phases of drug testing, except in the case of life-threatening disease (Food and Drug Administration 1977). This paternalistic move on the part of the federal government made it difficult, if not impossible, for studies of new drugs to be conducted on any woman under the age of 50, although women would be the prime recipients of prescriptions for these drugs once they were approved. Physicians would have no information about drug levels in women and how dosage might be modified to account for hormonal variations throughout the menstrual cycle.

As a result of increasing pressure following revelations in the late 1980's about the paucity of information about women's health, the NIH, the largest public grant-making body in the United States, instructed researchers applying for funding to include women and racial/ethnic minorities in all research studies. In 1990, the NIH established the Office of Women's Health Research; at the time the NIH was headed by the first woman to hold the position, Dr. Bernadine Healy. Despite the fanfare and visibility given this move, this office was poorly funded and not given grant-making power, allegedly because of the desire not to "ghettoize" women's health into one agency, but rather to encourage research on women in all of the Institutes. The wisdom of this approach remains to be examined. It is also worrisome that at the time of this writing, the Congressional Women's Caucus, which had been instrumental in calling for the creation of the Office of Women's Health Research and related measures, is unfunded in the wake of the Republican sweep of the 1994 congressional elections. The potential impact of this on the newly gained awareness of the need for women's health research will soon be seen.

The year 1991 proved pivotal for research on drugs requiring FDA approval. In that year the U.S. Supreme Court overturned the lower court ruling in favor of Johnson Controls, the lead battery manufacturer that had prohibited women under the age of 70 from employment unless they underwent sterilization (see Chapter 2). The Court stated that "categorical exclusion constituted sex discrimination, thus affirming that women are the appropriate parties to weigh risks and benefits and make informed decisions" (Chavkin 1994: 99). The implications of this ruling were not lost on the FDA, which in 1993 revised its 1977 restriction on the inclusion of fertile women in clinical trials that evaluated drugs, and now requires that they be included in order for a drug to be considered for approval. This landmark move is not, however, retroactive. As a result, we will likely never have the information we need about the different ways in which women (particularly those who are pregnant or at different phases of the menstrual cycle or their lives) handle hundreds of FDA-approved drugs they are already taking.

This brief review illustrates that the practice of excluding women from research studies was actually very short lived, lasting less than twenty years. Those regulations, therefore, cannot account for the paucity of information on women's health, though they certainly exacerbated it. Similarly, it would be naive to expect that we will see major advances now that these restrictions have been lifted. The reality is that attitudes of both researchers and potential female subjects must be changed. The former must consider researching issues of importance to women and their health, and the latter must become involved as participants in research studies.

What will women need in order to become interested in becoming subjects in research studies? There are both tangible and intangible needs that have not heretofore been acknowledged or addressed. In the former category, it must be remembered that participation in a research study requires time, usually during the day. For many women who work outside the home, this presents problems in terms of work, transportation, and child care. Offering payment may partially overcome these obstacles, but payments, if too large, may also be viewed as coercive. As an Institute of Medicine report asks, "Is it inappropriate to recruit poor, inner-city women into a study that will benefit society but that will cost them money and time, possibly jeopardize their work performance, and not offer a reasonable assurance of health benefit? Is the obligation to serve society through participation in studies one that accrues only to those for whom society is meeting the minimum need for food, clothing, and shelter?" (Institute of Medicine 1994: 121).

At a more theoretical level, one must ask what will motivate women to participate. Dr. Machelle Allen addresses this question with the view that participation in research appeals to the traditional construct of altruism and care. "Theoretically, participation in clinical trials, with its potential benefit to humanity, would be something highly acceptable to women" (Allen 1994). In our experience, women have different questions and expectations regarding their participation. For example, they seem to have more curiosity about why they were chosen and about the research results. "What did you learn about me?" and "How did I differ from other people in the study?" are commonly asked questions. In other words, they need not only information up front but also feedback after the study is completed. This, of course, is not to say that men don't share these interests, but that they less often express them.

There is considerable suspicion about the research process among women in general, and women of color in particular. There is the widespread sense that research is done by white males on women and minorities, who will be used as guinea pigs. These concerns must be addressed and alleviated by involving women in the decisions around what issues need to be researched and in formulating the questions to be asked. Sensitivity to issues of gender and culture is critical, not only in conceptualizing research studies but in considering the needs and wishes of the populations to be studied. Recruitment by peers sends the appropriate message and enhances the possibility of successful outcome.

This brings us to consideration of not only the gender of the research subject, but also that of the researcher. According to Bernadine Healy, former director of the NIH, female scientists are likely to choose different research problems to address, and to frame clinical problems differently, than do men (Healy 1991).

There is evidence that women are more effective than men in recruiting women subjects into research studies. According to the Institute of Medicine's recent report, "the low number of women scientists, particularly at the upper levels of the research hierarchy, is directly related to the level of women's participation in clinical studies and the amount of attention devoted to women's health concerns" (Institute of Medicine

1994: 112). Moreover, women researchers appear more effective in eliciting sensitive information from women subjects. Belenky et al. (1986) suggest that women are more likely than men to interact with study participants in the process of collecting information and to trust subjective responses in the interview process.

Some argue that the entire approach to clinical research, the "scientific method" itself, is inappropriate for addressing the health needs of women because it is based on stereotypic masculine values, such as individualism, achievement, mastery, and, especially, detachment. The traditional relationship between the researcher and the research subject is hierarchical, with the former in control. The value placed on impersonality and objectivity, it is said, renders science "value-free."

This position is challenged, not only by feminists, but by others. Stephen Jay Gould labels it the "illusion of objectivity through numbers." He objects to the tradition of trusting "hard" or objective data, regardless of their clinical relevancy, and cites the example of craniometry, the "scientific" measurement of the skull that yielded results that allowed "comfortable white males" to "prove" that blacks, women, and the poor are inferior by virtue of their smaller cranial dimensions, rather than challenging the accuracy of the methodology or considering alternative and more plausible explanations (Gould 1981).

The concept of science as "neutral" is itself open to debate. For example, in the process of investigating the epidemic of toxic shock syndrome in 1981, the committee of the Institute of Medicine of which I was a member was stymied by the absence of information in the medical literature about the normal bacterial content of the vagina during menses, despite an abundant literature on this subject for other times of the month. The reason for this important gap in the knowledge base rapidly became apparent: Physicians don't do pelvic examinations during menses. Although this practice is understandable when the object of the examination is obtaining a specimen for a Pap smear, it is absolutely the antithesis of a rational approach when the objective is to get a culture specimen, as bacteria grow best in the presence of blood. A plausible alternative explanation for the common prohibition against performing a pelvic examination during menses may be the long-standing culturally and religiously determined taboos against contact with menstruating women and the products of menstruation. Value-free, indeed!

The alternative to the traditional scientific method, espoused by many feminists, is one that is humanistic and subjective. It grows out of the "caring" roots of medical practice, according to Jevne and Oberle (1993). This approach argues for inclusion of the individual human experience and for attention to the environment and context in which the study is to be conducted. The opinions and perspective of prospective subjects would be sought in determining the focus of the research, designing it, and developing its instruments. "The search for insight and understanding of the needs of others is the central focus for most feminist studies" (Jevne and Oberle 1993: 203).

In my opinion, neither position is entirely right or wrong. Scientists must continue to use rigorous quantitative measures and analytic techniques if they are to have credibility in the scientific community, and if their findings are to be valid, reliable, and generalizable to other populations. On the other hand, the importance of inclusion of the women of a target population in the conceptualization of research is not only appropriate, but also a realistic prerequisite for facilitating their participation as research subjects.

This dual approach will surely enhance and enrich the research and is now beginning to be undertaken. The use of focus groups is growing in popularity. These are discussions with members of groups of stakeholders early in the research process to ascertain their views about the content and relevance of, as well as the potential problems with, a proposed study.

While the intellectual debate concerning research methodology continues, it is important that we do not lose sight of the goal, that of broadening and deepening our knowledge in order to improve the health of women. This requires education of legislators, industry leaders, medical and other science educators, health care providers, and insurers, as well as the public. Each has a critical role to play in ensuring that there will be funding for necessary research; facilitation, personnel, and resources for the required studies; and inquiring minds motivated to make new discoveries—and, most important, research subjects who will appreciate that their own best interests and those of their loved ones will be well served by their participation in studies.

Appendixes

The Ten Leading Causes of Death in Women at Each Life Stage (1994 data)

Ages 15–24
Accidents
Homicide
Cancer
Suicide
Heart disease
HIV/AIDS
Pneumonia
Pregnancy
Cerebrovascular disease

Ages 25–44
Cancer
Accidents
HIV/AIDS
Heart disease
Homicide
Suicide
Cerebrovascular disease
Liver disease
Diabetes mellitus
Pneumonia

Ages 45–65
Cancer
Heart disease

Cerebrovascular disease
Chronic obstructive pulmonary disease
Diabetes mellitus
Accidents
Liver disease
Pneumonia
Suicide
Nephritis

Ages 65 and Over

Heart disease
Cancer
Cerebrovascular disease
Pneumonia and influenza
Chronic obstructive pulmonary disease
Diabetes mellitus
Accidents
Atherosclerosis
Nephritis
Septicemia

Comprehensive Geriatric Assessment

Physical Health
    Traditional problem list
    Disease severity indicators
    Self-ratings of health and disability
    Quantifications of need for, and use of, medical services
    Disease-specific rating scales
Overall functional ability
    Activities of daily living scales (bathing, dressing, eating, toileting, transferring, and walking)
    Instrumental activities of daily living scales (household and money management, use of telephone, etc.)
Psychological health
    Cognitive function
    Affective function
Socioeconomic variables
    Social interactions network
    Social support needs and resources
    Quality of life assessment
    Economic resources and access
Environmental characteristics
    Environmental adequacy and safety
    Access to services (shopping, pharmacy, transportation, and recreation)

SOURCE: American Medical Association Council on Scientific Affairs, *Archives of Internal Medicine* 150: 2461. Copyright 1990, American Medical Association.

Glossary of Assisted Reproductive Technology Terms

Artificial insemination refers to the placement of semen into the vagina or reproductive tract by means other than sexual intercourse. Artificial insemination with husband's sperm (AIH) was developed for use when the male is unable to achieve intercourse or cannot ejaculate during intercourse. Currently, it is most frequently offered in combination with controlled ovarian stimulation for treatment of unexplained infertility. Direct placement of sperm into the uterine cavity (intrauterine insemination or IUI) is a modification of artificial insemination which is used when the normal passage of sperm through the uterine cervix is thought to be impaired by abnormal cervical mucus. In cases of severe male factor infertility, or where there is concern regarding hereditary disease by the husband, donor sperm may be used for the procedure, and therapeutic donor insemination (TID) offered.

Cryopreservation is a process of freezing a zygote, embryo, or sperm in liquid nitrogen at very low temperatures ($-196°$ Celsius), essentially suspending biologic activity. Cryopreservation of eggs is presently not efficient or effective.

Frozen embryo transfer (FET) refers to the transfer of a frozen embryo after a previous ART cycle. It is common for extra oocytes to be retrieved from women. This situation arises because transfer of excessive number of embryos, while leading to increased chances for multiple implantation, may also be associated with poorer obstetric outcomes and increased pregnancy complications. Most patients are, therefore, advised to accept only a limited number of embryos (usually from one to six, depending on age, and observed quality of the embryos) with any "spare" embryos of good quality stored in a frozen state. These cryopreserved embryos can be transferred at any subsequent cycle, without the additional expense or intervention of another ovarian stimulation and retrieval procedure. The chances of a successful pregnancy from frozen embryos thawed and transferred are again influenced by age of the patient, quality of embryos stored, and number of embryos transferred, but are reported in the range of 15-20% probability of delivered pregnancy per embryo transfer done.

Gamete intra-fallopian transfer (GIFT) was introduced soon after the advent of IVF. This technique involves steps similar to IVF up through the stage of gamete procurement. Instead of allowing for extracorporeal (outside of the body) fertilization, the freshly acquired eggs and sperm are immediately placed into the fallopian tubes where fertilization is hoped to occur. This procedure is used to treat women with minimal tubal disease, endometriosis, and unexplained infertility. Most programs offering GIFT report a success rate approximately 5-10% higher than IVF success rates in the same program.

In vitro fertilization (IVF) was the first ART procedure to employ laboratory manipulation of gametes in an effort to achieve pregnancy. As part of this procedure, the female patient undergoes intense ovarian stimulation to produce numerous mature eggs (referred to as controlled ovarian hyperstimulation). These eggs are collected by gentle needle aspiration during laparoscopy or during vaginal ultrasound. At the same time, the male partner produces a semen sample from which sperm will be obtained and processed. Eggs and sperm are subsequently combined to allow for fertilization. The fertilization process is usually successful, with approximately 60-75% eggs fertilized for most couples. Following two days of growth and development, three to four newly formed embryos are placed into the uterine cavity. Ten days to two weeks later, a pregnancy test is performed to determine whether successful implantation has occurred. This procedure is utilized in cases of tubal obstruction or damage, endometriosis, unexplained infertility, and in some cases of male infertility.

The overall probability of successful delivery per egg retrieval is influenced by a large number of variables, such as the age of the patients, the quality of the eggs, sperm, and embryos, number of embryos transferred, and the diagnosis associated with the patients' infertility. For women less than 40, with normal sperm, the average United States success rates are close to 20% deliveries per oocyte retrieval cycle attempted.

Intra-cytoplasmic sperm injection (ICSI) is a relatively new micromanipulation technique developed to help couples achieve fertilization, when there is a severe compromise in sperm numbers or function, or where there has been a failure to fertilize in a previous IVF attempt. This procedure is similar to regular IVF, up to the preparation of the sperm and eggs in the laboratory. The semen sample is prepared by centrifuging, or spinning the sperm cells through a special medium called Percoll. This solution separates live sperm from debris and most of the dead sperm. During a subsequent step, a single live sperm is selected and placed into a glass needle and is injected directly into the egg. This procedure overcomes many of the barriers to fertilization and allows those couples with little hope of achieving successful pregnancy to obtain fertilized embryos.

Oocyte (egg) aspiration is the harvesting of mature eggs from the ovaries. This is done either through the ultrasound-guided approach or through laparoscopy. The most common method of oocyte aspiration uses ultrasound to guide the aspirating needle into the ovaries in order to retrieve one or more eggs. The ultrasound probe and needle are placed into the vagina. Oocyte aspiration is generally first attempted using an ultrasound-guided approach. If it becomes apparent that an ultrasound-guided approach is not possible, the aspiration will be completed using a surgical laparoscopic approach. Laparoscopy involves placing a small telescope called a laparoscope inside the abdominal cavity through a small incision (cut in the skin) made next to the navel or belly button. Another incision is made in the lower abdomen above the pubic area to allow for the insertion of a suction needle to aspirate the eggs from the ovaries. The surgeon uses the laparoscope to locate the ovaries and guide the aspiration needle.

Oocyte donation is a procedure that may be employed where the recipient is unable to provide eggs, or unable to achieve embryos of sufficient quality to achieve implantation. It involves use of eggs provided from a donor woman. This method of ART may be combined with IVF, GIFT, or other similar procedures. The process involves at least three parties: the donor female, the recipient female, and the male. Because this procedure involves several different individuals, every effort must be made to ensure that each participant has a thorough understanding of the process through documented informed consent. As part of this procedure, the donor undergoes intense ovarian stimulation to develop multiple mature oocytes. Viable eggs are collected and then combined with sperm. The resultant fertilized eggs are placed into the uterus of the designated recipient. This method may be used for women who lack eggs due to ovarian failure or lack ovaries due to surgical removal. In addition, oocyte donation may be appropriate for patients concerned about genetic diseases.

Ovarian stimulation to develop multiple eggs is done by the use of fertility drugs. These are clomiphene citrate (Serophene or Clomid), human menopausal gonadotropin (hMG, or Pergonal), human follicle stimulating hormone (hFSH, or Metrodin), human chorionic gonadotropin (hCG, or Profasi), and gonadotropin releasing hormone-like drugs (such as Lupron). These drugs are used in various combinations to stimulate the development of multiple oocytes in the ovaries. While clomiphene citrate may be taken by mouth, as a pill, the rest require injection by needle and syringe, sometimes daily over a period of days or even several weeks. To insure the proper timing and dosage for these drugs, and proper timing for the oocyte aspiration procedure, frequent pelvic examinations, blood tests, and ultrasound tests are required.

Zygote intra-fallopian transfer (ZIFT) was developed as a modification of the GIFT procedure either initially or as a delayed GIFT. As part of the ZIFT process, eggs and sperm are obtained as described for IVF, combined in the laboratory, and observed for one day. When fertilization is successful, the resulting early embryo (called a zygote), is transferred directly into healthy fallopian tubes as a zygote intrafallopian transfer, or ZIFT.

SOURCE: Assisted Reproductive Technology: A systemwide task force report and recommendations to strengthen oversight and improve quality of care. University of California, Office of the President. March 1996.

DSM-IV Diagnostic Criteria for Anorexia Nervosa and Bulimia Nervosa

Anorexia Nervosa

A. Refusal to maintain body weight over a minimally normal weight for age and height (e.g., weight loss leading to maintenance of body weight 15% below that expected), or failure to make expected weight gain during period of growth, leading to body weight below 15% of that expected.
B. Intense fear of gaining weight or becoming fat, even though underweight.
C. Disturbance in the way in which one's body weight or shape is experienced, undue influence of body shape and weight on self-evaluation, or denial of the seriousness of current low body weight.
D. In postmenarchal females, amenorrhea, i.e., the absence of at least three consecutive menstrual cycles. (A woman is considered to have amenorrhea if her periods occur only following hormone, e.g., estrogen, administration.)

Restricting type: During the episode of anorexia nervosa, the person does not regularly engage in binge eating or purging behavior (i.e., self-induced vomiting or misuse of laxatives or diuretics).

Binge eating / purging type: During the episode of anorexia nervosa, the person regularly engages in binge eating or purging behavior (i.e., self-induced vomiting or the misuse of laxatives or diuretics).

Bulimia Nervosa

A. Recurrent episodes of binge eating. An episode of binge eating is characterized by both of the following:
    1) eating in a discrete period of time (e.g., within any 2-hour period) an amount of food that is definitely larger than most people would eat in a similar period of time in similar circumstances; and
    2) a sense of lack of control over eating during the episode (e.g., a feel-

ing that one cannot stop eating or control what or how much one is eating).

B. Recurrent inappropriate compensatory behavior to prevent weight gain, such as self-induced vomiting; misuse of laxatives, diuretics, or other medications; fasting; or excessive exercise.

C. The binge eating and inappropriate compensatory behaviors both occur, on average, at least twice a week for 3 months.

D. Self-evaluation is unduly influenced by body shape and weight.

E. The disturbance does not occur exclusively during episodes of anorexia nervosa.

Purging type: The person regularly engages in self-induced vomiting or the misuse of laxatives or diuretics.

Nonpurging type: The person uses other inappropriate compensatory behaviors, such as fasting or excessive exercise, but does not regularly engage in self-induced vomiting or the misuse of laxatives or diuretics.

SOURCE: American Psychiatric Association 1994. Reprinted with permission from the *Diagnostic and Statistical Manual of Mental Disorders, Fourth Edition.* Copyright 1994 American Psychiatric Association.

Recommended Daily Allowances

Adolescent Females

Energy intake: 2,200 calories

Protein: 44–46 g

Fat

    Less than 30 percent of total calories

    Less than 10 percent of total fats from saturated fatty acids

    Less than 300 mg cholesterol

Carbohydrates: More than 225 g (50 percent of calories)

Vitamins

    A: 800 micrograms

    D: 10 micrograms

    E: 8 mg (as alpha-tocopherol)

    K: 45–55 micrograms

    C: 50–60 mg

    Thiamin: 1.1 mg

    Riboflavin: 1.3 mg

    Niacin: 15 mg niacin equivalents

    B_6: 1.4–1.5 mg

    Folate: 150–80 micrograms

    B_{12}: 2.0 micrograms

    Biotin: 30–100 micrograms

    Pantothenic acid: 4–7 mg

Minerals

    Calcium: More than 1,200 mg

    Phosphorus: 1,200 mg

    Magnesium: 280 mg

    Iron: 15–18 mg

    Zinc: 12 mg

Copper: 1.5–3.0 mg
Manganese: 2.0–5.0 mg
Fluoride: 1.5–2.5 mg
Chromium: 50–200 micrograms
Molybdenum: 75–250 micrograms
Iodine: 150 micrograms
Selenium: 45–50 micrograms

Nonpregnant Women Ages 25–50

Energy intake: 2,200 calories
Protein: 50 g
Fat
    Less than 30 percent of total calories
    Less than 10 percent of total fats from saturated fatty acids
    Less than 300 mg cholesterol
Carbohydrates: More than 225 g (50 percent of calories)
Vitamins
    A: 800 micrograms
    D: 5 micrograms
    E: 8 mg (as alpha-tocopherol)
    K: 65 micrograms
    C: 60 mg
    Thiamin: 1.1 mg
    Riboflavin: 1.3 mg
    Niacin: 15 mg niacin equivalents
    B_6: 1.6 mg
    Folate: 180 micrograms
    B_{12}: 2.0 micrograms
    Biotin: 30–100 micrograms
    Pantothenic acid: 4–7 mg
Minerals
    Calcium: 800 mg
    Phosphorus: 800 mg
    Magnesium: 280 mg
    Iron: 15 mg
    Zinc: 12 mg
    Copper: 1.5–3.0 mg
    Manganese: 2.0–5.0 mg
    Fluoride: 1.5–4.0 mg
    Chromium: 50–200 micrograms
    Molybdenum: 75–250 micrograms
    Iodine: 150 micrograms
    Selenium: 55 micrograms

Pregnant Women

Energy intake: 2,520 calories in second and third trimesters
Protein: 60 g
Fat
    Less than 30 percent of total calories
    Less than 10 percent of total fats from saturated fatty acids
    Less than 300 mg cholesterol
Carbohydrates: More than 225 g (50 percent of calories)
Vitamins
    A: 800 micrograms
    D: 10 micrograms
    E: 10 mg (as alpha-tocopherol)
    K: 65 micrograms
    C: 70 mg
    Thiamin: 1.5 mg
    Riboflavin: 1.6 mg
    Niacin: 17 mg niacin equivalents
    B_6: 2.2 mg
    Folate: 400 micrograms
    B_{12}: 2.2 micrograms
    Biotin: 30–100 micrograms
    Pantothenic acid: 4–7 micrograms
Minerals
    Calcium: 1,200 mg
    Phosphorus: 1,200 mg
    Magnesium: 320 mg
    Iron: 30 mg
    Zinc: 15 mg
    Copper: 1.5–3.0 mg
    Manganese: 2.0–5.0 mg
    Fluoride: 1.5–4.0 mg
    Chromium: 50–200 micrograms
    Molybdenum: 75–250 micrograms
    Iodine: 175 micrograms
    Selenium: 65 micrograms

Lactating Women

Energy intake
    2,840 calories (first six months)
    2,710 calories (second six months)
Protein
    65 g (first six months)
    62 g (second six months)

Fat
  Less than 30 percent of total calories
  Less than 10 percent of total fats from saturated fatty acids
  Less than 300 mg cholesterol
Carbohydrates: More than 225 g (50 percent of calories)
Vitamins
  A
    1,300 micrograms (first six months)
    1,200 micrograms (second six months)
  D: 5 micrograms
  E
    12 mg (as alpha-tocopherol) (first six months)
    11 mg (second six months)
  K: 65 micrograms
  C
    95 mg (first six months)
    90 mg (second six months)
  Thiamin: 1.6 mg
  Riboflavin
    1.8 mg (first six months)
    1.7 mg (second six months)
  Niacin: 20 mg niacin equivalents
  B_6: 2.1 mg
  Folate
    280 micrograms (first six months)
    260 micrograms (second six months)
  B_{12}: 2.6 micrograms
  Biotin: 30–100 micrograms
  Pantothenic acid: 4–7 mg
Minerals
  Calcium: 1,200 mg
  Phosphorus: 1,200 mg
  Magnesium
    355 mg (first six months)
    340 mg (second six months)
  Iron: 15 mg
  Zinc
    19 mg (first six months)
    16 mg (second six months)
  Copper: 1.5–3.0 mg
  Manganese: 2.0–5.0 mg
  Fluoride: 1.5–4.0 mg
  Chromium: 50–200 micrograms

Molybdenum: 75–250 micrograms
Iodine: 200 micrograms
Selenium: 75 micrograms

Women Over 50

Energy intake: 1,900 calories
Protein: 50 g
Fat
    Less than 30 percent of total calories
    Less than 10 percent of total fat from saturated fatty acids
    Less than 300 mg cholesterol
Carbohydrates: More than 250 g (50 percent of calories)
Vitamins
    A: 800 micrograms
    D: 5 micrograms
    E: 8 mg (as alpha-tocopherol)
    K: 65 micrograms
    C: 60 mg
    Thiamin: 1.0 mg
    Riboflavin: 1.2 mg
    Niacin: 13 mg niacin equivalents
    B_6: 1.6 mg
    Folate: 180 micrograms
    B_{12}: 2.0
    Biotin: 30–100 micrograms
    Pantothenic acid: 4–7 mg
Minerals
    Calcium: 800 mg
    Phosphorus: 800 mg
    Magnesium: 280 mg
    Iron: 10 mg
    Zinc: 12 mg
    Copper: 1.5–3.0 mg
    Manganese: 2.0–5.0 mg
    Fluoride: 1.5–4.0 mg
    Chromium: 50–200 micrograms
    Molybdenum: 75–250 micrograms
    Iodine: 150 micrograms
    Selenium: 55 micrograms

SOURCE: National Research Council 1989.

Reference Matter

References

Abernathy DR, Greenblatt DJ, and Shader RI (1984). Imipramine disposition in users of oral contraceptive steroids. *Clin Pharmacol Ther* 35: 792–97.

Abrams RC and Alexopoulos GS (1987). Substance abuse in the elderly: Alcohol and prescription drugs. *Hosp Community Psychiatry* 38: 1285–87.

Adler NE and Tschann JM (1993). The abortion debate: Psychological issues for adult women and adolescents. In S Matteo, ed., *American women in the nineties: Today's critical issues*, pp. 193–212. Boston: Northeastern University Press.

Advance report of final mortality statistics, 1989 (1992). *Monthly Vital Statistics Report* 40(8) (Jan. 7): supp 2.

Ahlborg G and Bodin L (1991). Tobacco smoke exposure and pregnancy outcome among working women. *Am J Epidemiol* 133: 338–47.

Alan Guttmacher Institute (1976). 11 million teenagers: What can be done about the epidemic of adolescent pregnancy? Washington, D.C.: Planned Parenthood Federation of America, Inc.

——— (1993a). Preconception and prenatal care can improve birth outcomes. *Issues in Brief*. Mar.

——— (1993b). Reproductive health and health care reform: Special considerations. *Issues in Brief*. Aug.

Albanes D, Jones DY, Micozzo MS, et al. (1987). Associations between smoking and body weight in the US population: Analysis of NHANES II. *Am J Public Health* 77: 439–44.

Albertson AM, Tobolmann RC, and Marquart L (1997). Estimated dietary calcium intake and food sources for adolescent females, 1980–1992. *J Adolesc Health* 20 (Jan.): 20–26.

Allen M (1994). The dilemma for women of color in clinical trials. *J Am Med Wom Assoc* 49: 105–9.

Allen MG (1976). Twin studies of affective illness. *Arch Gen Psychiatry* 33: 1476–78.

Alpert MA, Sabetti M, Kushner M, et al. (1992). Frequency of isolated panic attacks and panic disorder in patients with the mitral valve prolapse disorder. *Am J Cardiol* 69: 1489–90.

Altman LK (1991). Men, women and heart disease: More than a question of sexism. *New York Times,* Aug. 6, national ed.

———— (1994). Flawed study raises questions on U.S. research. *New York Times,* Mar. 15, p. B11.

———— (1995). AIDS is now the leading killer of Americans from 25 to 44. *New York Times,* Jan. 31.

Alza Corporation (1986). Progestasert intrauterine progesterone contraceptive system. Product insert.

American Association of Retired Persons and U.S. Department of Health and Human Services, Administration on Aging (n.d.). A profile of Americans: 1990. PF3049(1290)D996.

American Association of University Women Educational Foundation (1991). Shortchanging girls / Shortchanging America. Washington, D.C.: American Association of University Women.

———— (1992). How schools shortchange girls. Washington, D.C.: American Association of University Women.

American Cancer Society (1992). Cancer facts and figures, 1992. Atlanta: American Cancer Society.

American College of Obstetricians and Gynecologists, Committee on Obstetrics (1988). ACOG committee opinion no. 64: Guidelines for vaginal delivery after a previous cesarean birth. Washington, D.C.: American College of Obstetricians and Gynecologists.

American College of Physicians (1991). Promotion and tenure of women and minorities on medical school faculties. *Ann Intern Med* 114: 63–68.

American Fertility Society Ethics Committee (1994). Ethical consideration of assisted reproductive technologies. *Fertil Steril* 62 (supp 1): 35S.

American Medical Association Center on Health Policy Research (1989). Income comparisons of male and female physicians. *SMS Report* 3: 3–4.

American Medical Association Council on Ethical and Judicial Affairs (1988). Ethical implications of age-based rationing of health care. Chicago: American Medical Association.

American Medical Association Council on Scientific Affairs (1990). White paper on elderly health. *Arch Intern Med* 150: 2459–72.

American Psychiatric Association (1986). *Diagnostic and statistical manual of mental disorders (DSM-III).* 3d ed. Washington, D.C.: APA Press.

———— (1994). *Diagnostic and statistical manual of mental disorders (DSM-IV).* 4th ed. Washington, D.C.: APA Press.

American School Health Association, Association for the Advancement of

Health Education, and Society for Public Health Education (1989). *The national adolescent student health survey: A report on the health of America's youth*. Oakland, Calif.: Third Party Publishers.

American woman: Progress, but... (1991). *Washington Spectator* 17(9): 1. May 1.

Anastos K, Charney P, Charon RA, et al. (1991). Hypertension in women: What is really known? *Ann Intern Med* 115: 287–93.

Anderson JE (1981). Prescribing of tranquilizers to women and men. *Can Med Assoc J* 125: 1229–32.

Andrews FM, Abbey A, and Halman LJ (1992). Is fertility-problem stress different? The dynamics of stress in fertile and infertile couples. *Fertil Steril* 57: 1247–53.

Angell M (1992). Breast implants—Protection or paternalism? *N Engl J Med* 326: 1695–96.

Angier N (1991). Women swell ranks of science, but remain invisible at the top. *New York Times*, May 21, p. C1.

——— (1992). Bedside manners improve as more women enter medicine. *New York Times*, June 21.

Angold A and Rutter M (1992). Effects of age and pubertal status on depression in a large clinical sample. *Dev & Psychopath* 4: 5–28.

Armstrong TJ and Chaffin DB (1979). Carpal tunnel syndrome and selected personal attributes. *J Occup Med* 21: 481–86.

Aro H and Taipale V (1987). The impact of timing of puberty on psychosomatic symptoms among fourteen- to sixteen-year-old Finnish girls. *Child Dev* 58: 261–68.

Association of American Medical Colleges (1994). *Women in Medicine Update* 8 (fall): 1.

Auclaire P and Schwartz IM (1986). *Overview: An evaluation of the effectiveness of intensive home-based services as an alternative to placement for adolescents and their families*. Minneapolis, Minn.: Hubert H. Humphrey Institute of Public Affairs.

Ayanian JZ and Epstein AM (1991). Differences in the use of procedures between men and women hospitalized for coronary artery disease. *N Engl J Med* 325: 221–25.

Bachrach LK, Guido D, Katzman DK, et al. (1990). Decreased bone density in adolescent girls with anorexia nervosa. *Pediatrics* 86: 440–47.

Bachrach LK, Katzman DK, Litt IF, et al. (1991). Recovery from osteopenia in adolescent girls with anorexia nervosa. *J Clin Endocrinol Metab* 72: 602–6.

Baldwin L-M, Hutchinson HL, and Rosenblatt RA (1992). Professional relationships between midwives and physicians: Collaboration or conflict? *Am J Public Health* 82: 262–64.

Barolsky SM, Gilbert CA, Farugui A, et al. (1979). Differences in electrocardiographic response to exercise of women and men: A non-bayesian factor. *Circulation* 60: 1021.

Barrett-Connor E, Brown WV, Turner J, et al. (1979). Heart disease risk factors and hormone use in postmenopausal women. *JAMA* 241: 2167–69.

Barrett-Connor E and Bush TL (1989). Estrogen replacement and coronary heart disease. *Cardiovasc Clin* 19: 159–72.

Barrett-Connor E and Kritz-Silverstein D (1993). Estrogen replacement therapy and cognitive function in older women. *JAMA* 269: 2637–41.

Barrett-Connor E, Kritz-Silverstein D, and Edelstein SL (1993). A prospective study of dehydroepiandrosterone sulfate (DHEAS) and bone mineral density in older men and women. *J Epidemiol* 137: 201–6.

Barrett-Connor E, Wilcosky T, Wallace RB, and Heiss G (1986). Resting and exercise electrocardiographic abnormalities associated with sex hormone use in women: The Lipid Research Clinics Program Prevalence Study. *Am J Epidemiol* 123: 81.

Bastian L, Bennett CL, and Adams J (1993). Differences between men and women with HIV-related pneumocystis carinii pneumonia: Experience from 3,070 cases in New York City in 1987. *J Acquired Immune Deficiency Syndromes* 6: 617–23.

Baumrind D (1987). A developmental perspective on adolescent risk taking in contemporary America. In CE Irwin, ed., *Adolescent social behavior and health: New directions for child development*, pp. 93–125. San Francisco: Jossey-Bass.

Becker RC (1990). Clinical highlights and future directions. *Cardiology* 77 (supp 2 [Cardiovascular disease in women]): 1–5.

Belenky MF, Clinchy BM, Goldberger NR, and Tarule JM (1986). *Women's ways of knowing: The development of self, voice, and mind.* New York: Basic Books.

Bell CA (1991). Female homicides in United States workplaces, 1980–1985. *Am J Public Health* 81: 729–32.

Bemmann KC (1994). Letter to President Clinton on behalf of American Medical Women's Association. Mar. 25.

Berdie J, Berdie M, Wexler S, et al. (1983). *An empirical study of families involved in adolescent maltreatment.* San Francisco: URSA Institute.

Berger A and Schaumberg HH (1984). More on neuropathy from pyridoxine abuse. *N Engl J Med* 311: 986–87.

Bergkvist L, Adami H-O, Persson I, et al. (1989). Prognosis after breast cancer diagnosis in women exposed to estrogens and estrogen-progesterone replacement therapy. *Am J Epidemiol* 130: 221–28.

Berk ML and Taylor AK (1984). Women and divorce: Health insurance coverage, utilization and health care expenditures. *Am J Public Health* 74: 1276–78.

Berkel H, Birdsell DC, and Jenkins H (1992). Breast augmentation: A risk factor for breast cancer? *N Engl J Med* 326: 1649–53.

Berkowitz AD and Perkins HW (1987). Recent research on gender differences in collegiate alcohol use. *J Am Coll Health* 36: 123–29.

Bernard AM, Hayward RA, Rosevear JS, and McMahon LF (1993). Gender and hospital resource use. *Evaluation Health Professions* 16: 177–89.

Bernstein L, Ross RK, and Henderson BE (1992). Prospects for the primary prevention of breast cancer. *J Epidemiol* 135: 142–52.

Bertollini R, DiLallo D, Spadea T, and Perucci CA (1992). Cesarean section rates in Italy by hospital payment mode: An analysis based on birth certificates. *Am J Public Health* 82: 257–61.

The best kept secret (1993). *New York Times Magazine*, June 10.

Bickel J (1988). Women in medical education: A status report. *New Engl J Med* 319: 1579–84.

——— (1995). Women applicants level off, faculty continue growth. *Academic Physician Scientist* Jan.: 5.

Blythe DA, Simmons RG, Bulcroft R, et al. (1981). The effects of physical development on self-image and satisfaction with body-image for early adolescent males. In RG Simmons, ed., *Research in community and mental health*, vol. 2, pp. 43–73. Greenwich, Conn.: JAI Press.

Borkowski M, Murch M, and Walker V, eds. (1983). *Marital violence: The community response*. London: Tavistock.

Borum ML (1996). Patient and physician gender may influence colorectal cancer screening by resident physicians. *J Women's Health* 5: 363–68.

Boston Women's Health Book Collective (1979). *Our bodies, ourselves*, 2d ed. New York: Simon & Schuster.

——— (1984). *The new our bodies, ourselves*. New York: Simon & Schuster.

Boston University Medical Center (1993). *News in Brief*. Oct. 31.

——— (1994). *News in Brief*. Feb. 4.

Bowker LH, Arbitell M, and McFerron JR (1988). On the relationship between wife beating and child abuse. In K Yllo and M Bograd, eds., *Feminist perspectives on wife abuse*. Newbury Park, Calif.: Sage.

Brack CJ, Orr DP, and Ingersoll G (1988). Pubertal maturation and adolescent self-esteem. *J Adolesc Health Care* 9: 280–85.

Bradford J, Ryan C, and Rothblum ED (1994). National lesbian health care survey: Implications for mental health care. *J Consult Clin Psychol* 62: 228–42.

Bremner WJ, Bagatell CJ, and Steiner RA (1990). Gonadotropin-releasing hormone antagonist plus testosterone: A potential male contraceptive. *J Clin Endocrinol Metab* 73: 465–69.

Brody JE (1991). Recognizing the demons of depression: The pain may be disguised in men. *New York Times*, Dec. 18, p. B11.

——— (1995). Cancer cases are up, but the future isn't bleak. *New York Times*, Feb. 1.

Brooks-Gunn J (1984). The psychological significance of different pubertal events to young girls. *J Early Adolesc* 4: 315–27.

Budoff PW (1987). Use of prostaglandin inhibitors in the treatment of premenstrual syndrome. *Clin Obstet Gynecol* 30: 453–64.

Buist A, Norman TR, and Dennerstein L (1990). Breastfeeding and the use of psychotropic medication: A review. *J Affective Disord* 19: 197–206.

——— (1993). Mianserin in breast milk (letter). *Br J Clin Pharmacol* 36: 133–34.

Burke K, Burke J, Regier D, and Rae D (1990). Age of onset of selected mental disorders in five community populations. *Arch Gen Psychiatry* 47: 511–18.

Calle EE, Miracle-McMahill HL, Thun MJ, and Heath CW Jr. (1994). Cigarette smoking and risk of fatal breast cancer. *Am J Epidemiol* 139: 1001–7.

Cancer and Steroid Hormone Study of the Centers for Disease Control and the National Institute of Child Health and Human Development (1987). The reduction in risk of ovarian cancer associated with oral contraceptive use. *N Engl J Med.* 316: 650–55.

Cannon LJ, Bernack EJ, and Walter SD (1981). Personal and occupational factors associated with carpal tunnel syndrome. *J Occup Med* 23: 255–58.

Cantos A, Neidig P, and O'Leary KD (1991). *Fear and injuries of women and men in a treatment program for domestic violence.* Stony Brook, N.Y.: Behavioral Science Association.

Carmen E, Rieker PP, and Mills T (1984). Victims of violence and psychiatric illness. *Am J Psychiatry* 141: 378–83.

Carnegie Task Force on Meeting the Needs of Young Children (1994). Starting points. New York: Carnegie Corporation of New York. Apr.

Carr PL, Friedman RH, Moskowitz MA, and Kazis LE (1993). Comparing the status of women and men in academic medicine. *Ann Intern Med* 119: 908–13.

Cartwright L (1987). Occupational stress in women physicians. In RL Payne and J Firth-Cozens, eds., *Stress in health professions*, pp. 71–87. Chichester, Eng.: Wiley.

Cary J, Hein K, and Dell R (1990). Theophylline disposition in adolescents with asthma. *Ther Drug Monit* 13: 309–13.

Cascardi M (1992). Marital aggression: Impact, injury, and health correlates for husbands and wives. *Arch Intern Med* 152: 1178–84.

Cawley M, Kostic J, and Cappello C (1990). Informational and psychological needs of women choosing conservative surgery / primary radiation for early stage breast cancer. *Cancer Nurs* 13: 90–94.

Center for Population Options (1992). *Teenage pregnancy and too-early childbearing: Public costs, personal consequences.* 6th ed. Washington, D.C.: Center for Population Options.

Centers for Disease Control (1990). Use of mammography—United States, 1990. *Mortality and Morbidity Weekly Report* 39: 621–30.

——— (1992a). Tobacco, alcohol and other drug use among high school students—United States, 1991. *Mortality and Morbidity Weekly Report* 41: 698–703.

———— (1992b). Surveillance summaries, p. 10, Fig. 9.

———— (1993a). *Mortality and Morbidity Weekly Report* 42: 4.

———— (1993b). *Mortality and Morbidity Weekly Report* 42: 18.

———— (1993c). Sexually transmitted diseases treatment guidelines. *Mortality and Morbidity Weekly Report* 42: 72.

———— (1993d). Rates of cesarean delivery—United States, 1991. *Mortality and Morbidity Weekly Report* 42: 285–89.

———— (1993e). Emergency department response to domestic violence—California, 1992. *Mortality and Morbidity Weekly Report.* 42: 617–19.

———— (1994a). *Mortality and Morbidity Weekly Report* 43: 132–37.

———— (1994b). Update: Impact of the expanded AIDS case definition for adolescents and adults on case reporting—United States, 1993. *Mortality and Morbidity Weekly Report* 43: 160–70.

———— (1994c). *Mortality and Morbidity Weekly Report* 43: 273–81. Apr. 22.

———— (1994d). Prevalence of overweight among adolescents—United States, 1988–91. *Mortality and Morbidity Weekly Report* 43: 818–21.

———— (1995a). *Mortality and Morbidity Weekly Report* 44: Sept. 22.

———— (1995b). State-specific pregnancy and birth rates among teenagers— United States, 1991–1992. *Morbidity and Mortality Weekly Report* 44: 677.

CEWAER (California Elected Women's Association for Education and Research), California Women's Health Project, and Center for Research on Women's and Children's Health of the California Public Health Foundation (1993). The health of California women. Berkeley, Calif.: CEWAER.

Chalker R and Whitmore KE (1990). *Overcoming bladder disorders.* New York: Harper and Row.

Chavkin W (1994). Women and clinical research. Editorial. *JAMWA* 49: 99–100.

Children's Defense Fund (1991). *The state of America's children.* Washington, D.C.: Children's Defense Fund.

Chouinard A, Annable L, and Steinberg S (1986). A controlled clinical trial of fluspirilene, a long-acting injectable neuroleptic, in schizophrenic patients with acute exacerbation. *J Clin Psychopharmacol* 6: 21–26.

Chrischilles EA, Foley DJ, Wallace RB, et al. (1992). Use of medications by persons 65 and over: Data from the established populations for epidemiologic studies of the elderly. *J Gerontol* 47: M137–44.

Chrischilles EA, Lemke JH, Wallace RB, and Drube GA (1990). Prevalence and characteristics of multiple analgesic drug use in an elderly study group. *J Am Geriatr Soc* 38: 979–84.

Chrischilles EA, Segar ET, and Wallace RB (1992). Self-reported adverse drug reactions and related resource use: A study of community-dwelling persons 65 years of age and older. *Ann Intern Med* 117: 634–40.

Christie KA, Burke JD, Reiger DA, et al. (1988). Epidemiologic evidence for early onset of mental disorders and higher risk of drug abuse in young adults. *Am J Psychiatry* 145: 971–75.

Clancy CM and Massion CT (1992). American women's health care: A patchwork quilt with gaps. *JAMA* 268: 1918–20.

Clark PI, Glasser SP, Lyman GH, et al. (1988). Relation of results of exercise stress tests in young women to phases of the menstrual cycle. *Am J Cardiol* 61: 197.

Clever LH, ed. (1988). Special issue: Women and medicine. *West J Med* 149 (Dec.): 734–40.

——— (1991). There's a long, long trail a-winding (editorial). *West J Med* 155: 540.

Clingempeel WG, Colyar JJ, Brand E, and Hetherington EM (1992). Children's relationships with maternal grandparents: A longitudinal study of family structure and pubertal status effects. *Child Dev* 63: 1404–22.

Cohn LD (1991). Sex differences in the course of personality development: A meta-analysis. *Am Psychol* 109: 252–66.

Colditz GA, Stampfer MJ, Willett WC, et al. (1990). Prospective study of estrogen replacement therapy and risk of breast cancer in postmenopausal women. *JAMA* 264: 2648–53.

Colditz G, Willett WC, Hunter DJ, et al. (1993). Family history, age, and risk of breast cancer: Prospective data from the Nurses' Health study. *JAMA* 270: 338–43.

Cole JR (1979). *Fair science: Women in the scientific community.* New York: Free Press.

Cole JR and Zuckerman H (1984). The productivity puzzle: Persistence and change in patterns of publication of men and women scientists. In P Maehr and MW Steinkamp, eds., *Advances in motivation and achievement,* 2: 217–58. Greenwich, Conn.: JAI Press.

Collins A, Freeman EW, Boxer AS, and Tureck R. (1992). Perceptions of infertility and treatment stress in females as compared with males entering in vitro fertilization treatment. *Fertil Steril* 57: 350–56.

Colton ME and Gore S (1991). *Adolescent stress: causes and consequences.* Hawthorne, N.Y.: Aldine de Gruyter.

Commonwealth Fund (1993). Survey of women's health. New York: Commonwealth Fund. July 14.

Corea G (1992). *The invisible epidemic.* New York: HarperCollins.

Corrao JM, Becker RC, Ockene IS, and Hamilton GA (1990). Coronary heart disease risk factors in women. *Cardiology* 77 (supp 2): 8–24.

Creinin MD and Vittinghoff E (1994). Methotrexate and misoprostol vs misoprostol alone for early abortion: A randomized controlled trial. *JAMA* 272: 1190–95.

Cromer BA, Frankel ME, Hayes J, and Brown RT (1992). Compliance with breast self-examination instructions in high school students. *Clin Pediatr* 31: 215–20.

Cutler WB, Friedmann E, Felmet K, and Genovese-Stone E (1992). Stress urinary incontinence: A pervasive problem among healthy women. *J Women's Health* 1: 259–66.

Daling JR, Malone KE, Voight LF, et al. (1994). Risk of breast cancer among young women: Relationship to induced abortion. *JNCI* 86: 1584–92.

Darney PD (1993). Who will do the abortions? *Women's Health Issues* 3: 158–61.

Datz FL, Christian PE, and Moore J (1987). Gender-related differences in gastric emptying. *Nucl Med* 28: 1204–7.

Davis DL (1991). Fathers and fetuses. *New York Times*, Mar. 1, national ed.

Decoufle P and Stanislewczyk K (1977). Retrospective survey of cancer in relation to occupation. NIOSH pub. no. 77-178. Cincinnati, Ohio: U.S. Department of Health, Education and Welfare, National Institute of Occupational Safety and Health.

De Krom MCTFM, Kester ADM, Knipschild PG, and Spaans F (1990). Risk factors for carpal tunnel syndrome. *Am J Epidemiol* 132: 1102–10.

Desmarais RL, Kaul W, Watson DD, and Beller GA (1993). Do false positive thallium-201 scans lead to unneccessary catheterization? Outcome of patients with perfusion defects on quantitative planar thallium–201 scintigraphy. *J Am Coll Cardiol* 21: 1058–63.

Devesa SS, Blot WJ, Stone BJ, et al. (1995). Recent cancer trends in the United States. *JNCI* 87: 175–82.

DiClemente R, Brown L, Beausoleil N, and Lodico M (1993). Comparison of AIDS knowledge and HIV-related sexual risk behaviors among adolescents in low and high AIDS prevalence communities. *J Adolesc Health* 14: 231–36.

Dietz W, Gortmaker W, and Cheung L (1985). Inactivity, diet, and the fattening of America. *Pediatrics* 75: 807–12.

Ditkoff EC, Crary WG, Cristo M, and Lobo RA (1991). Estrogen improves psychological function in asymptomatic postmenopausal women. *Obstet Gynecol* 78: 991–95.

Doebbert G, Riedmiller KR, and Kizer KW (1988). Occupational mortality of California women, 1979–1981. *West J Med* 149: 734–40.

Doll R, Gray R, Hafner B, and Peto R (1980). Mortality in relation to smoking: 22 years' observations on female British doctors. *Br Med J* 280: 967–71.

Dorn LD, Crockett LJ, and Petersen AC (1988). The relations of pubertal status to intrapersonal changes in young adolescents. *J Early Adolesc* 8: 405–19.

Dornbusch S, Carlsmith JM, Gross RT, et al. (1981). Sexual development, age, and dating: A comparison of biological and social influences upon one set of behaviors. *Child Dev* 52: 179–85.

Dubas JS, Graber JA, and Petersen AC (1991). The effects of pubertal development on achievement during adolescence. *Am J Educ* 99 (special issue: Development and education across adolescence): 444–60.

Duncan PD, Ritter PL, Dornbusch SM, et al. (1985). The effects of pubertal timing on body image, school behavior, and deviance. *J Youth Adolesc* 14 (special issue: Time of maturation and psychosocial functioning in adolescence: I): 227–35.

Dunne FP, Barry DG, Ferriss JB, et al. (1991). Changes in blood pressure during the normal menstrual cycle. *Clin Sci* 81: 515–18.

Early Breast Cancer Trialists' Collaborative Group (1988). Effects of adjuvant tamoxifen and of cytotoxic therapy on mortality in early breast cancer: An overview of 61 randomized trials among 28,896 women. *N Engl J Med* 319: 1681–92.

EDK Associates (1993). *Men beating women: Ending domestic violence—A qualitative and quantitative study of public attitudes on violence against women.* New York: EDK Associates.

Eisenberg C (1989). Medicine is no longer a man's profession. *New Engl J Med* 321: 1542–44.

Elders MJ, Perry CL, Eriksen M, and Giovino CA (1994). The report of the surgeon general: Preventing tobacco use among young people. *Am J Public Health* 84: 543–47.

Eley JW, Hill HA, Chen VW, et al. (1994). Racial differences in survival from breast cancer: Results of the National Cancer Institute Black/White Cancer Survival Study. *JAMA* 272: 947–54.

Elias M (1994). A new test for silicone reaction. *USA Today,* Jan. 7.

Ellinwood EH, Easier MES, Linnoila M, et al. (1983). Effects of oral contraceptives and diazepam-induced psychomotor impairment. *Clin Pharmacol Ther* 35: 360–66.

Endreson IM, Vaernes R, Ursin H, and Tönder O (1987). Psychological stress-factors and concentrations of immunoglobulins and complement components in Norwegian nurses. *Work Stress* 1: 365–76.

Engs RC and Hanson DJ (1990). Gender differences in drinking patterns and problems among college students: A review of the literature. *J Alcohol Drug Educ* 35: 36–47.

Erdwins CJ and Mellinger JC (1984). Midlife women: Relation of age and role to personality. *J Pers Soc Psychol* 47: 390–95.

Ericson A, Eriksson M, Kalen B, and Zetterstrom R (1987). Maternal occupation and delivery outcome: A study using central registry data. *Acta Paediatr Scand* 76: 512–18.

Ezzati TM, Massey JT, Waksberg J, et al. (1992). Sample design: Third National Health and Examination Survey. Hyattsville, Md.: U.S. Department of Health and Human Services, Public Health Service, Centers for Disease Control, National Center for Health Statistics.

Faludi S (1991). *Backlash: The undeclared war against American women.* New York: Crown.

Fieve RR, Go R, Dunner DL, and Ellston R (1984). Search for biological markers in a long-term epidemiologic and morbid risk study of affective disorders. *J Psychiatr Res* 18: 425–45.

Fincham FD and Bradbury TN, eds. (1990). *The psychology of marriage: Basic issues and applications.* New York: Guilford.

Fingerhut LA, Kleinman JC, and Kendrick JS (1990). Smoking before, during, and after pregnancy. *Am J Public Health* 80: 541–44.

Fiset C and LeBel M (1990). Influence of the menstrual cycle on the absorption and elimination of D-xylose. *Clin Pharmacol Ther* 48: 529–36.

Fisher LD, Kennedy JW, Davis KB, et al. (1982). Association of sex, physical size, and operative mortality after coronary artery bypass in the Coronary Artery Surgery Study (CASS). *J Thorac Cardiovasc Surg* 84: 334–41.

Flannery DJ, Rowe DC, and Gulley BL (1993). Impact of pubertal status, timing, and age on adolescent sexual experience and delinquency. *J Adolesc Res* 8: 21–40.

Fletcher SW, Black W, Harris R, et al. (1993). Report of the International Workshop on Screening for Breast Cancer. *JNCI* 85: 1644–56.

Flitcraft A (1990). Battered women in your practice? *Patient Care* 24: 107.

Follinstad DR, Brennan AF, Hause ES, et al. (1991). Factors moderating physical and psychological symptoms of battered women. *J Fam Violence* 6: 81–95.

Fontham ET, Correa P, Reynolds P, et al. (1994). Environmental tobacco smoke and lung cancer in nonsmoking women: A multicenter study. *JAMA* 271: 1752–59.

Food and Drug Administration (1977). General considerations for the clinical evaluation of drugs. DHEW publ. II FDA 77-3040. Washington, D.C.: U.S. Government Printing Office.

Forrest JD and Henshaw SK (1993). Providing controversial health care: Abortion services since 1973. *Women's Health Issues* 3: 152–57.

Franco K, Evans CL, Best AP, et al. (1983). Conflicts associated with physicians' pregnancies. *Am J Psychiatry* 140: 902–4.

Frank E, Winkleby MA, Altman DG, et al. (1991). Predictors of physicians' smoking cessation advice. *JAMA* 266: 3139–44.

Freedman JE (1994). Statement on behalf of the American Medical Women's Association to Subcommittee on Aging, Senate Committee on Labor and Human Resources. Mar. 9.

Freiman MP and Marder WD (1984). Changes in hours worked by physicians, 1970–1980. *Am J Public Health* 74: 1348–52.

Friedman LS, Ostermeyer EA, Lynch ED, et al. (1994). The search for BRCAI. *Cancer Res* 54: 6374–82.

Friedman M and Rosenman RH (1974). *Type A Behavior and Your Heart*. New York: Knopf.

Gabriel SE, O'Fallon WM, Beard CM, and Kurland LT (1995). Trends in the utilization of silicone breast implants, 1964–1991, and methodology for a population-based study of outcomes. *J Clin Epidemiol* 48: 527–37.

Ganske MG (1992). Are women doctors better for women? *McCalls*, Nov.

Garbarino J (1990). Adolescent victims of maltreatment. Paper prepared for the Office of Technology Assessment, U.S. Congress. Washington, D.C., Apr.

Garcia Coll C and de Lourdes Mattel M, eds. (1989). *The psychosocial development of Puerto Rican women*. New York: Praeger.

Gillick MR, Serrell NA, and Gillick LS (1982). Adverse consequences of hospitalization in the elderly. *Soc Sci Med* 16: 1033–38.

Given JE, Jones GS, and McMillen EL (1985). A comparison of personality characteristics between in vitro fertilization patients and other infertile patients. *J Vitro Fertil Embryo Transfer* 2: 49–54.

Gordon T, Kannel WB, Dawber TK, et al. (1975). Changes associated with quitting cigarette smoking: The Framingham Study. *Am Heart J* 90: 322–28.

Gortmaker S, Must A, Perrin J, et al. (1993). Social and economic consequences of overweight in adolescence and young adulthood. *N Engl J Med* 329: 1008–12.

Gortmaker S, Must A, Sobol AM, et al. (1996). Television viewing as a cause of increasing obesity among children in the United States, 1986–1990. *Arch Pediatr Adolesc Med* 150: 356–62.

Gould SJ (1981). *The mismeasure of man*. New York: W. W. Norton.

Grady D and Ernster V (1992). Does cigarette smoking make you ugly and old? *Am J Epidemiol* 135: 839–42.

Greenblatt DJ, Allen MD, Harmatz JS, and Shader RI (1980). Diazepam disposition determinants. *Clin Pharmacol Ther* 27: 301–12.

Greenland P, Reicher-Reiss H, Goldbourt U, and Behar S (1991). Israeli SPRINT investigators: In-hospital and l-year mortality in 1,524 women after myocardial infarction—comparison with 4,315 men. *Circulation* 83: 484–91.

Gross J (1994). Our bodies, but my hysterectomy. *New York Times*, June 26, national ed., p. 4: 1.

Gross TP and Schlesselman JJ (1994). The estimated effect of oral contraceptive use on the cumulative risk of epithelial ovarian cancer. *Obstet Gynecol* 83: 419–24.

Grossman MI, Kirsner JB, and Gillespie IA (1963). Basal and histalog stimulated gastric secretion in control subjects and in patients with peptic ulcer or gastric cancer. *Gastroenterology* 45: 14–26.

Gruchow HW, Anderson AJ, Barboriak JJ, et al. (1988). Postmenopausal use of estrogen and occlusion of coronary arteries. *Am Heart J* 115: 954–63.

Hadley J, Steinberg E, and Feder J (1991). Comparison of uninsured and privately insured hospital patients: Condition on admission, resource use, and outcome. *JAMA* 265: 374–79.

Haertel U, Heiss G, Filipiak B, and Doering A (1992). Cross-sectional and longitudinal associations between high density lipoprotein cholesterol and women's employment. *Am J Epidemiol* 135: 68–78.

Ham RJ (1988). *Am Geriatr Soc Newslett* (Dec. 17): 3.

Hamberger LK, Saunders DG, and Hovey M (1992). Prevalence of domestic violence in community practice and rate of physician inquiry. *Fam Med* 24: 283–87.

Hankey BF, Brinton LA, Kessler LG, and Abrams J (1991). Section 4: Breast. In BA Miller, LAG Reis, BF Hankey, et al., eds., *SEER cancer statistics review, 1973–90.* Bethesda, Md.: U.S. Department of Health and Human Services, Public Health Service, National Institutes of Health.

Hankinson SE, Hunter DJ, Colditz GA, et al. (1993). Tubal ligation, hysterectomy and risk of ovarian cancer. *JAMA* 270: 2813–18.

Hartmann H (1991). Women's health in the United States. Washington, D.C.: Institute for Women's Policy Research. July 12.

Hassink SS, Sheslow DV, DeLancey E, et al. (1996). Serum leptin in children with obesity: Relationship to gender and development. *Pediatrics* 98: 201–3.

Hatcher RA, Stewart F, Trussell J, et al. (1990). *Contraceptive technology, 1990–1992.* New York: Irvington.

Hayward C, Killen JD, Hammer LD, et al. (1992). Pubertal stage and panic attack history in sixth- and seventh-grade girls. *Am J Psychiatry* 149: 1239–43.

Hayward C, Killen JD, Wilson DM, Hammer LD, Litt IF, et al. (1997). The psychiatric risk associated with early puberty in adolescent girls. *J American Academy of Child and Adolescent Psychiatry* 36 (Feb.): 255–62.

Hazuda HP, Haffner SM, Stern MP, et al. (1986). Employment status and women's protection against coronary heart disease. *Am J Epidemiol* 123: 623–40.

Healy B (1991). The yentl syndrome. *New Engl J Med* 325: 274–76.

Hearn MT, Yuzpe A, Brown SE, and Casper RF (1987). Psychological characteristics of in vitro fertilization participants. *Am J Obstet Gynecol* 156: 269–74.

Heath GW, Pratt M, Warren CW, and Kann L (1994). Physical activity patterns in American high school students: Results from the 1990 Youth Risk Behavior Survey. *Arch Pediatr Adolesc Med* 148: 1131–36.

Hein K (1987). Developmental pharmacology in adolescents: The inauguration of a new field. *J Adol Health Care* 8: 8–35.

Heins M, Smock S, Marindale L, et al. (1977). Comparison of the productivity of women and men physicians. *JAMA* 237: 2514–17.

Hellinger FJ (1993). Women with AIDS receive fewer services than men with AIDS. *Res Activities* 171: 1–2. U.S. Department of Health and Human Services, Public Health Service.

Henderson V and Buckwalter J (1994). Cognitive deficits of men and women with Alzheimer's disease. *Neurology* 44: 90–96.

Henton J, Cate R, Koval J, et al. (1983). Romance and violence in dating relationships. *J Fam Issues* 4: 467–82.

Hicks DR, Martin JP, Getchell JP, et al. (1985). Inactivation of HTLV-III/LAV-infected cultures of normal human lymphocytes by nonoxynol-9 in vitro. *Lancet* 2: 1422–23.

Hillard PJA (1992). Oral contraception noncompliance: The extent of the problem. *Adv Contraception* 1 (supp): 13–20.

Himes NSE (1963). *Medical history of contraception*. New York: Gamut.

Hogan AJ, Solomon DJ, Bouknight RR, and Solomon CT (1991). Under-utilization of medical care services by HIV-infected women? Some preliminary results from the Michigan Medicaid Program (letter). *AIDS* 5: 338–39.

Holmbeck GN and Hill JP (1991). Rules, rule behaviors, and biological maturation in families with seventh-grade boys and girls. *J Early Adolesc* (special issue dedicated to the work of John P. Hill: II, Pubertal maturation and family relations): 236–57.

Homer CJ, James SA, and Siegel E (1990). Work-related psychosocial stress and risk of preterm, low birthweight delivery. *Am J Public Health* 80: 173–77.

Hopkins J, Marcus M, and Campbell SB (1984). Postpartum depression: A critical review. *Psychol Bull* 95: 498–515.

Horton JA, ed. (1992). *The women's health data book*. New York: Elsevier.

Hsia J (1993). Gender differences in diagnosis and management of coronary disease. *J Women's Health* 2: 349–52.

Hubert HB, Eaker D, Garrison RJ, and Castelli WP (1987). Life-style correlates of risk factor change in young adults: An eight-year study of coronary heart disease risk factors in the Framingham offspring. *Am J Epidemiol* 125: 812–31.

Humphrey JA, Stephens V, and Allen DF (1983). Race, sex, marijuana use, and alcohol intoxication in college students. *J Stud Alcohol* 44: 733–38.

Hunter DJ, Spiegelman D, Adami HO, et al. (1996). Cohort studies of fat intake and the risk of breast cancer—a pooled analysis. *N Engl J Med* 334: 356–61.

Inazu JK and Fox GL (1980). Maternal influence on the sexual behavior of teenage daughters. *J Fam Issues* 1: 81–102.

Institute of Medicine (1994). *Women and health research*. Washington, D.C.: National Academy Press.

Jacobs Institute of Women's Health (1992). *The women's health data book*. New York: Elsevier.

Jacobson A and Richardson B (1987). Assault experiences of 100 psychiatric inpatients: Evidence of the need for routine inquiry. *Am J Psychiatry* 144: 908–13.

Jamison KM and Flanagan TJ (1989). *Sourcebook of criminal justice statistics*. Washington, D.C.: U.S. Department of Justice, Bureau of Justice Statistics.

Jecker NS (1991). Age-based rationing and women. *JAMA* 226: 3012–15.

Jecker NS and Pearlman RA (1989). Ethical constraints on rationing medical care by age. *J Am Geriatr Soc* 37: 1067–75.

Jelic T, Wardlaw G, Ilich Z, et al. (1992). Timing of peak bone mass in Caucasian females and its implication for the prevention of osteoporosis. *J Bone Min Res* 75: 187.

Jermain DM (1992). Psychopharmacologic approach to postpartum depression. *J Women's Health* 1: 47–52.

Jessor R (1987). Problem behavior theory, psychosocial development, and adolescent problem drinking. *Br J Addict* 82: 331–42.

Jevne R and Oberle K (1993). Enriching health care and health care research: A feminist perspective. *Humane Med* 9: 201–6.

John EM, Savitz DA, and Shy CM (1994). Spontaneous abortions among cosmetologists. *Epidemiology* 5: 147–55.

Johnston LD, O'Malley PM, and Bachman JG (1993). National survey results on drug use from the Monitoring the Future study, 1975–1992. Vol. 2, College students and young adults. NIH pub. no. 93-3598. Rockville, Md.: National Institute on Drug Abuse.

Kaiser Foundation / Commonwealth Fund (1992). Report to the board of directors, Commonwealth Fund. Nov. 10.

Kandel D and Logan JA (1984). Patterns of drug use from adolescence to young adulthood: 1. Periods of risk for initiation, continued use, and discontinuation. *Am J Public Health* 74: 660–66.

Kaplan M (1983). A woman's view of DSM-III. *Am Psychol* 38: 786–92.

Karasek R, Gardell B, and Lindell J (1987). Work and non-work correlates of illness and behaviour in male and female Swedish white collar workers. *J Occup Behav* 8: 187–207.

Karasek RA and Theorell T (1990). *Healthy work*. New York: Basic Books.

Kashani JH, Orvaschel H, Rosenberg TK, et al. (1987). Psychopathology in a community sample of children and adolescents: A developmental perspective. *J Am Acad Child Adolesc Psychiatry* 28: 701–6.

Katz S, Branch LG, Branson MH, et al. (1983). Active life expectancy. *New Engl J Med* 309: 1218–24.

Kaufman NJ (1994). Smoking and young women: The physician's role in stopping an equal opportunity killer. *JAMA* 271: 629–30.

Kazis L, Carr P, Friedman R, and Moskowitz M (1993). Comparing the status of women and men in academic medicine. *Ann Intern Med* 119: 908–13.

Kegel AH (1951). Physiologic therapy for urinary stress incontinence. *JAMA* 146: 915–17.

Kelsey JL (1993). Breast cancer epidemiology: Summary and future directions. *Epidemiol Rev* 15: 256–63.

Kendall-Tackett K and Simon A (1988). Molestation and the onset of puberty: Data from 365 adults molested as children. *Child Abuse Negl* 12: 73–83.

Key TJA and Pike MC (1988). The role of oestrogens and progestogens in the epidemiology and prevention of breast cancer. *Eur J Cancer Clin Oncol* 24: 29–43.

Khan SS, Nessim S, Gray R, et al. (1990). Increased mortality of women in coronary artery bypass surgery: Evidence for referral bias. *Ann Intern Med* 112: 561–67.

Killen J, Hayward C, Litt I, et al. (1992). Is puberty a risk factor for eating disorders? *Am J Dis Child* 146: 323–25.

Killen JD, Taylor CB, Hayward C, et al. (1994). Pursuit of thinness and onset of eating disorder symptoms in a community sample of adolescent girls: A three year prospective analysis. *Int J Eating Disord* 16: 227–38.

Kiprowska I (1978). Women in ancient medicine. *J Am Med Wom Assoc* 33: 453–58.

Kirschstein RL (1991). Research on women's health. *Am J Publ Health* 81: 291–93.

Kjellstrand CM (1988). Age, sex and race inequity in renal transplantation. *Arch Int Med* 148: 1305–9.

Klebanoff MA, Shiono PH, and Rhoads GG (1990). Outcomes of pregnancy in a national sample of resident physicians. *New Engl J Med* 323: 1040–45.

Klein J and Litt IF (1981). Epidemiology of adolescent dysmenorrhea. *Pediatrics* 68: 661–64.

Kochanek KD and Hudson BL (1994). Advance report of final mortality statistics, 1992. *Monthly Vital Statistics Report* 43(6): supp.

Kolata G (1994). Support for lumpectomies reasserted. *New York Times*, Nov. 16.

Koran L and Litt IF (1988). A contemporary view of house staff well-being. *West J Med* 148: 97–101.

Krahn DD, Demitrack MA, Kurth C, et al. (1992). Dieting and menstrual irregularity. *J Women's Health* 1: 289–91.

Kritz-Silverstein D and Barrett-Connor E (1993a). Bone mineral density in postmenopausal women as determined by prior oral contraceptive use. *Am J Public Health* 83: 100–102.

———— (1993b). Early menopause, number of reproductive years, and bone mineral density in postmenopausal women. *Am J Public Health* 83: 983–88.

Kritz-Silverstein D, Wingard DL, and Barrett-Connor E (1992). Employment status and heart disease risk factors in middle-aged women: The Rancho Bernardo study. *Am J Public Health* 82: 215–19.

Kyvik S (1990). Motherhood and scientific productivity. *Social Studies of Science* 20: 149–60. London: Sage.

LaRosa JH (1988). Women, work, and health: Employment as a risk factor for coronary heart disease. *Am J Obstet Gynecol* 158: 1597–1605.

———— (1990). Executive women and health: Perceptions and practices. *Am J Public Health* 1450–54.

Laurent SL, Garrison CZ, Thompson SJ, et al. (1992). An epidemiologic study of smoking and primary infertility in women. *Fertil Steril* 57: 565–72.

LaVecchia C, Negri E, Franceschi S, et al. (1995). Olive oil, other dietary fats and the risk of breast cancer. *Cancer Causes Control* 6: 545–50.

Lazovich DA, White E, Thomas DB, and Moe RE (1991). Underutilization of breast-conserving surgery and radiation therapy among women with Stage I or II breast cancer. *JAMA* 266: 3433–38.

Lazovich DA et al. (1994). *New York Times*, Mar. 15, national ed.

Lennane KJ and Lennane RJ (1973). Alleged psychogenic disorders in women—a possible manifestation of sexual prejudice. *N Engl J Med* 288: 288–92.

Lerner RM (1985). Adolescent maturational changes and psychosocial development: A dynamic interactional perspective. *J Youth Adolesc* 14 (special issue: Time of maturation and psychosocial functioning in adolescence: II): 355–72.

Lewis M (1985). Older women and health: An overview. *Women and Health* 10: 1–16.

Lewit S (1970). Outcome of pregnancy with intrauterine device. *Contraception* 2: 47–57.

Liberati A, Patterson WB, Biener L, and McNeil BJ (1987). Determinants of physicians' preferences for alternative treatments in women with early breast cancer. *Tumori* 73: 601–9.

Licciardone JC, Brownson RC, Chang JC, and Wilkins JR (1990). Uterine cervical cancer risk in cigarette smokers: A meta-analytic study. *Am J Prev Med* 6: 274–81.

Linn S, Carroll M, Johnson C, et al. (1993). High-density lipoprotein cholesterol and alcohol consumption in U.S. white and black adults: data from NHANES II. *Am J Public Health* 83: 811–16.

Lipsitz IA, Nyquist RP, Wei JY, and Rowe J (1983). Postprandial reduction in blood pressure in the elderly. *N Engl J Med* 309: 81–83.

Lissner L, Bengtsson C, Lapidus L, and Bjorkelund C (1992). Smoking initiation and cessation in relation to body fat distribution based on data from a study of Swedish women. *Am J Public Health* 82: 273–75.

Litt IF (1988). The health of adolescent women in the 1980s. *West J Med* 149 (special issue: Women and medicine): 696–99.

——— (1991). The interaction of pubertal and psychosocial development during adolescence. *Pediatrics Rev* 12: 249–55.

——— (1993). Health issues for women in the 1990s. In S Matteo, ed., *American women in the nineties*. Boston: Northeastern University Press.

——— (1996). Pregnancy in adolescence. Editorial. *JAMA* 275: 1030.

Litt IF, Cuskey WR, and Rudd S (1980). Identifying the adolescent at risk for contraceptive noncompliance. *J Pediatr* 96: 742–45.

Litt IF and Schonberg SK (1975). Medical complications of drug abuse in adolescents. *Med Clin North Am* 59: 1445–52.

Lock M (1991). Contested meanings of the menopause. *Lancet* 337: 1270–72.

Loop FD, Golding LR, MacMillan JP, et al. (1983). Coronary artery surgery in women compared with men: Analysis of risks and long-term results. *J Am College of Cardiol* 1: 383–90.

Louie AK, Lewis TB, and Lannon RH (1993). Use of low-dose fluoxetine in major depression and panic disorder. *J Clin Psychiatry* 54: 435–38.

McAlister A, Perry C, and Maccoby N (1979). Adolescent smoking: Onset and prevention. *Pediatrics* 63: 650–58.

MacArthur C, Lewis M, and Knox EG (1991). Health after childbirth. *Br J Obstet Gynaecol* 98: 1193–95.

McCarthy M (1990). The thin ideal, depression and eating disorders in women. *Behav Res Ther* 28(2): 205–15.

McCormack A, Janus M, and Burgess A (1986). Runaway youths and sexual victimization: Gender differences in an adolescent runaway population. *Child Abuse Negl* 10: 387–96.

MacDonald I (1956). Gastric activity during the menstrual cycle. *Gastroenterology* 30: 602–7.

McDowell MA, Briefel RR, Alaimo K, et al. (1994). Energy and macronutrient intakes of persons ages 2 months and over in the United States: Third national health and nutrition examination survey, Phase 1, 1988–91. *Advance Data* 255 (Oct. 24).

McGoldrick K (1986). Wife-beating: Everyday mayhem and murder (editorial). *J Am Med Wom Assoc* 41: 35.

McGrath E, Keita GP, Strickland BR, and Russo NF, eds. (1990). *Women and depression: Risk factors and treatment issues.* Washington, D.C.: American Psychological Association.

McIntosh JL, Hubbard RW, and Santos JF (1981). Suicide among the elderly: A review of issues with case studies. *J Gerontol Soc Work* 4: 63–74.

McLeer SA and Anwar R (1989). A study of battered women presenting in an emergency department. *Am J Public Health* 79: 65–66.

MacLeod L (1980). *Wife battering in Canada: A vicious circle.* Ottawa: Canadian Advisory Council on the Status of Women.

MacLeod SM, Giles HG, Bengert B, et al. (1979). Age and gender-related differences in diazepam pharmacokinetics. *J Clin Pharmacol* 19: 15–19.

Marcus R, Drinkwater B, Dalsky G, et al. (1992). Osteoporosis and exercise in women. *Med Sci Sports Exerc* 24 (supp): S301–7.

Martins R, Holzapfel S, and Baker P (1992). Wife abuse: Are we detecting it? *J Women's Health* 1: 77–80.

Matthews KA, Wing RR, Kuller LH, et al. (1990). Influence of natural menopause on psychological characteristics and symptoms of middle-aged healthy women. *J Consult Clin Psychol* 58: 345–51.

Maxson WS (1987). The use of progesterone in the treatment of PMS. *Clin Obstet Gynecol* 30: 465–77.

May PA (1987). Suicide among American Indian youth: A look at the issues. *Children Today* 16: 22–25.

Mazure CM, Takefman JE, Milki AA, and Polan ML (1992). Assisted reproductive technologies: II, Psychologic implications for women and their partners. *J Women's Health* 1: 275–81.

Mead M (1928). *Coming of age in Samoa.* New York: Morrow.

Medical Letter (1992). 34: 109.

Medical Research International and SART (1992). In vitro fertilization-embryo transfer (IVF-ET) in the United States: 1990 results from the IVF-ET registry. *Fertil Steril* 57: 15–24.

Meilahn EH, Becker RC, and Corrao JM (1995). Primary prevention of coronary heart disease in women. *Cardiology* 86(4): 286–98.

Melton LJ III (1990). Screening for osteoporosis. *Ann Intern Med* 112: 516–28.

Meyers JK, Weisman MM, and Tischler GL (1984). Six-month prevalence of psychiatric disorders in three communities. *Arch Gen Psychiatry* 41: 959–67.

Milham S Jr. (1983). *Occupational mortality in Washington State, 1950–1979.* NIOSH pub. no. 83-116. Cincinnati, Ohio, and Buffalo, N.Y.: U.S. Department of Health and Human Services, National Institute of Occupational Safety and Health.

Milki AA, Mazure CM, Takefman JE, and Polan ML (1992). Assisted reproductive technologies: I, Medical alternatives for women and their partners. *J Women's Health* 1: 267–73.

Minnesota Women's Fund (1990). Reflections at risk: Growing up female in Minnesota.

Mitchell JH, Tate C, Raven P, et al. (1992). Acute response and chronic adaptation to exercise in women. *Med Sci Sports Exerc* 24 (supp): S258–65.

Mitchell JL, Tucker J, Loftman PO, and Williams SB (1992). HIV and women: Current controversies and clinical relevance. *J Women's Health* 1: 35–39.

Monthly Vital Statistics Report (1993). 42(4) (Sept. 30): supp. U.S. Department of Health and Human Services.

Moore D (1988). Body image and eating behavior in adolescent girls. *Am J Dis Child* 142: 1114–18.

Morantz-Sanchez RM (1985). *Sympathy and science.* New York: Oxford University Press.

Morin GD (1990). Seasonal affective disorder: The depression of winter. *Arch Psych Nursing* 4: 182–87.

Morrison L (1988). The battering syndrome: A poor record of detection in the emergency department. *J Emerg Med* 6: 521.

Morse RM (1988). Substance abuse among the elderly. *Bull Menninger Clin* 53: 259–68.

Muller C (1991). *Health care and gender.* New York: Russell Sage.

Murphy JF, Dauncey M, Newcombe R, et al. (1984). Employment in pregnancy: Prevalence, maternal characteristics, perinatal outcome. *Lancet* 1: 1163–66.

Must A, Jacques P, Dallal G, et al. (1992). Long-term morbidity and mortality of overweight adolescents: A follow-up of the Harvard Growth Study of 1922–1935. *N Engl J Med* 327: 1350–55.

National Center for Health Statistics (1985). Vital and health statistics: Current estimates from the National Health Interview Survey: United States, 1982. U.S. Department of Health and Human Services pub. no. PHS 85-1578. Washington, D.C.: National Center for Health Statistics.

—— (1991). Health, United States, 1990. U.S. Department of Health and Human Services pub. no. PHS 91-1232. Hyattsville, Md.: Public Health Service.

National Girls Initiative (1990). Flyer. New York: Ms. Foundation for Women.

National Research Council (1989). *Recommended dietary allowances.* 10th ed. Washington, D.C.: National Academy Press.

Nelson DE, Giovino GA, Shopland DR, et al. (1995). Trends in cigarette smoking among U.S. adolescents, 1974 through 1991. *Am J Publ Health* 85: 34–40.

Newberger EH, Barken SE, Lieberman ES, et al. (1992). Abuse of pregnant women and adverse birth outcome: Current knowledge and implications for practice. *JAMA* 267: 2370–72.

Newcomb PA, Storer BE (1995). Postmenopausal hormone use and risk of large-bowel cancer. *J National Cancer Institute* 87: 1067–71.

Noble, Barbara Presley (1994). *New York Times,* May 1, national ed.

Nolen-Hoeksema S (1990). *Sex differences in depression.* Stanford, Calif.: Stanford University Press.

Notelovitz M (1989). Estrogen replacement therapy: Indications, contraindications, and agent selection. *Am J Obstet Gynecol* 161: 8–17.

Notman MT and Nadelson C (1973). Medicine: A career conflict for women. *Am J Psychiatry* 130: 1123–27.

Notman MT, Salt P, and Nadelson C (1984). Stress and adaptation in medical students: Who is most vulnerable? *Compr Psychiatry* 25: 355–66.

Nyamathi A, Bennett C, Leake B, et al. (1993). AIDS-related knowledge, perceptions, and behaviors among impoverished minority women. *Am J Public Health* 83: 65–71.

Offer D, Ostrove E, Howard KI, et al. (1989). *The teenage world: Adolescents' self-image in ten countries.* New York: Plenum.

Office of Technology Assessment (1991). Adolescent health. 2 vols. OTS-H-468. Apr. Washington, D.C.: GPO.

Older Women's League (1991). *Critical condition.* Washington, D.C.: Older Women's League.

Olsen L and Holmes W (1983). *Youth at risk: Adolescents and maltreatment.* Boston: Center for Applied Social Research.

Ontario Medical Association, Committee on Wife Assault (1991). Reports on wife assault: A medical perspective: Approaches to treatment of the male batterer and his family. Toronto.

Paikoff RL, Brooks-Gunn J, and Warren MP (1991). Effects of girls' hormonal status on depressive and aggressive symptoms over the course of one year. *J Youth Adolesc* 20 (special issue: The emergence of depressive symptoms during adolescence): 191–215.

Palinkas LA, Wingard DL, and Barrett-Connor E (1990). Chronic illness and depressive symptoms in the elderly: A population-based study. *J Clin Epidemiol* 43: 1131–41.

Passannante MR and Nathanson CA (1987). Women in the labor force: Are sex mortality differences changing? *J Occup Med* 29: 21–28.

Pathak DR and Whittemore AS (1992). Combined effects of body size, parity, and menstrual events on breast cancer incidence in seven countries. *Am J Epidemiol* 135: 153–68.

Pearce DM (1993). Something old, something new: Women's poverty in the 1990s. In S Matteo, ed., *American Women in the Nineties*, pp. 79–97. Boston: Northeastern University Press.

Pechansky R and Thomas JW (1981). The concept of access: Definition and relationship to consumer satisfaction. *Med Care* 19: 127–40.

Perkins HW (1992). Gender patterns in consequences of collegiate alcohol abuse: A 10-year study of trends in an under-graduate population. *J Stud Alcohol* 53(5): 458–62.

Pfeffer MA, Braunwald E, Moye LA, et al. (1992). Effect of captopril on mortality and morbidity in patients with left ventricular dysfunction after myocardial infarction: Results of the survival and ventricular enlargement trial. *N Engl J Med* 327: 669–77.

Pfeiffer J (1985). Girl talk–boy talk. *Science*. Feb.: 58–63.

Pharmaceutical Manufacturers Association (1991). New medicines in development for women. Dec. Washington, D.C.: Pharmaceutical Manufacturers Association.

Phibbs CS, Mark DH, Luft HS, et al. (1993). Choice of hospital for delivery: A comparison of high-risk and low-risk women. *Health Serv Res* 28: 201–22.

Pierce JP (1989). International comparisons in trends in cigarette smoking prevalence. *Am J Public Health* 79: 152–57.

Pierce JP, Lee L, and Gilpin EA (1994). Smoking initiation by adolescent girls, 1944 through 1988: An association with targeted advertising. *JAMA* 271: 608–11.

Pirie PL, Murray DM, and Leupker RV (1991). Gender differences in cigarette smoking and quitting in a cohort of young adults. *Am J Public Health* 81: 324–27.

Pitt B (1975). Psychiatric illness following childbirth. *Br J Psychiatry Spec* 9: 409–15.

Pitts FN, Winokur S, and Stewart MA (1961). Psychiatric syndromes, anxiety symptoms and response to stress in medical students. *Am J Psychiatry* 118: 333–40.

Pitts T and Steiner H (1994). Unpublished data. Department of Child Psychology, Stanford University, Stanford, CA.

Powers J and Eckenrode J (1988). The maltreatment of adolescents. *Child Abuse Negl* 12: 189–99.

Prendergast ML (1994). Substance use and abuse among college students: A review of recent literature. *J Am Coll Health* 43: 99–113.

Prentice RL, Kakar F, Hursting S, et al. (1988). Aspects of the rationale of the Women's Health Trial. *JNCI* 80: 802–14.

Prien RF and Cole JO (1978). The use of psychopharmacological drugs in the aged. In WG Clark and J del Guidice, eds., *Principles of psychopharmacology*. 2d ed. New York: Academic.

Raman SV (1995). Study dispels myths about breasts. *Stanford Daily*, Feb. 1.

Randolph AG, Washington AE, and Prober CG (1993). Cesarean delivery for women presenting with genital herpes lesions: Efficacy, risks, and costs. *JAMA* 270: 77–82.

Regier D (1990). *J Psychiatric Res* 24 (supp. 2): 3–14.

Reichel W (1965). Complications in the care of 500 elderly hospitalized patients. *J Am Geriatr Soc* 13: 973–81.

Repetti RL, Matthews KA, and Waldron I (1989). Employment and women's health: Effects of paid employment on women's mental and physical health. *Am Psychol* 11: 1394–1400.

Retzky SS and Rogers RM (1995). Urinary incontinence in women. *Clinical Symposia* 47: 28.

Rice DP and Feldman JJ (1983). Living longer in the United States: Demographic changes and health needs of the elderly. *Milbank Mem Fund Q* 61: 362–96.

Ridker PM, Vaughan DE, Stampfer MJ, et al. (1994). Association of moderate alcohol consumption and plasma concentration of endogenous tissue-type plasminogen activator. *JAMA* 272: 929–33.

Rierdan J, Koff E, and Stubbs ML (1987). Depressive symptomatology and body image in adolescent girls. *J Early Adol* 7: 205–16.

Rincke C (1981). The professional identities of women physicians. *JAMA* 245: 2419–21.

Risch H, Howe G, Jain M, et al. (1993). Are female smokers at higher risk for lung cancer than male smokers? A case-control analysis by histologic type. *Am J Epidemiol* 138: 281–93.

Rogers AS (1994). A research agenda for the study of therapeutic agents in adolescents. *J Adolesc Health* 15: 672–78.

Rohan TE, Howe GR, Friedenreich CM, et al. (1993). Dietary fiber, vitamins A, C, and E, and risk of breast cancer: A cohort study. *Cancer Causes and Control* 4: 29–37.

Rosen CJ, Holick MF, and Millard PS (1994). Premature graying of hair is a risk marker for osteopenia. *J Clin Endocrinol Metab* 79: 854–57.

Rosenberg HM, Burnett C, Maurer J, and Spirtas R (1993). Mortality by occupation, industry, and cause of death: 12 reporting states, 1984. *Monthly Vital Statistics Report* 42(4): supp. Hyattsville, Md.: National Center for Health Statistics.

Rosenberg MJ, Davidson AJ, Chen J-H, et al. (1992). Barrier contraceptives and sexually transmitted diseases in women: A comparison of female-dependent methods and condoms. *Am J Public Health* 82: 669–74.

Rounsaville B, Weissman M, Prusoff B, and Herceg-Baron R (1979). Process of psychotherapy among depressed women with marital disputes. *Am J Orthopsychiatry* 49: 505–10.

Russo J and Russo IH (1987). Biology of disease: Biological and molecular bases of mammary carcinogenesis. *Lab Invest* 57: 112–37.

Rutter M (1994). Resilience: Some conceptual considerations. *Contemp Pediatr* 11: 36–46.

Sabiston DC (1988). Surgical treatment of coronary artery disease. In JB Wyngaarden and LH Smith, eds., *Cecil Textbook of Medicine*, 18th ed., pp. 337–40. Philadelphia: W. B. Saunders.

Sandler RS, Sandler DP, Comstock GW, et al. (1988). Cigarette smoking and the risk of colorectal cancer in women. *JNCI* 80: 1329–33.

Saurel-Cubizolles MJ, Subtil D, and Kaminski M (1991). Is preterm delivery still related to physical working conditions in pregnancy? *J Epidemiol Community Health* 45: 29–34.

Savin-Williams RC (1990). *Gay and lesbian youths: Expressions of identity.* Washington, D.C.: Hemisphere.

Schappert SM (1993). Office visits to psychiatrists: United States, 1989–90. *Advance Data* 237: 1–16.

Schemo DJ (1994). Chemical plants seen as a factor in breast cancer. *New York Times*, Apr. 13, p. A1.

Schermerhorn GR, Colliver J, Verhulst S, and Schmidt E (1986). Factors that influence career patterns of women physicians. *J Am Med Wom Assoc* 41: 74–87.

Schnorr TM, Grajewski BA, Hornung RW, et al. (1991). Video display terminals and the risk of spontaneous abortion. *New Engl J Med* 324: 727–33.

Schoenborn CA and Boyd G (1989). Smoking and other tobacco use, United States. Vital Health Statistics, series 10, no. 169. U.S. Department of Health and Human Services pub. no. (PHS)j89-1597. Hyattsville, Md.: National Center for Health Statistics.

Schultz DL (1990). Risk, resiliency, and resistance: Current research on adolescent girls. Survey for the Ms. Foundation Funding Initiative for Girls. New York: Ms. Foundation.

Seachrist L (1994). Disparities detailed in NCI division. *Science* 264: 340.

Seligman MEP (1975). *Helplessness: On depression, development and death.* San Francisco: Freeman.

Shafer MA (1994). Sexually transmitted diseases in adolescents. *Adolesc Health Update* 6(2): 1–7.

Shaller JG (1990). The advancement of women in academic medicine. *JAMA* 264: 1854–55.

Sheehy G (1992). *The silent passage.* New York: Random House.

Sherwin BB (1988). Affective changes with estrogen and androgen replacement therapy in surgically menopausal women. *J Affective Disord* 14: 177–87.

Sichieri R, Everhart JE, and Roth H (1991). A prospective study of hospitalization with gallstone disease among women: Role of dietary factors, fasting period, and dieting. *Am J Publ Health* 81: 880–84.

Silbereisen RK, Petersen AC, Albrecht HT, and Kracke B (1989). Maturational timing and the development of problem behavior: Longitudinal studies in adolescence. *J Early Adolesc* 9 (special issue: Early adolescent transitions): 247–68.

Simpson GM, Yadalam KG, Levinson DF, et al. (1990). Single dose pharmacokinetics of fluphenazine after fluphenazine decanoate administration. *J Clin Psychopharmacol* 10: 417–21.

Singh GK, Matthews TJ, Clarke SC, et al. (1995). Annual summary of births, marriages, divorces, and deaths: United States, 1994. *Monthly Vital Statistics Report* 43(13). Hyattsville, Md: National Center for Health Statistics.

Smith DE, Lewis CE, Caveny JL, et al. (1994). Longitudinal changes in adiposity associated with pregnancy. *JAMA* 271: 1747–51.

Smith JM, Kucharski LT, and Oswald WT (1979). Tardive dyskinesia: Effect of age, sex, and criterion level of symptomatology on prevalence estimates. *Psychopharmacol Bull* 15: 69–71.

Smith RB, Divoll M, Gillespie WR, and Greenblatt DJ (1983). Effect of subject age and gender on the pharmacokinetics of oral triazolam and temazepam. *J Clin Psychopharmacol* 3: 172–76.

Smith S, Rinehard VS, Ruddock VE, and Schiff I (1987). Treatment of premenstrual syndrome with alprazolam: Results of a double-blind, placebo-controlled randomized crossover clinical trial. *Obstet Gynecol* 70: 37–43.

Sohrabji F, Miranda RC, and Toran-Allerand CD (1994). Estrogen differentially regulates estrogen and nerve growth factor receptors in RNAs in adult sensory neurons. *J Neuroscience* 14: 459–71.

Solomon DH (1988). New issues in geriatric care. *Ann Intern Med* 108: 718–32.

Sorensen R (1973). *Adolescent sexuality in contemporary America.* New York: World Books.

Stampfer MJ, Colditz GA, Willett WC, et al. (1991). Postmenopausal estrogen therapy and cardiovascular disease: Ten-year follow-up from the Nurses' Health Study. *N Engl J Med* 325: 756–62.

Stark E and Flitcraft A (1988). Violence among intimates: An epidemiologic review. In VB Van Hasselt, RL Morrisson, AS Bellack, and M Hersen, eds., *Handbook of family violence*, pp. 293–317. New York: Plenum.

———— (1991). Spouse abuse. In ML Rosenberg and MA Fewley, eds., *Violence in America: A public health approach*, p. 1389. New York: Oxford University Press.

Steel K, Gertman PM, Creslenzi C, and Anderson J (1981). Iatrogenic illness on a general medical service at a university hospital. *N Engl J Med* 304: 638–41.

Stein JA and Fox SA (1990). Language preference as an indicator of mammography use among Hispanic women. *JNCI* 82: 1715–16.

Steinberg L (1988). Reciprocal relation between parent-child distance and pubertal maturation. *Dev Psychol* 24: 1–7.

Sterling TD and Weinkam JJ (1976). Smoking characteristics by type of employment. *J Occup Med* 18: 743–54.

Stets J and Straus MA (1990). Gender differences in reporting marital violence and its medical and psychological consequences. In MA Straus and RJ Gelles, eds., *Physical violence in American families: Risk factors and adaptations in 8,145 American families*. New Brunswick, N.J.: Transaction.

Storz N and Green W (1983). Body weight, body image and perception of fad diets in adolescent girls. *J Nutr Educ* 15: 15–19.

Straus M and Gelles R (1986). Societal change and change in family violence from 1975–85 as revealed in two national surveys. *J Marriage Fam* 48: 465–79.

Straus M, Gelles R, and Steinmetz S (1980). *Behind closed doors: Violence in the American family*. New York: Doubleday.

Sullivan JM, Vander Zwaag R, Hughes JP, et al. (1988). Postmenopausal estrogen use and coronary atherosclerosis. *Ann Intern Med* 108: 358–63.

———— (1990). Estrogen replacement and coronary artery disease: Effect on survival in postmenopausal women. *Arch Intern Med* 150: 2557–62.

Surgeon General of the United States (1986). Surgeon General's Report. Washington, D.C.

Tang M, Jacobs D, Stern Y, et al. (1996). Effect of oestrogen during menopause on risk and age at onset of Alzheimer's disease. *Lancet* 348: 429–32.

Tannen D (1990). *You just don't understand: Women and men in conversation*. New York: William Morrow and Ballantine.

Taylor DC and Ounsted C (1989). Gender and survival. Letter, *Lancet* 1: 1444.

Teenage tobacco use: Data estimates from the teenage attitudes and practices survey, United States, 1989 (1993). *Advance Data* 224.

Theorell T, Orth-Gomer K, and Eneroth P (1990). Slow-reacting immunoglobulin in relation to social support and changes in job strain: A preliminary note. *Psychosom Med* 52: 511–16.

Thom MH and Studd JW (1980). Procedures in practice: Hormone implantation. *Br Med J* 280: 648–50.

Thomas DB (1991). Oral contraceptives and breast cancer: Review of the epidemiological literature. In Institute of Medicine, Division of Health Promotion and Disease Prevention, *Oral contraceptives and breast cancer*. Washington, D.C.: National Academy Press.

Thompson FE and Dennison BA (1994). Dietary sources of fats and cholesterol in US children aged 2 through 5 years. *Am J Public Health* 84: 799–806.

Tobin JN, Wassertheil-Smoller S, Wexler JP, et al. (1987). Sex bias in considering coronary bypass surgery. *Ann Intern Med* 107: 19–25.

Topical treatment for bacterial vaginosis (1992). *Med Lett Drugs Ther* 34: 109.

Trichopoulos D, MacMahon B, and Cole P (1972). The menopause and breast cancer risk. *JNCI* 48: 605–13.

Trotter RT (1982). Ethnic and sexual patterns of alcohol abuse: Anglo and Mexican-American college students. *Adolescence* 17: 305–25.

Trussell J et al. (1990). A guide to interpreting contraceptive efficacy studies. *Obstet Gynecol* 76: 558–67.

Trussell J, Sturgen K, Strickler J, and Dominik R (1994). Comparative contraceptive efficacy of the female condom and other barrier methods. *Fam Plann Perspect* 26: 66–72.

Tsai C-L and Liu T-K (1992). Osteoarthritis in women: Its relationship to estrogen and current trends. *Life Sci* 50: 1737–44.

Tucker L and Bagwell M (1991). Television viewing and obesity in adult females. *Am J Public Health* 81: 908–11.

Uemurea D and Pisa Z (1988). Trends in cardiovascular disease mortality in industrialized countries since 1950. *World Health Stat Q* 41: 115–77.

Ursin H, Mykletun R, Tönder O, et al. (1984). Psychological stress-factors and concentration of immunoglobulins and complement components in humans. *Scand J Psychol* 25: 340–47.

U.S. Bureau of the Census (1990). Poverty in the United States. Washington, D.C.: GPO.

U.S. Department of Health and Human Services (1980). Office on Smoking and Health. The health consequences of smoking for women. A report of the Surgeon General. Rockville, Md.: Public Health Service.

——— (1987a). The health consequences of involuntary smoking. A report of the Surgeon General. U.S. Department of Health and Human Services / Centers for Disease Control pub no. 89-8411. Washington, D.C.: GPO.

——— (1987b). Smoking and health: A national status report. A report to Congress. USDHHS HHS/PHS/CDC 87-8396. Washington, D.C.: GPO.

——— (1993). 1992 BRFSS summary prevalence report. Atlanta: U.S. Department of Health and Human Services, Public Health Service.

Van Egeren LF (1992). The relationship between job strain and blood pressure at work, at home, and during sleep. *Psychosomatic Medicine* 54: 337–43.

Vaughan VC III (1996). Care of the child with a fatal illness. In Behrman RE, Kliegman RM, and Arvin AM, eds., *Nelson Textbook of Pediatrics*, 15th ed. Philadelphia: W. B. Saunders.

Vital and Health Statistics: Current estimates from the National Health Interview Survey: United States, 1982 (1985). Washington, D.C.: Public Health Service, National Center for Health Statistics. U.S. Department of Health and Human Services pub. no. (PHS) 85-1578.

Vollmann RF (1977). The menstrual cycle. In *Major problems in obstetrics and gynecology*, vol. 7, pp. 1–193. Philadelphia: W. B. Saunders.

Wald A, Van Thiel DH, Hoechstetter L, et al. (1981). Gastrointestinal transit: The effect of the menstrual cycle. *Gastroenterology* 80: 1497–1500.

Waldron I and Herold J (1986). Employment, attitudes toward employment, and women's health. *Women and Health* 11: 79–98.

Waldron I and Jacobs J (1988). Effects of labor force participation on women's health: New evidence from a longitudinal study. *J Occup Med* 30: 977–83.

Walker LE (1984). *The battered woman syndrome*. New York: Springer.

Walker LEA and Browne A (1985). Gender and victimization by intimates. *J Pers* 53: 179–95.

Wallace JP, Inbar G, and Ernsthausen K (1994). Lactate concentrations in breast milk following maximal exercise and a typical workout. *J Women's Health* 3: 91–96.

Wallis LA, Gilder H, and Thaler H (1981). Advancement of men and women in medical academia: A pilot study. *JAMA* 246: 2350–53.

Ward S, Heidric S, and Wolberg W (1989). Factors women take into account when deciding upon type of surgery for breast cancer. *Cancer Nurs* 12: 344–51.

Warner R (1978). The diagnosis of antisocial and hysterical personality disorders: An example of sex bias. *J Nerv Ment Dis* 166: 839–45.

Wentz AC (1994). Waking up the U.S. to the "morning-after" pill. *J Women's Health* 3: 81–82.

Whitcup SM and Miller F (1987). Unrecognized drug dependence in psychiatrically hospitalized elderly patients. *J Am Geriatr Soc* 35: 297–301.

Willett WC and Ascherio A (1994). Trans fatty acids: Are the effects only marginal? *Am J Public Health* 84: 722–24.

Williamson DF, Mandans J, Anda RD, et al. (1991). Smoking cessation and severity of weight gains in a national cohort. *N Engl J Med* 324: 739–45.

Wing RR, Matthews KA, Kuller LH, et al. (1991). Weight gain at the time of menopause. *Arch Intern Med* 151: 97–102.

Winokur G and Tanna V (1969). Possible role of x-linked dominant factor in manic depressive disease. *Dis Nervous System* 30: 89–94.

Women in Pediatrics (1983). *Pediatrics* (supp).

Woolhandler S and Himmelstein DY (1988). Reverse targeting of preventive care due to lack of health insurance. *JAMA* 259: 2872–74.

Worcester N (1988). October is domestic violence month: The network news. *Psychiatr Clin North Am* 2: 1.

World Health Organization (1981). Health care in the elderly: Report of the technical group on use of medicaments by the elderly. *Drugs* 22: 279–94.

Wyngaarden JB and Smith LH, eds. (1988). *Cecil Textbook of Medicine*. 18th ed. Philadelphia: W. B. Saunders.

Yonkers KA, Kando JC, Cole JO, and Blumenthal S (1992). Gender differences in pharmacokinetics and pharmacodynamics of psychotropic medication. *Am J Psychiatry* 149: 587–95.

Zane N (1988). *In our own voices*. New York: PEER.

Zappert L and Weinstein H (1985). Sex differences in the impact of work on physical and psychological health. *Am J Psychiatry* 142: 1174–78.

Zemsky B (1991). Coming out against all odds: Resistance in the life of a young lesbian. *Women Ther* 11, 3/4 (Sept.): 185–200.

Index

Library of Congress Cataloging-in-Publication Data

Litt, Iris F.
  Taking our pulse: The health of America's women / Iris F. Litt
    p.   cm.
  Includes bibliographical references and index.
  ISBN 0-8047-2828-3 (cloth)—ISBN 0-8047-3137-3 (pbk.)
  1. Women—Health and hygiene.   I. Title.
RA778.L816   1997
362.1'082—dc21   97-9512
                                                      CIP

∞ This book is printed on acid-free, recycled paper.

Original printing 1997
Last figure below indicates year of this printing:
06 05 04 03 02 01 00 99 98 97